The Platelet in Health and Disease

The Platelet in Health and Disease

Edited by Clive P. Page PhD
Department of Pharmacology, King's College, University of London

OXFORD
BLACKWELL SCIENTIFIC PUBLICATIONS
LONDON EDINBURGH BOSTON
MELBOURNE PARIS BERLIN VIENNA

Editorial Offices:
Osney Mead, Oxford OX2 0EL
25 John Street, London WC1N 2BL
23 Ainslie Place, Edinburgh EH3 6AJ
3 Cambridge Center, Cambridge
Massachusetts 02142, USA
54 University Street, Carlton
Victoria 3053, Australia

Other Editorial Offices:
Arnette SA
2, rue Casimir-Delavigne
75006 Paris
France

Blackwell Wissenschaft
Meinekestrasse 4
D-1000 Berlin 15
Germany

Blackwell MZV
Feldgasse 13
A-1238 Wien
Austria

First published 1991

Set by Setrite Typesetters, Hong Kong
Printed and bound in Great Britain
by Hartnolls Ltd, Bodmin, Cornwall

DISTRIBUTORS

Marston Book Services Ltd
PO Box 87
Oxford OX2 0DT
(*Orders*: Tel. 0865 791155
Fax: 0865 791927
Telex: 837515)

USA
Mosby-Year Book, Inc.
11830 Westline Industrial Drive
St Louis, Missouri 63146
(*Orders*: Tel: 800 633–6699)

Canada
Mosby-Year Book, Inc.
5240 Finch Avenue East
Scarborough, Ontario
(*Orders*: Tel: 416 298–1588)

Australia
Blackwell Scientific Publications
(Australia) Pty Ltd
54 University Street
Carlton, Victoria 3053
(*Orders*: Tel: 03 347–0300)

British Library
Cataloguing in Publication Data

Page, Clive P.
The platelet in health & disease.
1. Man. Blood. Platelets
I. Title
612.117

ISBN 0–632–02714–2

Contents

List of Contributors

Christopher M. Athayde, *Division of Biomedical Sciences, King's College, Campden Hill Road, London W8 7AH, UK*

G. Burton, *Human Reproduction Unit, Royal North Shore Hospital of Sydney, St Leonards, NSW 2065, Australia*

Keith D. Butler, *Ciba-Geigy Pharmaceuticals, Wimblehurst Road, Horsham, West Sussex, RH12 4AB, UK*

J. Stewart Cameron, *Clinical Science Laboratories, Guy's Tower, Guy's Hospital, London Bridge SE1 9RT, UK*

Maria B. Donati, *Istituto di Ricerche Farmacologiche Mario Negri, Consorzio Mario Negri Sud, Via Nazionale, 66030 Santa Maria Imbaro, Italy*

Paolo Gresele, *Istituto di Semeiotica Medica, University of Perugia, Medical School, Perugia, Italy*

Caroline M. Herd, *Department of Pharmacology, King's College, London University, Chelsea Campus, Manresa Road, London SW3, UK*

Michel Joseph, *Centre d'Immunologie et de Biologie Parasitaire, Unité mixte INSERM 167 – CNRS 624, Institut Pasteur, Lille, France*

John E. Kaplan, *Department of Physiology and Cell Biology, Albany Medical College, Albany, New York 12208, USA*

Richard F. Levine, *Veterans Administration, Medical Centre, 50 Irving Street, NW, Washington DC 20422, USA*

Asrar B. Malik, *Department of Physiology and Cell Biology, Albany Medical College, Albany, New York 12208, USA*

John F. Martin, *Wellcome Research Laboratories, Beckenham BR3 3BS and Department of Medicine, King's College School of Medicine, London SE5 9PJ, UK*

Gillian R. May, *Department of Pharmacology, King's College, London University, Chelsea Campus, Manresa Road, London SW3, UK*

Philip K. Moore, *Department of Pharmacology, King's College, London University, Chelsea Campus, Manresa Road, London SW3, UK*

Chris O'Neill, *Human Reproduction Unit, Royal North Shore Hospital of Sydney, St Leonards, NSW 2065, Australia*

Clive P. Page, *Department of Pharmacology, King's College, London University, Chelsea Campus, Manresa Road, London SW3, UK*

Andreina Poggi, *Istituto di Ricerche Farmacologiche Mario Negri, Consorzio Mario Negri Sud, Via Nazionale, 66030 Santa Maria Imbaro, Italy*

D.M. Saunders, *Human Reproduction Unit, Royal North Shore Hospital of Sydney, St Leonards, NSW 2065, Australia*

Michael C. Scrutton, *Division of Biomolecular Sciences, King's College, Campden Hill Road, London W8 7AH, UK*

David P. Tuffin, *ICI Pharmaceuticals, Mereside, Alderley Park, Macclesfield, Cheshire SK10 4TG, UK*

Preface

It is now widely accepted that platelets are important blood elements involved in haemostatic events, which when inappropriately activated contribute to a number of thrombotic and cardiovascular disorders. However, it is less widely appreciated that platelets have other physiological roles and that inappropriate activation of platelets can also contribute to a range of other pathophysiological states not normally associated with thrombosis. An example of this is provided by the growing evidence that platelets can possess IgE receptors and participate both in allergic defence mechanisms and contribute to various types of allergic inflammatory disorders. This book has attempted to bring together a group of internationally recognized authorities to discuss platelets in health and disease in the broadest context, rather than just concentrating on the role of this blood element in thrombosis and haemostasis. Basic chapters on platelet production and the types of receptors and cellular transduction mechanisms possessed by platelets have also been included as these are areas of platelet research where considerable advances have been made over the last few years. It is hoped that this book will provide a useful overview to scientists and clinicians alike with either an active or general interest in the biological significance of platelets in health and disease.

Clive Page

1: Evidence in Favour of the Lungs and Against the Bone Marrow as the Site of Platelet Production

John F. Martin and Richard F. Levine

Introduction

Ever since Wright established the megakaryocyte as the cell of origin of the blood platelets, most haematologists have believed that platelets are shed in the bone marrow. The mechanism of platelet formation is debated, and there are several theories extant: pseudopodia, demarcation membranes, and physical fragmentation (Wright, 1910; Paulus *et al.* 1979; Radley & Scurfield, 1980; Trowbridge *et al.* 1982). These proposals are not all mutually exclusive, but they are, save for the third, generally presumed to occur either within, or adjacent to, the marrow sinusoids. The existence of multiple concepts and the absence of a consensus are due to the lack of definitive and convincing observations of platelet production. The failure to demonstrate clearly and reproducibly the mechanism of platelet shedding may indicate that morphologists have been observing the wrong organ. We argue below that there is little objective data supporting a marrow origin of platelets, and growing evidence in favour of the process occurring within the pulmonary microvasculature.

Evidence for and against a marrow origin of platelets

If scientific opinion is to be based upon evidence, then there is little evidence that platelets are produced in the bone marrow. Only two facts have been quoted in favour of thrombopoiesis in the marrow: the presence of megakaryocyte naked nuclei and a cinematographic study of megakaryocytes in the bone marrow (Kinosita & Ohno, 1961). The number of nuclei without cytoplasm (naked nuclei), which are found in the bone marrow after biopsy, is probably very low. However, there are no published data of quantification. Since megakaryocytes mature in the bone marrow, the presence of naked nuclei in the marrow certainly implies that the cytoplasm of the megakaryocyte has left the nucleus in the marrow. However, this does not mean that platelets were produced in this process.

When thrombopoiesis was accelerated by destroying circulating platelets in an animal model, large pieces of megakaryocyte cytoplasm were seen in the circulation apparently without nuclei (Fig. 1.1) (Slater *et al.* 1983). Tinggaard Pedersen

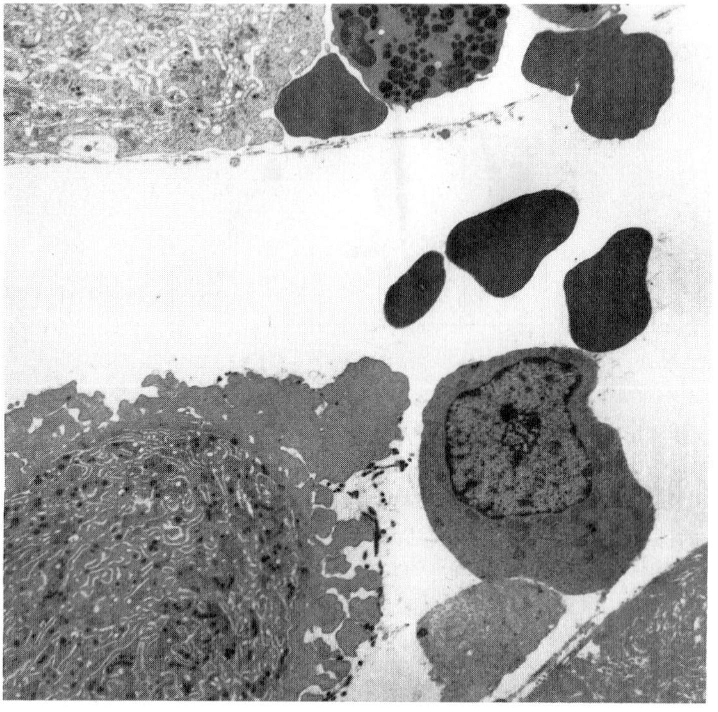

Figure 1.1 A transmission electron micrograph showing rabbit bone marrow (above) separated from the venous sinusoid by the parasinusoidal membrane. A large piece of megakaryocyte cytoplasm is seen in the venous sinusoid (bottom left). A red cell is seen leaving the bone marrow (top right). (Magnification ×2100.)

(1978) has also shown that cytoplasmic fragments of megakaryocytes circulate without nuclei. Figure 1.2 shows that the whole of a megakaryocyte's cytoplasm can have a tenuous attachment to its nucleus. Therefore, the presence of naked nuclei within the marrow does not necessarily imply that platelets have been produced there. Circumstantial evidence suggests that they have remained behind when anucleate megakaryocyte cytoplasm has entered the venous circulation.

Kinosita and Ohno (1961) have made a film which they claim shows bone marrow production of platelets from a megakaryocyte. This film is not now apparently available for viewing. However, a description does exist. They inserted a glass window into the femur of a rabbit and filmed a megakaryocyte shedding part of its cytoplasm on the glass window. However, they would have been unaware that megakaryocytes spread on glass, and what they observed may have been associated with that phenomenon. The same film, however, did show whole megakaryocytes being carried away in the blood.

The idea that platelets bud from megakaryocytes is first stated in Wright's paper of 1910. Although he saw buds and pseudopods arising from marrow megakaryocytes he also saw them in the spleen and in circulating megakaryocytes in blood vessels. He states '... (my observations) have led me to the conclusion that such small portions of giant cell cytoplasm, and also the small pseudopods, by separation from the cell become the blood platelets'. The paper describes a mechanism of platelet production, but does not contain definitive evidence about the marrow being the site.

When the marrow of the accelerated platelet production model in the rabbit is examined by electron microscopy, one can indeed see buds associated with megakaryocytes (Fig. 1.3). However, these buds protrude through the para-sinusoidal membrane that separates the bone marrow from the blood venous system. Furthermore they do not appear to contain granules. In Figure 1.3 a whole mature megakaryocyte can be seen in the venule. It is plausible that the buds are associated with movement of the megakaryocyte from the marrow to the venule. The presence of buds or pseudopods on the surface of marrow megakaryocytes does not necessarily imply platelet production in the marrow. There is, therefore, no evidence that platelets are produced in the bone marrow.

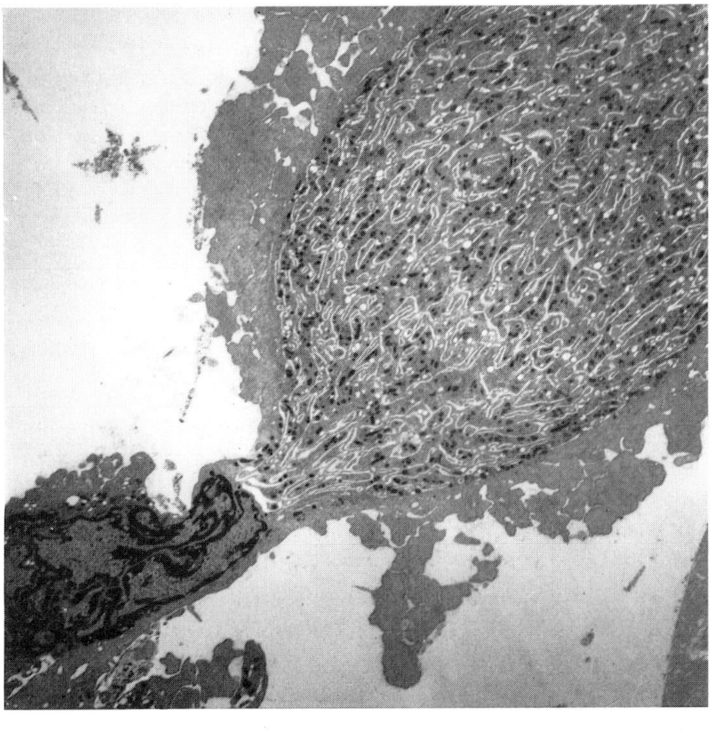

Figure 1.2 Transmission electron micrograph of rabbit bone marrow showing an amoeboid megakaryocyte barely connected to its nucleus. (Magnification ×2100.)

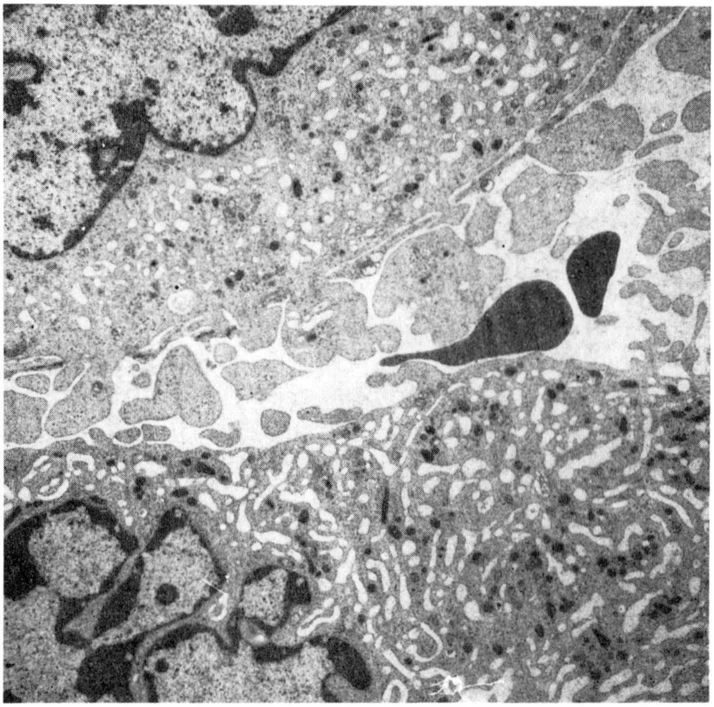

Figure 1.3 Transmission electron micrograph of rabbit bone marrow. A mature megakaryocyte is shown with processes protruding between sinusoidal cells. The processes could be interpreted as platelets budding off. However, they are more likely to be associated with the passage of megakaryocytes into the sinus space as they enter the venous system. This is supported by the presence of a mature megakaryocyte within the sinusoidal space. (Magnification ×3500.)

Evidence for platelet production in the lungs

The lungs are the second organ, after the marrow, in numerical content of megakaryocytes. The megakaryocytes present in all other tissues are probably only passing through in the circulation. Ever since 1894, scientists have debated the origins and functions of the pulmonary megakaryocytes. Howell and Donohue (1937) were the first to propose that platelet production occurs in the lungs. In 1965 Kaufman and coworkers connected the vascular supply of the lungs of dogs in series, and found that the distal lung contained very few megakaryocytes (Kaufman *et al.* 1965). This surgical preparation demonstrated that not only was the circulation the source of the pulmonary megakaryocytes, but also that the lung was an effective filter of the circulating megakaryocytes. Several workers have shown that maturing marrow megakaryocytes can enter the sinusoids with their cytoplasm intact. In addition, numerous investigators have documented circulating megakaryocytes in humans and in animals. Furthermore, an increase in the number of circulating megakaryocytes has been reported in several conditions, such as inflammation, cancer and bleeding, which are sometimes associated with secondary thrombocytosis. When there is a demand for increased platelet production the number of pulmonary megakaryocytes increases (Aabo & Hansen, 1978; Breslow *et al.* 1968; Hasen & Aabo, 1978; Hume *et al.* 1964; and Sharnoff, 1959).

In an important study, Tinggaard Pedersen counted the megakaryocytes entering and exiting from the lungs in humans (Tinggaard Pedersen, 1978). This was accomplished using megakaryocytes isolated by cytofiltration from blood samples obtained during cardiac catheterizations from the pulmonary artery and the aorta. The numbers of megakaryocytes he found entering the lungs seemed sufficient to provide most of the new platelets needed for normal steady state turnover. Other groups using similar methods have found a comparable range of data. This work might have made a greater impact had greater numbers of megakaryocytes been found, and had those in passage to the lungs had ample cytoplasm which could be the source of new platelets. However, in these reports only half of the central venous megakaryocytes had any cytoplasm at all and few had 'normal' amounts.

More recently, a new study has obtained even more compelling data in favour of pulmonary production of platelets. Using special media known to preserve megakaryocytes and more effective isolation methods than in the earlier work, Levine *et al.* found many more megakaryocytes with intact cytoplasm in the pulmonary arteries than reported previously but, as before, very few in the aortic samples. These circulating intact megakaryocytes had large amounts of mature cytoplasm (average megakaryocyte volume = 34 000 fl). With data on the patients' cardiac outputs, they extrapolated the measured data to an average of 40×10^6 intact megakaryocytes per day entering and being trapped in the lungs. The amount of megakaryocyte cytoplasm involved seems too great not to be used in platelet formation. In fact, the total volume of cytoplasm in these megakaryocytes corresponded to the amount required for steady state platelet production in these patients. (This conclusion is supported by previous indirect evidence from man and rat obtained by Trowbridge *et al.* 1984.)

The data were replicated in a second set of 20 patients undergoing catheterization. In this set, samples of pulmonary microvascular blood were also taken, using a new technique which involves retrograde aspiration through an inflated balloon catheter. In blood from the lung capillaries and small arterioles, intact megakaryocytes occurred with 12-times the frequency found in the main pulmonary arteries. This increment is a clear demonstration of filtration of intact megakaryocytes in the small vessels of the lungs. Importantly, the sizes of megakaryocytes recovered using this technique, were no different from those entering the lungs. These data therefore fail to confirm the concept of platelet production by binary division. By this hypothesis, Trowbridge and colleagues (Trowbridge *et al.* 1982; Trowbridge & Harley, 1984) suggested that megakaryocytes entered the pulmonary circulation with high kinetic energy derived from the right ventricle. They would then impact against the bifurcations of the dividing pulmonary arteries. The process was to explain the log normal distribution of platelet volume by a physical fragmentation process. Although Levine's more recent results argue against such a binary division process proceeding with repeated division of the pulmonary artery, they do not exclude the possibility of physical forces contributing to platelet production deep in the vasculature. The most simple inference from the recovery of intact megakaryocytes this deep in the microvasculature, is that transformation of the megakaryocyte cytoplasm into platelets, if it does take place in the lungs, must occur at, or distal to, the site of wedging. The wedging must occur in vessels as small as, or smaller in diameter, than the megakaryocytes. Specific morphometric data on this site and the degree of megakaryocyte deformability in this location is presently lacking. The wider conclusion from this work is that if such large numbers of mature megakaryocytes are delivered intact to the pulmonary capillaries, do not appear in the arterial circulation and do not continually accumulate in the lungs, they are either converted into platelets there or phagocytosed *in toto*.

If platelets are produced by circulating megakaryocytes in the lung, an explanation of how platelet formation occurs in the fetus is necessary. Term infants normally have the same range of platelet counts as adults, but negligible pulmonary perfusion as fetuses. Levine and colleagues have also carried out a study which examined circulating megakaryocytes going to, and returning from, the placenta. Megakaryocytes were isolated by elutriation from blood samples obtained from the umbilical arteries and veins of term infants, at routine Caesarian sections after the clamping of the cord. A large differential between the arterial and venous megakaryocyte counts was found, indicating a continual and high rate of megakaryocyte filtration in the placenta (approximately 20×10^6 per day). Although the megakaryocytes are smaller in a fetus than in an adult, the megakaryocyte numbers and sizes are still consistent with fetal production of platelets occurring in the placenta, as originally proposed by Martin and colleagues (Martin *et al.* 1983).

Bases for persistence in belief in a marrow locus of platelet production

The primary reason for the delay in accepting the concept of platelet production in the lungs, has been the lack of better evidence than exists for marrow production. Apparently, few haematologists are aware that megakaryocytes are routinely found in the circulation. This is probably because the absolute incidence of circulating megakaryocytes is quite low. In addition, most blood cell examination is performed on samples drawn from the antecubital fossa vein, which drains an area in adults in which little active marrow is found. By light microscopic observations of lung sections, Howell and Donohue (1937) drew conclusions about platelet shedding from megakaryocyte pseudopods in pulmonary vessels, similar to the descriptions of Wright in the marrow sinusoids (Wright, 1910). However, more recent light microscopic studies have not provided any clear evidence of platelet production, only of apparent pseudopods in the pulmonary microvasculature. There is only a single electron micrographic study known to us of megakaryocytes in the lungs. That report, using both scanning and thin-section technology, showed some sizeable megakaryocytes in the pulmonary microvasculature but shed no light on possible platelet production.

The other major reason for persistent belief in a marrow site is tradition. Wright's conclusions about the fact, mechanism and site of platelet production by marrow megakaryocytes have been largely accepted *in toto* and passed down from teacher to student for 80 years. Indeed, a contemporary account illustrates the force of Wright's insights and observations: 'To one who has had the opportunity of examining the preparations of Dr J.H. Wright, the last word seems to have been said on the subject of the origin of the blood-platelets and the function of the bone marrow giant cell, the megolokaryocyte [sic].' Wright's establishment of the lineage relationship of the megakaryocyte and platelets, and of the origin of platelet organelles and cytoplasm in the megakaryocytes, have been extensively confirmed and even amplified by modern morphologic, immunologic and biochemical studies. As in the above quote by Bunting, a continued belief in Wright's concept of platelet formation may be simply an extrapolation of acceptance beyond these two, now proven, concepts. His third major hypothesis was that platelets are formed from megakaryocyte cytoplasm detached from the cell in the marrow sinusoids: 'All or most of the cytoplasm of the giant cell is given off to the blood stream and the nucleus degenerates. The more or less naked nucleus is often carried by the blood stream to the lungs where it lodges in the capillaries.' Wright's hypothesis does not allow for the finding of so many intact megakaryocytes in the lungs and is thus contradicted by the earlier and the more recent data.

It has been assumed that the locus of platelet production is the same as the site of megakaryocyte precursor multiplication and differentiation; that these cells carry out all their functions at the site of their birth. An analogy may have been made with the established production of blood leukocytes and erythrocytes, which occurs entirely within the marrow. In mammalian red cell formation, the cytoplasm usually sheds its nucleus within the marrow. In a sense, platelets also shed their nuclei. However, megakaryocytes are very different from other blood cell precursors. Megakaryocytes are polyploid and unique to mammals. In addition, unlike other lineages in which a precursor cell divides to produce two daughter cells, each megakaryocyte may produce about 3000 essentially similar cells. One hypothesis states that the formation of such a large number of platelets from a mature megakaryocyte is the consequence of, or mediated by, pent-up cytokinesis forces accumulated during polyploidization. What controls this process is quite unknown. Clearly, platelet formation is far more complicated than the production of white cells and red cells, and may require circumstances not found in the marrow.

Why the lungs?

The lungs are the first capillary bed confronting the circulating megakaryocytes, at a time in their travels when they are moving at increasing speed generated by the right ventricle. Major consequences appear inevitable from the large sizes of these intact megakaryocytes (mean diameter 40 μm, range as high as 88 μm). Although megakaryocytes demonstrate considerable deformability as they enter the circulation through small pores in the sinusoidal walls, considerably greater forces are exerted on them as they arrive in the pulmonary microvasculature at much greater speeds than those with which they leave the marrow. A rapid and significant change in shape and/or size must occur to avoid obstruction of the small vessels, especially because of the number of such interactions (averaging 28 000 per minute). The recent data cited above make it likely that the megakaryocytes do not survive this interaction intact, although they are apparently filtered or caught in small vessels prior to the actual transformation.

In addition to the greater shear forces on megakaryocytes in the pulmonary microvasculature, compared to those in the marrow, there may be other special conditions in the lungs that may prove to be necessary for platelet production. There are a number of substances for which the lung is a major or superior source and these substances could be important in the final phase of megakaryocyte maturation. For example, the lung is an excellent source of a maturation factor, megakaryocyte potentiator, and other growth factors. Because the endothelial cell content of the lungs in general is so much greater than that of the marrow, and comprises a significant part of the microvasculature, large quantities of prostacyclin and nitric oxide could be available. The microvasculature is also where the oxygen content of the blood increases abruptly. However, no data yet exists to establish the role(s) of any of these substances in platelet production. Interestingly, in general these remarks seem equally applicable to the placenta.

Requirements for proof of a pulmonary site of platelet production

An effort must be made to examine the living pulmonary microvasculature by sophisticated morphologic means, such as video-phase microscopy or electron microscopy after high-pressure perfusion fixation. In addition, methods must be devised to identify, label and collect newly-formed platelets.

Although the platelet count difference across the pulmonary circulation has shown an increase in the pulmonary vein, this is not evidence to support pulmonary platelet production (Martin *et al.* 1987). In a study of 13 patients, the mean platelet count in the pulmonary artery was 200 ± 21 and 212 ± 22 in the pulmonary vein. Using a one-tailed paired t-test this increase approached statistical significance ($P < 0.06$). In these patients the femoral artery platelet count was 221 ± 16 and the femoral vein count was 195 ± 16; a significant decrease ($P < 0.04$). It is tempting to attribute this increase in platelet count across the pulmonary circulation, which has been described previously by other authors (Sharnoff & Scardino, 1960), as evidence of pulmonary platelet production. However, it can be calculated that in normal pulmonary platelet production a difference of only 0.01% in platelet count across the pulmonary circulation would be expected, if all platelets were produced in the lungs. Such a difference would not be measurable by present platelet counting techniques. This suggests that sampling bias, or other artefacts such as dehydration of the blood as it passes through the lungs, may account for the apparent platelet count differences across the pulmonary circulation.

Even the criteria by which pulmonary platelet production could be proved beyond reasonable doubt are not clear. This original field requires both technical and intellectual application, not only because it is one of the most fascinating areas of vascular biology, but also because the site and production mechanisms of megakaryocyte transformation into platelets will probably be a source of human disease as yet unsuspected.

Acknowledgment

J.F. Martin is British Heart Foundation Professor of Cardiovascular Science.

References

Aabo, K. & Hansen, K.B. (1978) Megakaryocytes in pulmonary blood vessels. I. Incidence at autopsy, clinicopathiological relations especially to disseminated intravascular coagulation. *Acta Pathol Microbiol Scand* Section A, **86**, 285–291.

Breslow, A., Kaufman, R.M. & Lawsky, A.R. (1968) The effect of surgery on the concentration of circulatory megakaryocytes and platelets. *Blood* **32**, 382–401.

Hasen, K.D. & Aabo, K. (1978) Megakaryocytes in pulmonary blood vessels. Relations to malignant haematological diseases especially leukaemia. *Acta Pathol Microbiol Scand* Section A, **86**, 293–295.

Howell, W.H. & Donahue, D.P. (1937) The production of blood platelets in the lung. *J Exp Med* **65**, 177–204.

Hume, R., West, J.T., Malmgren, R.A. & Chu, E.A. (1964) Quantitative observation of circulating megakaryocytes in the blood of patients with cancer. *N Engl J Med* **270**, 111–117.

Kaufman, R.M., Airo, R., Pollack, S., Crosby, W.H. & Doberneck, R. (1965) Origin of pulmonary megakaryocytes. *Blood* **25**, 767–775.

Kinosita, R. & Ohno, S. (1961) Biodynamics of thrombopoiesis. In Johnson, S.A., Monto, R.W., Rebuck, J.W. & Horn, R.C. (eds) Blood platelets, pp. 611–616. Little & Brown, Boston.

Martin, J.F., Slater, D.N. & Trowbridge, E.A. (1983) Abnormal intrapulmonary platelet production: a possible cause of vascular and lung disease. *Lancet* **i**, 793–796.

Paulus, J.M., Bury, J. & Grosdent, J.C. (1979) Control of platelet territory development in megakaryocytes. *Blood Cells* **5**, 59–88.

Radley, J.M. & Scurfield, G. (1980) The mechanism of platelet release. *Blood* **56**, 996–999.

Sharnoff, J.G. (1959) Increased pulmonary megakaryocytes — probable role in postoperative thromboembolism. *J Am Med Assoc* **169**, 688–691.

Sharnoff, J.G. & Scardino, V. (1960) Platelet count differences in blood of the rabbit right and left heart ventricles. *Nature* **187**, 334–335.

Slater, D.N., Trowbridge, E.A. & Martin, J.F. (1983) The megakaryocyte in thrombocytopenia: a light and electronmicroscope study supporting the theory that all platelets are produced in the lungs. *Thromb Res* **31**, 163–176.

Tinggaard Pedersen, N. (1978) Occurrence of megakaryocytes in various vessels and their retention in the pulmonary capillaries in man. *Scand J Haematol* **21**, 369–375.

Trowbridge, E.A. & Harley, P.J. (1984) A computer model of the random binary sequential division of megakaryocyte cytoplasm to produce platelets. *Phys Med Biol* **29**, 1447–1487.

Trowbridge, E.A., Martin, J.F. & Slater, D.N. (1982) Evidence for a theory of physical fragmentation of megakaryocytes, implying that all platelets are produced in the pulmonary circulation. *Thromb Res* **28**, 461–475.

Trowbridge, E.A., Martin, J.F., Slater, D.N., Kishk, Y.T., Harley, P.J., Warren, C.W. & Woodcock, B. (1984) The origin of platelet count and volume. *Clin Phys Physiol Meas* **5**, 145–170.

Wright, J.H. (1910) The histogenesis of the blood platelets. *J Morphol* **21**, 263–278.

2: The Platelet Surface Membrane: Ultrastructure, Receptor Binding and Function

David P. Tuffin

The ability of human circulating blood platelets to adhere to damaged vessel endothelium and the exposed subendothelial connective tissue matrix *in vivo*, and to respond rapidly in stirred plasma to a variety of excitatory agonists including adenosine-5′-diphosphate (ADP), 5-hydroxytryptamine (5-HT), adrenaline, collagen or thrombin *in vitro*, has been recognized for many years. Moreover, although these cells are clearly capable of playing a central role in haemostasis by adherence at the sites of vessel wall damage, by the formation of aggregates, and the exposure of pro-coagulant surface phospholipid domains, the view has strengthened that the activation of circulating platelets might also contribute significantly to a number of other inflammatory and immune response-based disease conditions.

Despite much attention, the mechanisms by which the circulating quiescent platelet becomes activated, and the sequence of events which govern the unique nature of its response, have, until relatively recently, remained poorly understood. However, detailed information gained from careful morphological studies coupled with refined analytical techniques, ligand receptor binding studies and in particular molecular biology, has begun to shed considerable new light on the process. This is especially true of events at the platelet surface membrane, which collectively govern agonist–receptor binding, stimulus–response coupling, cell shape change, and ultimately, exposure of adhesive proteins and the formation of aggregates.

Platelet surface membrane ultrastructure

Prior to stimulation, the resting circulating platelet formed by cytoplasmic fragmentation from megakaryocytes in bone marrow or lung (Chapter 1) is discoid in shape with an equatorial diameter of 3–4 μm and a thickness of approximately 1 μm (White, 1987a). Electron microscopy of this non-nucleated cell reveals extensive invagination of the surface membrane comprising an open canalicular system continuous with the plasma membrane surface, which forms an interconnecting network of canaliculi distributed throughout the cell (Fig. 2.1). Unique to the platelet amongst circulating blood cells, and distinct from the intracellular dense tubular system, the canaliculi provide ready access to the interior of the platelet for plasma proteins and other substances, whilst also facilitating secretion from the amine and protein-storage granules during the release reaction (White, 1974).

The surface glycoproteins

At the surface membrane, the platelet possesses a substantial exterior coat or glycocalyx. Analytical studies employing a combination of specific labelling (lactoperoxidase-iodination; [^{125}I]diazotized di-iodosulphanilic acid), free-flow electrophoresis, and high-resolution sodium dodecyl sulphate-polyacrylamide gel electrophoresis (SDS-PAGE), under reducing and non-reducing conditions, established that this dense layer (some 20 nm thick) is rich in glycoproteins of at least ten different types (Table 2.1). Of these, glycoprotein Ib (GpIB), which exists as a complex of the disulphide-linked GpIbα and GpIbβ subunits with GpIX (Du *et al.* 1987; Fox *et al.* 1988a) is the most prominent periodic acid-Schiff (PAS)-staining component (Phillips & Agin, 1977), whilst the GpIIb–IIIa complex is the most abundant, and the only glycoprotein also detected in trace amounts on intracellular membrane (Hack & Crawford, 1984). It has become clear that the platelet surface glycoproteins play a primary role in the adhesion of platelets to exposed subendothelial matrix proteins, interaction with ligands such as collagen or thrombin, and exposure of fibrinogen receptors to facilitate aggregation (see George *et al.* 1985; Nurden, 1987) such that they merit detailed attention later in this review. Indeed, two inherited platelet functional disorders, Bernard–Soulier syndrome and Glanzmann's thrombasthenia, are caused by a congenital deficiency in the surface membrane glycoproteins Ib and IIb–IIIa complex respectively (Phillips *et al.* 1975; Nurden & Caen, 1978; Clemetson *et al.* 1982).

Of particular significance, evidence has also emerged that certain of the platelet glycoproteins belong to the family of cell surface adhesion polypeptides termed I-SCAM proteins or integrins. This superfamily comprises at least ten related cell–cell and cell–matrix adhesion proteins, which have been classified by structure into three groups.

1 The very late activation (VLA) antigens, first identified on lymphocytes.
2 The cytoadhesins.
3 The leucocyte adhesion (Leu–Cam) proteins (Hynes, 1986; Ginsberg *et al.* 1988).

Members of (1) and (2), but not (3), have been identified on the platelet surface membrane. Structurally, all are heterodimeric glycoproteins consisting of an α-subunit which frequently contains heavy and light chains, and a β-subunit possessing intrachain disulphide bonds. Within each group, the β-subunit appears common and the α-subunit is variable.

The platelet glycoproteins as a group are membrane-spanning polypeptides, each comprising a short C-terminal cytoplasmic region, a transmembrane segment of hydrophobic residues, and a relatively large N-terminal extracellular domain. They are therefore structurally equipped to serve as transmembrane receptor

Table 2.1 Biochemical characterization of the human platelet surface glycoproteins

Glycoprotein	Apparent M_r (approx.)	Isoelectric point (range)	PAS staining
Ia†	150–165 000	5.3–6.0	±
Ib*	170 000	—	+
Ibα	135–150 000‡	5.0–5.8	+
Ibβ	21–23 000	6.4–7.0	±
Ic*	148 000	—	?
Icα	134 000	—	?
Icβ	27 000	—	?
IIa†	125–135 000	5.5–5.7	+
IIb*	142 000‡	—	+
IIbα	115 130 000	5.3–6.1	+
IIbβ	25–28 000	5.1–5.6	±
IIIa†	90–95 000‡	5.2–5.8	+
IIIb(IV)	88–97 000	5.2–5.4	+
V	80–85 000	6.0–6.5	–
IX	22 000	—	–

Data in the table is compiled from platelet membrane preparations analysed by single or improved resolution two-dimensional sodium dodecyl sulphate polyacrylamide gel electrophoresis either alone (Phillips & Agin, 1977; George 1978; Kinoshita *et al.* 1979) or in combination with isoelectric focussing (Hack & Crawford, 1984) from which the isoelectric point values are derived. By generally accepted nomenclature, the Roman numerals and lettering are used to delineate the glycoproteins by rank order or molecular weight, whereas the α and β-subscripts are used to represent the subunits of respective glycoproteins evident after full reduction with mercaptoethanol or dithiothreitol. It should be noted that many of the platelet surface glycoproteins possess intermolecular and intramolecular disulphides. In the former case (*) reduction reveals the presence of smaller subunits the molecular weight sum of which approximates to the parent molecule, whilst in the latter case (†), reduction induces an apparent increase in molecular weight resulting from decreased electrophoretic mobility. For this reason, only apparent molecular weight ranges and isoelectric point values are quoted. For the purposes of this table, the degree of staining obtained using the periodic acid–Schiff reaction (PAS) is graded only as strong (+), weak (±) or absent (–).

‡ Partial or complete cDNA and amino acid sequence data for GpIbα (Titani *et al.* 1987; Lopez *et al.* 1987b), GpIIb (Loftus *et al.* 1987) and GpIIIa (Fitzgerald *et al.* 1987) is now available (see text).

proteins, being tightly anchored within the lipid bilayer through interaction with the hydrophobic segment. The existence of potential glycosylation sites based on available sequence data indicates that carbohydrate is present only in the N-terminal domains, thus influencing both tertiary structure and ligand binding in the extracellular environment. Conversely, the shorter intracellular regions may contain amino acid sequences which provide linkage to cytoskeletal proteins such as actin-binding protein (ABP) (in the case of GpIb–IX) or actin filaments

(GpIIb–IIIa). The significance of these observations with respect to the binding of individual ligands and physiological function is considered further below.

Membrane lipid components

The human platelet surface membrane, 7–9 nm in diameter, is a typical bilayer membrane composed of protein, lipid and carbohydrate. The membrane lipids are predominantly phospholipids (approximately 75%) and neutral lipid (20%) with a small amount of glycolipid also present (Shattil & Cooper, 1978). Early methods for studying mixed-membrane fractions, prepared from platelets lysed by sonication, glycerol or freeze-thawing, involved high-speed density-gradient centrifugation of the lysates in Ficoll or sucrose. Analysis of the separated cytoplasmic and granule-derived membrane obtained by these methods, has shown that overall, phosphatidylcholine and sphingomyelin make up more than half the membrane phospholipid present, the remainder being phosphatidylserine, phosphatidylethanolamine, and phosphatidylinositol (Barber & Jamieson, 1970; Kaulen & Gross, 1973). Glycosphingolipids and ceramides are present in low amounts (Tao *et al.* 1973) but their function is unknown, although intriguingly, the disialogangliosides GD2 and GD3 have been postulated to be present in a divalent cation complex with surface glycoproteins on neuroblastoma and human melanoma cells, and to play a significant role in the ability of these cells to interact with fibronectin or vitronectin via the Arg–Gly–Asp recognition peptide (Cheresh *et al.* 1987).

From a more refined comparison of surface and intracellular platelet membranes using high-voltage free-flow electrophoresis, some interesting differences in lipid composition have emerged. In particular, the intracellular membranes are largely devoid of sphingomyelin compared to the surface membrane, the latter also being relatively richer in phosphatidylserine (Lagarde *et al.* 1982). It is also apparent that the cholesterol:phospholipid ratio of the surface membrane fraction is some two-fold greater that of the intracellular membranes (Menashi *et al.* 1981). The differences may reflect a surface membrane requirement in the platelet for increased rigidity and decreased fluidity (Shattil & Cooper, 1976).

The cell and membrane cytoskeleton

The cytoskeleton of the circulating platelet, responsible for both the maintenance of normal morphometry (i.e. the discoid shape) in the unstimulated cell, and the alterations in cell shape induced by activation, is comprised predominantly of a circumferential band of microtubules (White & Sauk, 1984) and abundant cytosolic actin microfilaments (Boyles *et al.* 1985). Tubulin, a heterodimer of two α and β-subunit polypeptides, each with a molecular weight of approximately 55 000, is the major microtubular protein. The tubulin subunits polymerize to form bundles which, in turn, aggregate to make up the characteristic tube-like tertiary structure of the protein. These are associated with a number of high molecular weight

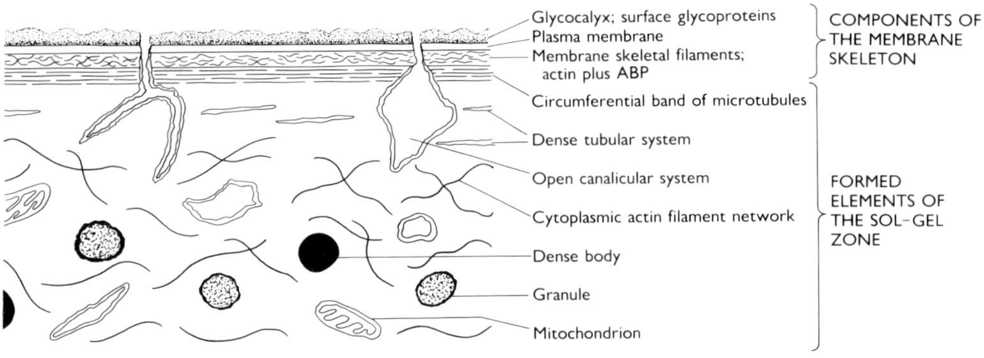

Figure 2.1 Key features of the membrane skeleton and sol–gel zone in the human platelet (drawing not to scale). For detailed electron microscopy studies encompassing both the appearance of quiescent discoid platelets and the considerable organizational changes which occur on activation, see White (1987a). (ABP = actin-binding protein.)

(300 000) microtubule associated proteins (MAPs) related, but not identical to, those described in other tissues. Although the process is as yet poorly understood, cytosolic calcium concentration and calmodulin appear important in the control of tubulin polymerization, with MAPs probably influencing the interaction of microtubules with other cytoskeletal proteins.

Actin, in both its filamentous and non-filamentous forms, has been estimated to constitute 20–30% of total platelet protein (Rosenberg *et al.* 1981a; Fox *et al.* 1984). Circular dichroism spectra show that platelet actin is present in quiescent platelets in both the polymeric F form and the soluble subunit G form, as is true of skeletal muscle actin (Landon *et al.* 1977); in contrast, the molar ratio of actin:myosin is much higher than in smooth or skeletal muscle tissue. However, a considerable proportion of the monomeric actin is associated in a stoichiometric I:I complex with the low molecular weight protein profilin. Termed profilactin, this complex effectively acts as a storage pool of actin monomer, dissociating rapidly when platelets are stimulated (Markey *et al.* 1981).

A considerable number of other structural proteins have been identified in the human platelet cytoskeleton (Table 2.2), many of which are able to bind to actin filaments, including ABP, P235 (related to the erythrocyte protein talin) and α-actinin. Recent *in vitro* data indicates that the organization (assembly or destabilization) and function of actin microfilaments is largely dictated by the association of actin with the above proteins, although vinculin, gelsolin and tropmyosin are also strongly implicated (for a detailed review see Fox, 1987). For example, if purified preparations of ABP and actin are incubated together, the cytoskeletal complex re-forms (Rosenberg *et al.* 1981b). Similarly, addition of ABP to solutions of actin, which also contain the troponin-tropomyosin complex, causes formation of very viscous gels, whilst α-actinin is reported to be capable of crosslinking dissociated actin into gels (Schollmeyer *et al.* 1978).

Table 2.2 Properties of platelet membrane cytoskeletal proteins

Protein	M_r	Properties	References
Actin (20–30%)	43 000	β and γ isoforms predominate Activates myosin Mg^{2+}ATPase	Landon *et al.* (1977)
Actin-binding protein (8%)	250 000 (dimer)	Crosslinks actin filaments	Schollmeyer *et al.* (1978) Rosenberg *et al.* (1981a)
Myosin (2–3%)	200 000 20 000 16 000	2 heavy chains } subunit complex 2 light chains 2 light chains Polymerizes with actin during the aggregatory process Contractile	Adelstein *et al.* (1971) Pollard *et al.* (1977)
P235 (3–8%)	235 000 (dimer)	Talin-like globular protein Cleaved by calcium-dependent protease	Collier & Wang (1982)
α-actinin (3%)	100 000	Rod-like protein. Crosslinks actin filaments? Links filament bundles to plasma membrane	Rosenberg *et al.* (1981b) Landon & Olomucki (1983)
Profilin	16 000	Inhibits actin polymerization by association with actin (1:1 complex) to form profilactin	Markey *et al.* (1981)
Tropomyosin	30 000	Multiple isoforms. Major components Tm4(α) *and* Tm5 (β) Forms stable coils. Regulates association of actin filaments.	Cote *et al.* (1978)
Gelsolin	91 000	Regulates actin filament length	Lind *et al.* (1982)
Vinculin	130 000	No effect on actin assembly May influence linkage of actin filament bundles to membrane?	Koteliansky *et al.* (1984)
Spectrin	235 000 240 000	Two subunits Present only in small amounts Regulates the organization of membrane skeleton?	Fox *et al.* (1987)
Caldesmon	147 000 150 000	Two subunits Regulates interaction of actin with myosin? Calmodulin sensitive	Pho *et al.* (1986)

The reported estimated proportion of total platelet protein is shown in parentheses for some of the major protein components. Actin and those proteins which bind to it account for some 50% of total platelet protein.

Preliminary evidence for the existence and structure of a platelet surface membrane cytoskeleton (analagous to that of the erythrocyte) has accrued steadily from a combination of biochemical and morphological studies. As a general rule, it appears that the majority of the proteins now viewed as candidate linkage proteins between actin microfilaments and the surface plasma membrane (e.g. ABP, vinculin, P235 and α-actinin) are potential substrates for a cytosolic calcium-dependent protease (see later). Indeed, it has been claimed that proteolysis of certain platelet proteins, including ABP, leads to the failure of platelets to form pseudopodia (Nachmias *et al.* 1979). Moreover, the cytoskeletal proteins actin, ABP and myosin, with associated elements such as tropomyosin and α-actinin, are present in the surface membrane fraction but virtually absent from preparations of intracellular membranes (Hack & Crawford, 1984). The findings correlate with histological observations that platelets possess a network of actin filaments situated just below the surface membrane bilayer which appears to function specifically as a membrane skeleton, in addition to the cytoplasmic population of actin filaments (Fox, 1985a,b).

The major protein components of the membrane cytoskeleton are now recognized as being actin, ABP and the GpIb–IX complex, although in Triton X-100 platelet lysates, actin filaments are also reported to associate with the GpIa–IIa complex and an as yet unidentified high molecular weight glycoprotein (Fox, 1985b). Actin-binding protein and GpIb co-isolate on anti-GpIb antibody affinity-chromatography columns (Okita *et al.* 1985), and from immunocytochemical experiments employing antibodies directed against ABP and the α-subunit of GpIb, it is clear that these proteins are distributed in the membrane cytoskeletal layer (Fox *et al.* 1988b). A scheme has been proposed (Fox & Boyles, 1988) in which microfilaments of actin, crosslinked by ABP, are in turn attached to the plasma membrane, primarily via binding domains on the cytosolic carboxy terminal region of the GpIb–IX complex as shown in Fig. 2.2 (Solum & Olsen, 1984; Fox, 1985b). Interaction of the membrane cytoskeleton with both surface membrane components such as GpIb–IX and microtubular proteins within the cell, may therefore play a key role in regulating the shape of the surface membrane, and hence maintaining the discoid shape of the unstimulated platelet in circulation (White, 1984). Furthermore, it appears conceivable that changes in the membrane cytoskeletal structure could markedly influence surface membrane receptor conformation, and membrane functions such as the ability of GpIb to bind to von Willebrand factor (vWF), platelet spreading, or the exposure of surface procoagulant phospholipid (Coller, 1981; Fox, 1985b; Fox & Boyles, 1988).

Activation-induced structural changes

The stimulation of platelets by exposure to foreign surfaces, or following addition of excitatory agonists to stirred platelet suspensions *in vitro*, causes a remarkable reorganization of both the surface and internal cell cytoskeleton. The platelets

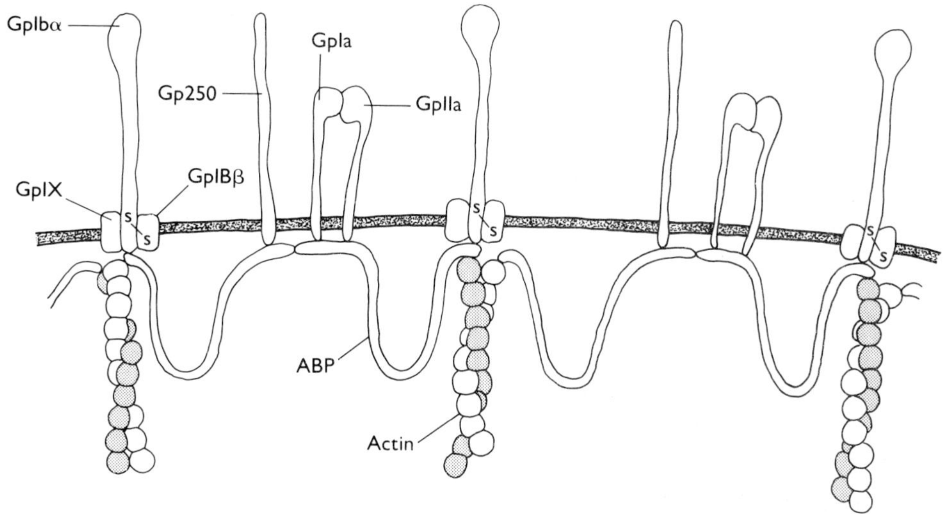

Figure 2.2 Possible functional relationship between platelet membrane cytoskeletal proteins and surface glycoprotein receptors. In the model, actin-binding protein (ABP) is postulated to serve as a linkage protein between actin filaments and glycoproteins such as the GpIb–Ix complex or GpIa–IIa. An as yet unidentified glycoprotein (Gp250) is also shown (see text). (From Fox & Boyles, 1988.)

rapidly lose their discoid shape, becoming more spherical in appearance, and extend short and long pseudopodia (White, 1987a; 1987b). This transformation is largely driven by altered organization of the cytoskeletal actin filamentous network as demonstrated in early studies of platelet morphology (Sixma & Molenaar, 1966). The degree of actin polymerization increases, and in the presence of ABP and α-actinin, the actin molecules assemble into filaments (Schollmeyer *et al.* 1978). In turn, the filaments become crosslinked, aligned into bundles and associated with newly phosphorylated myosin (Gonella & Nachmias, 1981).

The precise biochemical mechanisms responsible for the processes of actin polymerization and the assembly of filaments into parallel associations or bundles, which occurs during platelet shape change and pseudopod formation, remain to be fully elucidated. It has been suggested that an early critical step is the activation of a calcium-sensitive protease enzyme capable of hydrolyzing ABP and P235. A more recent report claims that this may also be the case for a third protein called spectrin (Table 2.2), present in only low amounts, but which is again closely associated with platelet membrane-bound actin, and in the erythrocyte is known to link actin filaments to plasma membrane glycoproteins (Fox *et al.* 1987b). This hypothesis is attractive, since it may explain how the removal of transmembrane connections and the disruption of the membrane cytoskeleton, presumed necessary to allow shape change and formation of pseudopods, is achieved. The time course for the hydrolysis of ABP, P235 and spectrin *in vitro* is rapid and appears compatible. Indirect supportive evidence obtained from the study of Bernard–Soulier syndrome platelets indicates that these cells, which lack the surface membrane GpIb, are considerably more deformable than normal platelets (White *et al.* 1984).

Internally, equally dramatic changes in the platelet cytoskeleton occur on activation. Granules, which in the unstimulated platelet are dispersed throughout the cytoplasm, become more concentrated in the centre of the cell through a contractile interaction of actin with myosin (Pollard *et al.* 1977; Painter & Ginsberg, 1984). The visible coils of the microtubular apparatus constrict into tight rings and also move to the central zone of the cell, whilst the open canalicular system appears to dilate and contains granule-stored secretory substances (White, 1984, 1987b). Comparison of these extensive cytoskeletal modifications in the presence and absence of taxol, an agent which blocks disassembly of microtubular proteins, reveals that microtubular disassembly and subsequent reassembly is not a prerequisite for the centralization of coils and organelles in the aggregating platelet as was first thought. Rather the coils of the microtubules remain intact throughout an intracellular contractile response driven by the assembly of actin into filaments and bundles (White & Rao, 1983; White & Sauk, 1984). The elegant cascade of metabolic events in the activated platelet (consequent on agonist-receptor binding), which accompanies the above changes in membrane and cytosolic skeletal proteins, is described in Chapter 3 of this volume.

The interaction of platelets with connective tissue proteins

The adhesion and aggregation of circulating blood platelets at sites of exposed vascular subendothelial matrix following vascular injury, is the first and critical event in the process of haemostasis, thrombus formation, and ultimately, vessel repair. The platelet response is dependent on a complex array of multiple-linked interactions which occur either directly between platelet surface membrane glycoproteins and vessel wall constituents, or indirectly via the vWF glycoprotein. Direct adhesion of platelets to collagen fibrils has been studied in most detail, but interactions with other proteins such as fibronectin or laminin may also be of importance. Human vWF is a high molecular weight oligomeric plasma protein synthesized, stored (in the Weibel–Palade bodies) and secreted by vascular endothelial cells, which can act as a bridge between the platelet membrane and subendothelial collagen (Sakariassen *et al.* 1979, 1986). At low-shear forces in large vessels, the interaction of platelets with the vessel wall is predominantly vWF-independent and supported by primary platelet binding sites for collagen fibrils (Santoro, 1986). However, under conditions of high shear accompanied by turbulent flow at arterial bifurcations, damage sites, or in smaller vessels and capillaries, a secondary or reinforcing vWF-dependent mechanism assumes importance (Stel *et al.* 1985; Turitto *et al.* 1985). The adhesion of platelets to collagen in the solid phase (spreading) under low or high shear, and the responses of stirred platelet suspensions to the addition of collagen fibrils (shape change, aggregation and secretion) can each be demonstrated *in vitro* (Baumgartner, 1977; Shadle & Barondes, 1982). Although physiologically complementary in the haemostatic process, the basic mechanisms responsible for vWF-dependent and independent platelet interactions with matrix proteins such as collagen, can thus be separated for study, and are best considered in this fashion.

Adhesion of platelets to collagen: the role of GpIa–IIa

Platelets are able to adhere to monomeric collagen via a cation-dependent mechanism (Santoro, 1986), but it has been recognized for some years that optimal platelet adhesion and stimulation is only achieved by collagen when in its natural triple-helical conformation and associated into a stable fibrillar form. Under these conditions, collagen types I and III (interstitial), IV (basement membrane), V (pericellular) and VI (pepsin-resistant), all of which are present in the vessel wall, appear capable of inducing platelet aggregation (Barnes, 1985; Morton *et al.* 1987). Carefully conducted cleavage experiments using cyanogen bromide (CNBr), in which peptides were renatured to restore the triple-helical form and polymerized to impose quaternary structure before the examination of aggregating activity, have shown that the α 1(I) and α 2(I)-chains of type I collagen both aggregate platelets through multiple discrete reactive sites present in the polypeptide, rather than via one specific reactive domain (Fitzsimmons *et al.* 1986). In contrast, parallel experiments with type III collagen reveal a highly reactive site at a single locus in the protein, which in type I collagen is essentially inactive (Morton *et al.* 1987). It is also clear from these and earlier studies that important charged residues are present at the collagen reactive sites, and further treatment of CNBr cleaved peptides from types I and III collagen with amino acid-modifying reagents specific for arginyl or lysyl residues has facilitated the identification of putative reactive sequences (Morton *et al.* 1987).

At the platelet surface membrane, convincing evidence for a population of specific high-affinity receptors for collagen has proved difficult to obtain. Various reports have implicated fibronectin, glucosyl transferase, complement component C1S, Factor XIII and GpIIb. None of these hypotheses have withstood rigorous examination. Chiang and colleagues have identified a PAS-positive M_r 65 000 protein from Triton-solubilized platelet membranes with apparent high affinity for the α 1(I)-chain of chick skin collagen (Chiang *et al.* 1982). Polyclonal and monoclonal antibodies raised against this protein selectively inhibit type I collagen-induced aggregation and the adhesion of platelets to an artificial collagen matrix (Chiang *et al.* 1987). Support for the concept that one of the major platelet surface glycoproteins might be the collagen receptor, gained additional credibility from two important observations. Firstly, Niewenhuis *et al.* (1985) identified a patient with a haemorrhagic disorder and extended bleeding time whose platelets responded normally to all agonists except collagen, and expressed only 15–25% of the normal level of membrane GpIa. Secondly, adhesion of platelets to polystyrene dishes coated with rat skin type I collagen was shown to depend on binding of an M_r 160 000 single polypeptide which demonstrated electrophoretic behaviour identical to that of GpIa (Santoro, 1986).

Whilst it remains unclear whether the polypeptide reported by Chiang *et al.* (1982) is related to GpIa, the identity of the platelet collagen receptor has been finally resolved by the observation that a monoclonal antibody, P1H5, prepared against the human fibroblast class II extracellular matrix receptor (ECMR II) which specifically inhibits the adhesion of human fibroblasts to collagen (Wayne & Carter, 1987) *also* inhibits the adhesion of human platelets to collagen types I and III (Kunicki *et al.* 1988). Extracellular matrix receptor II is a heterodimeric cell surface glycoprotein which contains α and β-subunits, each of approximate M_r 140 000, and is expressed on many cell types including fibroblasts, vascular endothelial cells and platelets. Moreover, it is now recognized as being homologous with the human T-cell VLA-2 antigen (estimated M_r 165 000/130 000) which, interestingly, had earlier been demonstrated on the platelet surface membrane by Hemler *et al.* (1987). Since some evidence already existed that platelet GpIa can be present as a membrane complex with GpIIa, and, in a separate study, a second monoclonal antibody 12F1 specific for the α_2-subunit of the VLA-2 heterodimer immunoprecipitated a collagen-binding protein isolated from platelet membranes and cross-reacted with platelet GpIa (Pischel *et al.* 1987a, 1987b; Santoro *et al.* 1988), it is apparent that the GpIa–IIa complex, which functions as the collagen adhesion receptor on the platelet, is synonymous with VLA-2/ECMR II (Table 2.3) and is thus a member of the integrin superfamily of cell surface receptors (Hynes, 1986; Hemler *et al.* 1987, 1988).

The von Willebrand receptor: GpIb–IX complex

Glycoprotein Ib, possessing an apparent M_r of 170 000 on SDS-polyacrylamide gels (Table 2.1) consists of two subunits: GpIbα (143 000) and GpIbβ (22 000). Binding studies that employ monoclonal antibodies indicate that some 20–25 000 molecules of GpIb are expressed on the surface membrane of each platelet (Coller *et al.* 1983b; Berndt *et al.* 1985). The purification of GpIb from platelet lysates proved difficult to achieve due to hydrolysis, and early reports consequently focussed on the resultant hydrolytic fragment glycocalicin, a high molecular weight (135 000) polypeptide cleaved from GpIbα close to its carboxy terminal by a calcium-activated protease present in platelets (Tsuji *et al.* 1983). More recently, purified α and β-subunits have been successfully obtained (Berndt *et al.* 1985), the amino acid sequence of the vWF-binding domain elucidated (Handa *et al.* 1986; Titani *et al.* 1987) and finally, the entire GpIbα subunit cDNA cloned (Lopez *et al.* 1987).

When immunoprecipitation or immunoelectrophoretic techniques were initially employed, GpIb was found to co-purify with a second low molecular weight glycoprotein, GpIX (22 000), and it has since become clear that it exists in a non-covalently bound stoichiometric 1:1 complex with GpIX at the platelet surface membrane (Berndt *et al.* 1985; Du *et al.* 1987). The GpIb polypeptide is a 610 amino acid heterodimer with the α and β-subunits linked by disulphide bonds, discrete hydrophilic and hydrophobic (membrane-spanning) regions, and leucine-rich repeat sequences in the extracellular amino-terminal vWF binding region (Fig. 2.3). Furthermore, data from Lopez *et al.* (1987) indicate that the α and β-subunits of GpIb are encoded by different DNA sequences on separate genes, rather than arising from post-translational modification of a single precursor protein. The α-subunit contains the bulk of the bound carbohydrate. It should be noted that the sequence data for GpIbα shows no homology with that of the adhesion receptors belonging to the integrin family (Table 2.3), but the domain in the glycocalicin-elongated hydrolytic fragment containing seven tandem leucine-rich repeats of a 24 amino acid sequence is homologous with those present in leucine-rich α_2-glycoprotein.

Recent elegant electron microscopy studies employing rotary shadowing (Fox *et al.* 1988a) have further shown that the GpIb–IX complex is a highly rod-like, asymmetrical structure approximately 60 nm in length with the glycocalicin fragment

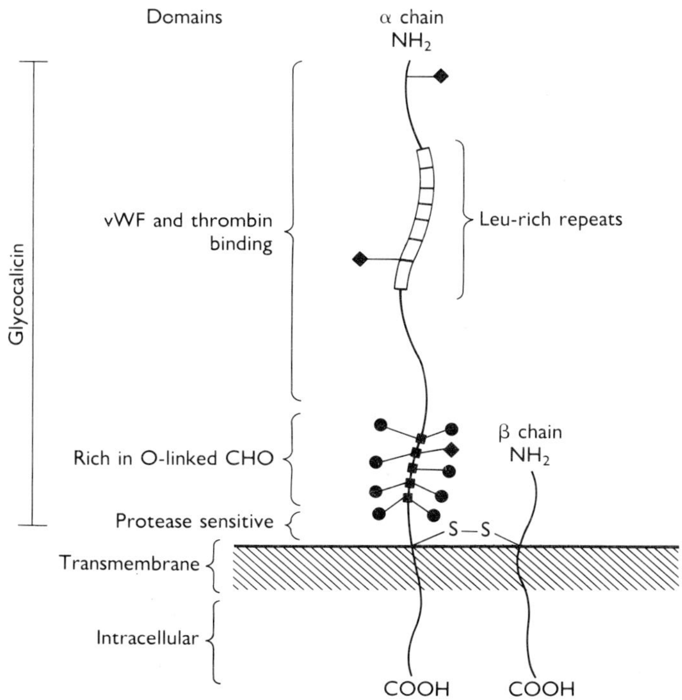

Figure 2.3 Structural organization of the α and β-subunits of GpIb. Possible O-linked and N-linked glycosylation sites are shown as solid circles and diamonds respectively, with Leu-rich domains (open bars) and the repeats of nine amino acids (closed bars) as indicated. The approximate position of the site cleaved by an endogenous calcium-activated protease to release the α-subunit fragment glycocalicin is also shown. (Reproduced with permission from Lopez *et al.* 1987.)

Table 2.3 Role of the platelet glycoproteins

Glycoprotein	Integrin nomenclature	Ligand(s)	Function
GpIa–IIa GpIb–IX GpIc–IIa GpIc–IIa	VLA-2 ($\alpha_2\beta$) – VLA-5 ($\alpha_5\beta$) VLA-6 ($\alpha_6\beta$)	Collagen vWF Fibronectin Laminin	Binding sites for subendothelial matrix adhesive proteins. Important in attachment of platelets to exposed tissue damage sites. Functional on quiescent circulating platelets. VLA-2 synonymous with ECMRII. Part of receptor/recognition site for thrombin (GpIb)?
GpIIb–IIIa	IIb–IIIa (Cytoadhesin)	Fibrinogen vWF fibronectin	Supports formation of platelet aggregates Competent receptors exposed by agonist stimulation
GpIV	–	Thrombospondin	Co-clusters with GpIIb–IIIa on aggregation Stabilizes binding of fibrinogen. Cell–cell surface interaction

largely constituting the elongated zone. Small (N-terminus) and large (C-terminus) globular domains correspond to the extracellular vWF binding (GpIbα) and membrane-insertion regions respectively. GpIbβ and GpIX are associated with GpIbα in the larger globular domain. The postulated actin-binding region of the complex (Fox, 1985b; Okita *et al.* 1985) is presumed to also reside at the membrane-spanning C-terminal end of the GpIb–IX complex. Interestingly, the GpIbβ subunit terminal domain is reported to be phosphorylated in the presence of elevated intracellular concentrations of cyclic AMP, the significance of which remains unclear (Wyler *et al.* 1986).

Initial evidence that GpIb constitutes the platelet receptor for vWF arose from the study of patients with Bernard–Soulier syndrome. This rare congenital bleeding disorder, which typically combines the presence of enlarged platelets, a decreased platelet survival time, and resultant thrombocytopoenia, is characterized by compromised platelet adhesion to damaged subendothelium despite no detectable change in circulating vWF levels. The platelets from such patients do, however, aggregate normally in stirred suspensions following addition of ADP, collagen or arachidonic acid. That the abnormality primarily involves a deficiency in the membrane content of GpIb and its hydrolysed fragment glycocalicin, was first established using SDS-PAGE more than a decade ago (Nurden & Caen, 1978). Subsequent studies have demonstrated the absence of the entire GpIb–IX complex (Clemetson *et al.* 1982). In addition, antibodies directed against GpIb prevent the adhesion of platelets to a vWF-containing collagen matrix and block ristocetin-induced platelet agglutination (George *et al.* 1984; Berndt *et al.* 1985; Sakariassen *et al.* 1986).

The incubation of platelet suspensions with leucocyte elastase causes a rapid loss of the response to vWF which parallels cleavage of an M_r 45 000 glycopeptide from GPIb. Antibodies specific for this N-terminal fragment in the GpIbα chain also inhibit vWF binding (Handa *et al.* 1986). From these observations and recent sequence data (Titani *et al.* 1987) the vWF-binding domain on GpIbα has been established as extending from His-1 (N-terminal residue) to Arg-290. This region of the molecule is actually poorly glycosylated, but contains the leucine-rich tandem repeats referred to above, and possesses three intrachain disulphide loops (Fig. 2.3). Although it appears certain that the platelet membrane deficiency in GPIb–IX complex thus accounts for decreased binding of Bernard–Soulier patient platelets to subendothelium, the situation remains complex. For example, vWF will still bind to Bernard–Soulier syndrome platelets, which indicates a second interactive site unrelated to the GPIb–IX complex (Ruggeri *et al.* 1983).

Platelet receptors for fibronectin and laminin: GpIc–IIa

The relatively recent identification of the GpIa–IIa complex (VLA-2) as the platelet receptor for collagen has been accompanied by a second line of evidence which indicates the presence on platelet surface membranes of two further members of the VLA-heterodimer adhesion receptor family. This derives from the detailed study of GpIc and GpIIa, and a possible functional relationship between these glycoproteins and the adherence to the connective tissue proteins fibronectin and laminin, which may be of considerable physiological importance (Ill *et al.* 1984; Houdijk & Sixma, 1985). Although fibronectin clearly interacts with GpIIb–IIIa (see below) this observation does not explain why unactivated platelets which lack competent GpIIb–IIIa receptors still demonstrate normal adhesion to artificial surfaces coated with fibronectin, or indeed laminin (Ill *et al.* 1984; Plow *et al.* 1985a). The data clearly suggest the presence of additional binding sites for such proteins distinct from GpIIb–IIIa.

Expression on the platelet surface of a glycoprotein immunologically related to the fibronectin receptor on fibroblasts was initially reported by Giancotti *et al.* (1986, 1987). This glycoprotein, like the fibroblast receptor, consists of two separate M_r 160 000 and 138 000 polypeptide chains in a non-covalently linked complex, and is believed to interact with fibronectin via the Arg–Gly–Asp tripeptide (Giancotti *et al.* 1988). Considerable evidence is now available which suggests that the heterodimer VLA-5 is the fibronectin receptor on other cells, based on work with fibroblasts, an osteosarcoma cell line and human placental tissue (Pytela *et al.* 1985; Argraves *et al.* 1987; Takada *et al.* 1987). The belief that the platelet surface membrane GpIc–IIa complex not only functions as a receptor for fibronectin, but is actually VLA-5, has been confirmed by elegant immunoblotting experiments on platelet lysates using a rabbit antiserum prepared against affinity column purified human placental VLA-5, and from V8 protease mapping of partially purified platelet glycoproteins using SDS-PAGE (Hemler *et al.* 1988).

Moreover, in a further series of experiments, a combination of preclearing of α_2 (GpIa), α_5 (GpIc) and β (GpIIa) VLA subunits, coupled with immunoblotting and V8 protease treatments, revealed a second polypeptide also derived from GpIc, and specifically recognized by the monoclonal antibody GoH3 (Sonnenberg *et al.* 1987; Hemler *et al.* 1988). The function of this second polypeptide, which again co-exists with the common VLA β-subunit (GpIIa), and has consequently been termed VLA-6 ($\alpha_6\beta$) by current nomenclature, was initially unclear. However, it is now established that VLA-6 is the platelet receptor for laminin since GoH3 prevents adherence of platelets to microtitre plates coated with laminin, but not type I collagen, fibronectin or fibrinogen (Sonnenberg *et al.* 1988). The adhesion of platelets to laminin observed in the absence of platelet activation resembles collagen adhesion in terms of its cation dependence, being supported by 2.0 mM Mn^{2+}, Mg^{2+} or Co^{2+}, but unlike the interaction of fibrinogen or fibronectin with GpIIb–IIIa, is independent of Ca^{2+} concentration and is therefore functional on resting platelets. Moreover, the interaction of platelets with laminin does not occur via the Arg–Gly–Asp recognition peptide, and is not affected by antibodies to GpIa.IIa or GpIIb–IIIa (Sonnenberg *et al.* 1988).

In summary, therefore, the glycoprotein on human platelets hitherto designated GpIc (Table 2.1) consists of two distinct glycoproteins, each of which like GpIa associates in a heterodimeric complex with a common β-subunit (GpIIa). These two GpIc polypeptides correspond to α_5 and α_6 in the integrin nomenclature, represent the platelet receptors for fibronectin and laminin respectively (Table 2.3), and are not resolved by traditional SDS-PAGE analysis under the standard reducing / non-reducing conditions generally employed, as they co-migrate.

Platelet surface membrane excitatory and inhibitory receptors

In recent years the major excitatory and inhibitory surface membrane receptors of the human platelet have been extensively characterized. Moreover, in certain cases the platelet receptor to a particular agonist has been the first to be pharmacologically defined in detail, and has consequently become the reference against which possible subtypes have been explored in other tissues e.g. thromboxane A_2 (TXA_2), platelet activating factor (PAF). That this should have occurred resulted not only from a decade of intense interest in the pharmacological manipulation of the platelet aggregatory response, but also from the ready availability and relative ease of preparation of these cells coupled with the advent of high specific activity radioligands for each of the principle platelet receptor populations so far identified. Nevertheless, a word of caution is necessary since receptor binding studies are not without pitfalls regarding technique and the correct interpretation of data. Many of the platelet ligand binding studies reported have employed widely differing assay methodology, including the use of whole cells or membrane preparations in association with a range of incubation conditions or temperatures (4 °C–37 °C), and subsequent separation of bound ligand from free by centrifugation or filtration.

Perhaps not surprisingly, multiple binding site isotherms (two or three component) have been widely reported which, in a number of cases, probably reflects either incorrect Scatchard analysis or problems with high levels of non-specific binding and uptake rather than true binding-site heterogeneity or phenoma such as site–site co-operativity. An example is discussed briefly for PAF below.

For the purposes of the present review, therefore, only high affinity platelet binding sites will be generally considered, a remarkable level of agreement for which has been achieved in the case of most ligands. Each has largely satisfied the series of criteria necessary before a binding site may be considered a true receptor site. The criteria include: (i) stereospecific, saturable and reversible binding of ligand; (ii) evidence of high affinity binding; (iii) concentration-dependent displacement of ligand by drug; and (iv) correlation between agonist affinity *in vitro* and pharmacological potency (i.e. correlation of receptor occupancy with response).

Since binding sites have been recognized in some biological systems which do not induce a physiological response (termed 'acceptor sites'), despite demonstrating high affinity, saturability, reversibility and stereospecificity, it is particularly important to satisfy criteria (iii) and (iv). In general, it appears from binding studies with excitatory and inhibitory agonists that receptor densities of a few hundred sites per platelet are the rule, notable exceptions being TXA_2 or prostacyclin (PGI_2/PGE_1) with some 1000–3000 sites per platelet, and the 5-HT_2 and adrenaline (β_2) sites with rather fewer (i.e. <100).

Platelet α and β-adrenoceptors

It is well established that the *in vitro* aggregatory response of the human platelet to adrenaline is mediated via α_2-adrenoceptors. Adrenaline-induced responses are blocked by the potent and selective α_2-antagonist yohimbine, whereas the α_1-antagonists prazosin or indoramin are only weakly active. Moreover, full aggregatory responses can be induced with a selective α_2-agonist UK 14304, but not with phenylephrine or methoxamine (Hsu *et al.* 1979; Grant & Scrutton, 1980). Radioligand binding experiments have shown that the non-selective α-agonist ligand [^{3}H]dihydroergocryptine ([^{3}H]DHE) is displaced significantly more potently by the α_2 selective antagonist yohimbine than by prazosin (Elliott & Grahame-Smith, 1982). In turn, [^{3}H]yohimbine binds to platelets with higher affinity and a lower degree of non-specific binding than [^{3}H]DHE (Motulsky & Insel, 1982a). Each platelet possesses between 200 and 300 α_2-adrenoceptors as defined by [^{3}H]yohimbine binding (Kerry *et al.* 1984; Table 2.4) whereas [^{3}H]DHE binds to approximately 50% more sites. The explanation for this is currently unclear, but [^{3}H]DHE binding to the additional sites is not displaced by α_1-adrenoceptor selective drugs (Motulsky & Insel, 1982a; Boon *et al.* 1983).

Detailed studies carried out to further define the α_2-adrenoceptor on platelets and in other tissues, by comparing the rank order of potency of a large number of agonists and antagonists across different binding assays, have provided evidence for at least two subpopulations. The platelet α_2-adrenoceptor (characterized by a low affinity for prazosin) has been tentatively designated α_2A, and a second α-adrenoceptor present in rat lung and human caudate nucleus, which possesses some 40-fold greater affinity for prazosin, is designated as α_2B (Bylund *et al.* 1988).

The existence of heterogeneity amongst α_2-adrenoceptors became unequivocably established with the cloning and sequencing of the genes which encode the α_2-adrenoceptors of the human platelet (Kobilka *et al.* 1987a) and human kidney (Regan *et al.* 1988). Predicted amino acid sequences for these two receptor proteins possess considerable homology in the membrane-spanning domains (Fig. 2.4) but are individually unique, whilst the genes are located on separate chromosomes, these being chromosome 10 (referred to as the platelet α_2-C10 receptor) and chromosome 4 (kidney α_2-C4 receptor) respectively. When the cloned platelet α_2-adrenoceptor was expressed in *Xenopus* oocytes and membranes prepared, [^{3}H]yohimbine bound with high affinity (K_D 2.5 nM) and competitive displacement of binding was observed in the antagonist potency order rauwolscine (K_i:3.5 nM) > yohimbine (4.4 nM) > idazoxan (18 nM) > phentolamine (27 nM) > prazosin (880 nM), in close agreement with previous studies on the platelet α_2-receptor.

Comparison of the predicted amino acid sequence for the human platelet α_2-adrenoceptor protein with those for the closely related β_1 and β_2-adrenoceptors from a human placenta cDNA library (Kobilka *et al.* 1987b; Frielle *et al.* 1987) reveals that its size (450 amino acids) is similar to both β_1 (477) and β_2 (413). Seven characteristic sequences of hydrobic residues, each 26 amino acids in length, are present and are flanked by hydrophilic charged residues. These hydrophobic sequences, believed to comprise the membrane-spanning domain of the protein, and capable of forming a bundle of seven α-helices (Fig. 2.4), are strikingly conserved amongst all receptors coupled to guanine nucleotide regulatory proteins which have been cloned to date, such that they have been designated the R_7G receptor family (Dohlman *et al.* 1987). Two possible N-linked glycosylation sites are present (asparagine residues 10 and 14). No potential phosphorylation sites are evident close to the C-terminus, but in the third cytoplasmic loop a total of 19 serine and threonine residues are present, with at one point four consecutive serine residues (296–299). The greatest sequence homology with the β_1 and β_2 receptor proteins (29 residues) is observed in the membrane-spanning region, with little evident in the C-terminal (intracellular) or N-terminal (extracellular) regions. Since the α_2, β_1 and β_2-adrenoceptors all bind adrenaline, it is tempting to speculate that this apparent homology in the membrane-spanning domains may represent the sequences responsible for ligand binding and coupling to the G-proteins G_i or G_s respectively. There is some evidence from studies with chimeric α_2/β_2-adrenoceptors that coupling to G-proteins is dictated by the fifth and sixth hydrophobic domains, whilst agonist binding is largely influenced by the seventh

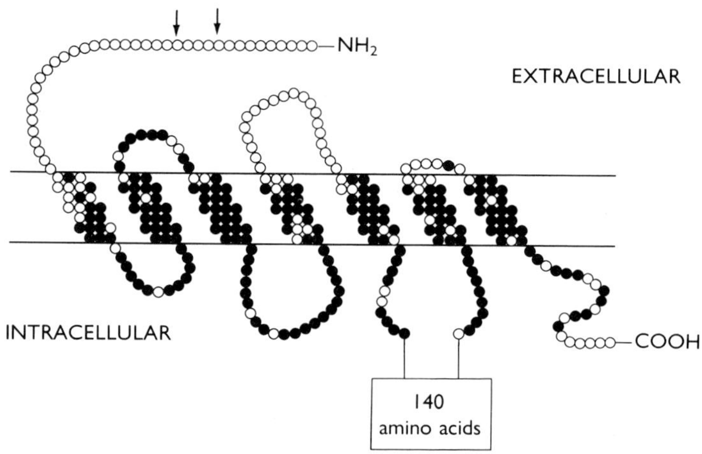

Figure 2.4 Proposed model for organization of the human platelet α_2-C10 adrenoceptor in the plasma membrane, based on published sequence data (Kobilka *et al.* 1987a). Homology with the human kidney α_2-C4 adrenoceptor (Regan *et al.* 1988) is indicated by closed circles. The seven transmembrane-spanning helices (defined by maxima in hydropathy plots) are a common feature of other adrenergic and muscarinic receptor proteins sequenced to date, leading to the descriptor 'R_7G' for this family of membrane spanning G-protein linked receptor proteins. Potential extracellular glycosylation sites at asparagine residues 10 and 14 are indicated (↓).

hydrophobic domain (Kobilka *et al.* 1988). However, more stringent site-directed mutagenesis studies, which should further define the loci that dictate agonist selectivity or coupling to G-proteins, are currently awaited.

In addition to an excitatory α_2-adrenoceptor, the human platelet does also possess a population of inhibitory β-adrenoceptors. Various studies have shown that both adrenaline (in the presence of the α-adrenoceptor antagonist phentolamine) and the β-adrenoceptor agonist isoprenaline inhibit aggregatory responses to a number of agonists including ADP, collagen or vasopressin (Mills & Smith, 1972; Jakobs *et al.* 1978; Kerry & Scrutton, 1983). Moreover, the platelet inhibitory adrenoceptor has been identified as being of the β_2-subtype, since the inhibitory activity of isoprenaline is blocked by ICI 118551 but not atenolol, whilst aggregatory responses to vasopressin are inhibited by the β_2-selective agonists salbutamol or terbutaline in a concentration-dependent manner (Kerry & Scrutton, 1983). Ligand binding studies with [^{125}I]pindolol indicate that human platelets express some five-fold fewer β_2 than α_2-adrenoceptors (Table 2.5).

The contribution of membrane α_2 and β_2-adrenoceptors to circulatory platelet function remains poorly understood. Marked variation exists across the mammalian species with respect to the pharmacological effects of either adrenaline or inhibitory β_2-agonists on platelets, which has been attributed to differences in binding affinities and respective α_2 or β_2-adrenoceptor density (Kerry *et al.* 1984). Moreover, competitive experiments with Gpp(NH)p (a guanosine triphosphate (GTP) analogue) suggest that in the human platelet the β_2-adrenoceptor may be relatively

Table 2.4 Low molecular weight excitatory platelet agonists

Agonist	Radioligand	High affinity receptor density (sites per platelet)	Receptor subtype	Selective antagonists	Binding study bibliography
Adrenaline	[^{3}H]dihydroergocryptine [^{3}H]yohimbine	300–500 200–300	α_2A-adrenoceptor	Yohimbine Rauwolscine	Elliot & Grahame-Smith, 1982 Kerry *et al.* 1984
ADP	[β-^{32}P]2-azido-ADP [β-^{32}P]2-methylthio-ADP	500 400–1200	P_2	ATP 2-chloro-ATP	MacFarlane *et al.* 1983
Serotonin	[^{3}H]ketanserin [^{3}H]spiroperidol [^{125}I]2-iodo-lysergic acid	<50	S_2(5-HT_2)	Ketanserin Ritanserin Spiperone	Leysen *et al.* 1981 McBride *et al.* 1987
PAF	[^{3}H]C_{18}-PAF	200–300	PAF_1	WEB 2086 L-659989	Kloprogge & Akkerman 1984 Tuffin *et al.* 1985
Thromboxane A_2	[^{3}H]U44069 [^{125}I]PTA-OH	2000	No subclassification at present	EPO92 13-azapinane TXA_2	Armstrong *et al.* 1983 Mais *et al.* 1985
Vasopressin	[^{125}I]vasopressin	74–100	V_1	Peptide analogues	Haslam & Rosson, 1972 Scrutton *et al.* 1986
Thrombin*	[^{125}I]thrombin	300–700	Receptor identity unknown	—	Tollefsen *et al.* 1974 Majerus *et al.* 1976 Martin *et al.* 1976

* Although a polypeptide agonist, preliminary evidence suggests that α-thrombin activates the platelet via a discrete excitatory receptor which can be selectively blocked by low molecular weight antagonists (see Ruda *et al.* 1988).

Table 2.5 Low molecular weight inhibitory platelet agonists

Agonist	Radioligand	High affinity receptor density (sites per platelet)	Receptor subtype	Selective antagonists	Binding study bibliography
Adrenaline	$[^{125}I]$iodopindolol $[^{125}I]$iodocyanopindolol	<100	β_2-adrenoceptor	ICI118551 Butoxamine	Kerry & Scrutton, 1983
Adenosine	$[^{3}H]$5-ethyl carboxamide adenosine (NECA)	Not known	A_2	Theophylline	Haslam *et al.* 1978
PGD_2	$[^{3}H]PGD_2$	210 100	DP	AH6809	Cooper & Ahern, 1979 Siegl *et al.* 1979a.
PGI_2 (PGE_1)	$[^{3}H]PGI_2$ $[^{3}H]PGE^1$	1000–3000	IP	None published	Siegl *et al.* 1979b. Eggerman *et al.* 1987 Schafer *et al.* 1979

poorly coupled to adenylyl cyclase via G_s (Barnett *et al.* 1985). With respect to tachyphylaxis, homologous densitization of either α or β-adrenoceptors has been widely reported for different tissues (Motulsky & Insel, 1982b) and this phenomenon is also true of the platelet α_2-adrenoceptor (Cooper *et al.* 1978). The biochemical sequence of events responsible has been particularly closely studied in certain tissues for the case of β-adrenoceptors (Harden, 1983; Sibley & Lefkowitz, 1985). Although the initial binding of an agonist causes activation of adenylyl cyclase via G_s, continued exposure results in phosphorylation of the receptor protein by a β-adrenoceptor-specific kinase, and consequent uncoupling from G_s (Strasser *et al.* 1986). With the advent of adrenoceptor sequence data, speculation concerning the site of phosphorylation has focussed on the serine-rich C-terminus. However, there is some evidence from site-directed mutagenesis studies indicating that desensitization can occur normally despite deletions in the C-terminal region of β-adrenoceptors, and moreover, that the α_2-adrenoceptor also appears to be a good substrate for the kinase despite the absence of serine residues in its abbreviated C-terminal sequence (Benovic *et al.* 1987; Strader *et al.* 1987; Kobilka *et al.* 1988). Finally, the β-adrenoreceptor becomes sequestered from the membrane in an internalized form unable to bind ligand, although the view that the receptor may be dephosphorylated and recycled remains tenable (Strasser *et al.* 1986). Returning to the platelet, whilst pharmacological desensitization of the α_2-adrenoceptor-mediated response can be reproducibly demonstrated, evidence pertaining to the mechanism in this cell is currently conflicting. It remains to be firmly established whether extended incubation of platelets with agents such as adrenaline or clonidine *in vitro* induces a decrease in receptor number (Cooper *et al.* 1978; Karliner *et al.* 1982), a change in coupling to inhibition of adenylyl cyclase via G_i, or even either of these options (Motulsky *et al.* 1986). From the above considerations, it appears possible that interactive relationships between platelet α_2 and β_2-adrenoceptors (perhaps heterologous desensitization), and indeed, between adrenaline and other physiological agonists (i.e. pharmacological potentiation), are more likely mechanisms through which functional platelet responses may be influenced by catecholamines.

The adenosine-5′-diphosphate (ADP) receptor

Adenosine-5′-diphosphate-induced shape change, aggregation and secretion by human platelets is inhibited in a competitive manner by the related nucleotides ATP (adenosine triphosphate) and AMP (adenosine monophosphate). However, the stereospecificity requirements of the platelet purinergic (P_2) receptor (Table 2.4) differ substantially from those of nucleotide receptors on other smooth muscle tissues (Burnstock *et al.* 1983). A further complication is provided by the observation that adenosine itself inhibits ADP-induced aggregatory responses non-competitively via a distinct population of adenosine (A_2) receptors (Table 2.5) linked to adenylyl cyclase (Haslam & Cusack, 1981). At present, neither P_2 nor A_2 receptors on platelets are fully characterized, although the former has been the object of considerable attention since ADP appears to play an important role in physiological activation.

Affinity labelling experiments with intact platelets have tentatively identified the ADP receptor as a single M_r 100 000 surface membrane protein which can be covalently modified by 5′-*p*-fluorosuphonylbenzoyladenosine (FSBA; Bennett *et al.* 1978). Some 200 binding sites per platelet are present at the onset of inhibition of ADP-induced shape change with this agent, which is claimed to selectively inhibit ADP responses, and also to act as a weak partial agonist at higher concentrations (Figures *et al.* 1987). However, since FSBA can be hydrolysed by platelets to *p*-fluorosulphonylbenzoic acid and adenosine (Bennett *et al.* 1978; Colman & Figures, 1984), and thus may not be specific for the ADP receptor, these data require verification.

Attempts to further characterize the platelet ADP receptor via radioligand-binding assays have also been fraught with problems. Measurement of steady-state binding has been complicated by rapid metabolism of the ligand, dilution of the ligand due to ADP release from dense storage granules in the presence of cell activation, and problems with non-specific binding and ligand trapping (Haslam & Cusack, 1981). Nevertheless, these problems have been largely overcome in experiments using the ligands [β-^{32}P]2-azido-ADP and [β-^{32}P]2-methylthio-ADP, which reveal the existence of between 400 and 1200 high affinity sites per platelet with competitive displacement of ligand by antagonists in the expected potency order ATP>AMP>UDP (MacFarlane *et al.* 1983).

5-Hydroxytryptamine

The ability of human platelets to respond to 5-hydroxytryptamine (5-HT, serotonin), to accumulate this agonist in dense granule storage sites via a specific surface membrane uptake receptor, and to secrete 5-HT has prompted considerable clinical interest regarding the relevance of these processes and their use as markers in patients suffering from migraine attacks or psychiatric disorders. A possible role for platelet 5-HT in control of stenosed coronary artery blood flow has also become evident. However, the co-existence of surface membrane pharmacological and uptake receptors, together with secretion of 5-HT from activated cells and high levels of non-specific binding in some studies has, as with ADP, served to complicate interpretation of radioligand binding study data.

Initial binding experiments with normal or formaldehyde-fixed human platelets employing 5-[^{14}C]HT as ligand suggested the presence of at least 2–300 specific high affinity binding sites per platelet (Kim *et al.* 1980), but later reports using [^{3}H]ketanserin, [^{3}H]spiroperidol or the high specific activity ligand [^{125}I]2-iodo-lysergic acid diethylamide revised estimates downwards to <50 sites per human platelet (Table 2.4) (Leysen *et al.* 1981; McBride *et al.* 1987). Good agreement with respect to dissociation constant (K_D) values in the range 1–2 nM has been achieved. Ligand binding to cat and human platelet membranes is competitively displaced by the 5-HT_2 antagonists ritanserin or ketanserin. In one study, the density of the 5-HT_2 binding sites on human platelet membranes significantly correlated ($P \leq 0.001$) with the observed degree of potentiation of ADP-induced threshold aggregatory responses by a fixed (10 μM) concentration of 5-HT (McBride *et al.* 1987).

Oligonucleotide probes based on sequence data for the 5-HT_{1C} receptor have been successfully employed to clone the 5-HT_2 receptor by screening a rat forebrain cDNA library (Pritchett, 1988). Ligands such as kitanserin, mianserin and spiperone bind with expected high affinity (1–2 nM) to this 5-HT_2 receptor expressed in human embryonic kidney cells. From modelling studies based on primary sequence data, the 5-HT_2 receptor conforms to the previously established structural pattern for other G-protein coupled adrenergic and muscarinic receptors (R_7G family). Notably, seven hydrophobic membrane spanning sequences can again be identified, with a long C-terminal intracellular segment, and a large intracellular loop between membrane-spanning domains V and VI. The membrane-spanning domains not only possess considerable sequence homology with 5-HT_{1A} and 5-HT_{1C} receptors as might be predicted (e.g. 78% overall homology with 5-HT_{1C}), but in certain highly conserved parts of the polypeptide such as transmembrane segment II, also with other G-protein coupled receptors such as the α_2-adrenoceptor described above (Hartig, 1989).

Lower affinity (μM) uptake receptors, responsible for the accumulation of 5-HT in the circulating platelet, are present in substantially greater numbers. Studies with 5-[^{14}C]HT or 5-[^{3}H]HT suggest as many as 10–30 000 sites per platelet (Peters & Grahame-Smith, 1980). [^{3}H]imipramine binding to human platelets (Demushkin *et al.* 1987) may be associated with, but is not a direct marker of, the platelet uptake receptor (Langer & Raisman, 1983). Since 5-HT is strongly implicated in the local control of vascular tone and enhances the sensitivity of platelets to other agonists, whilst circulating levels of 5-HT and receptor binding parameters alter in different disease states, clarification of the relationship between 5-HT uptake, stimulation and secretion in platelets merits further attention.

Eicosanoid excitatory agonists: prostaglandin H_2, thromboxane A_2 and platelet activating factor

The platelet is able to synthesize a potent array of eicosanoid excitatory agonists in concert, comprising prostaglandin H_2(PGH_2), thromboxane A_2 (TXA_2) and platelet activating factor (PAF), each capable of initiating and propagating the aggregatory response. Therapeutic interest in the modulation of platelet responses to these agents through the inhibition of synthesis or surface membrane receptor blockade has proved intense. Study of PGH_2 and TXA_2 receptors and responses was initially hampered by the short half-life of these agonists in aqueous medium. This problem has been overcome by the synthesis of stable analogues of PGH_2,

TXA_2 mimetics such as pinane TXA_2 (PTA_2) and carbocyclic TXA_2 (CTA_2) and most recently, the *de novo* synthesis (Bhagwat *et al.* 1985b) and pharmacological characterization of TXA_2 itself (Bhagwat *et al.* 1985a,b; Bunting *et al.* 1987).

An explanation for the initially paradoxical finding that TXA_2 receptor antagonists demonstrate substantially more potent anti-aggregatory activity than TXA_2 synthase inhibitors, has been provided by the steadily accumulating evidence that PGH_2, TXA_2 and their stable analogues each bind with varying affinity to the same human platelet receptor population (Armstrong *et al.* 1983; Mais *et al.* 1985; Narumiya *et al.* 1986). In these experiments binding to the PGH_2/TXA_2 receptor has been estimated in whole washed platelet preparations by employing [^{3}H]9,11-epoxymethano-PGH_2 ([^{3}H]U44069), [^{3}H]11,9-epoxymethano-PGH_2 ([^{3}H]U46619) and more recently, [^{125}I]9,11-dimethylmethano-11,12-methano-16-(3-iodo-4-hydroxyphenyl)-13,14-dihydro-13-aza-15 α,β-tetranor-TXA_2 ([^{125}I]PTA-OH) as high affinity ligands.

Multicomponent binding isotherms have been observed, but there is good agreement for binding to a population of high affinity sites with values for dissociation constants in the low nanomolar range and B_{max} values indicating approximately 2000 sites per platelet (Table 2.4). Rank order potency for the displacement of ligand from the high affinity site by a range of analogues of both PGH_2 and TXA_2 correlates closely with relative activity as agonists or antagonists in platelet aggregation studies.

Interestingly, exposure of washed platelets to potent agonists such as U46619 or SQ26655 causes a rapid desensitization to subsequent addition of agonist. Recent data suggests that the mechanism for this effect is the uncoupling of the receptor from a G-protein (i.e. an event analogous to that proposed for adrenoceptor desensitization — see earlier), rather than any immediate down regulation of receptor affinity or number (Murray & Fitzgerald, 1989). Solubilization of the platelet membrane PGH_2/TXA_2 binding site in its active form using a detergent, has enabled a preliminary M_r estimation of 140000 for the receptor-detergent complex (Burch *et al.* 1985) but otherwise, little is known.

Although it has been reported that the relative antagonist potency of a series of 13-azapinane analogues of TXA_2 differs between platelets and vascular smooth muscle, suggesting receptor heterogeneity (Mais *et al.* 1988), more exhaustive studies across a number of species and smooth muscle or platelet preparations provide no justification for invoking subtypes of the PGH_2/TXA_2 receptor at the present time (Jones *et al.* 1987). An initial claim that CTA_2 possesses agonist properties on vascular smooth muscle, but behaves as a pure antagonist at the platelet receptor, has not been substantiated (Burke *et al.* 1983). Indeed, a range of potent, novel antagonists such as BM13177, SQ29548, EP092 and ICI192605 possess comparable antagonist activity against responses in platelets, vascular and bronchial smooth muscle *in vitro*.

Platelet activating factor (PAF-acether; 1-0-alkyl-2-acetyl-sn-glycero-3-phosphorylcholine) is both synthesized and metabolized in the platelet by rapid conversion from and to its immediate precursor lyso-PAF by acetyl transferase and acetyl hydrolase respectively (Kramer *et al.* 1984; Touqui *et al.* 1985). [^{3}H]PAF has been shown to bind to specific high affinity receptor sites on human platelets (Kloprogge & Akkerman, 1984; Tuffin *et al.* 1985), with close agreement on K_D values and estimates of the number of sites per platelet (Table 2.4). The curious early observation that platelets from the rat do not respond to PAF is explained by the absence of high affinity platelet PAF receptors in this species. Total synthesis of PAF itself, and subsequently a range of close analogues, has enabled definition of the precise stereospecific and conformational requirements for agonist binding to the platelet PAF receptor. In particular, the chiralty of C_2 is important. There is an absolute requirement for the R-stereoisomer for full agonist activity since the S-stereoisomer is orders of magnitude less active. (R)-C_{18}-PAF inhibits high affinity [^{3}H]C_{18}-PAF binding to washed human platelets on an equimolar basis, whereas (R)-C_{16}-PAF appears significantly more potent, closely correlating with its five-fold greater relative aggregatory potency *in vitro* and *in vivo* (Tuffin *et al.* 1985). Racemic (R,S)-C_{18}-PAF exhibits half the inhibitory potency of the active (R)-isomer, whilst lyso-C_{18}-PAF is inactive at concentrations two orders of magnitude above those at which (R)-C_{18}-PAF maximally inhibits binding (Tuffin & Wade, 1987). Binding of [^{3}H]PAF is reported to be influenced by incubation medium concentrations of monovalent (Na^+, Li^+) and divalent (Mg^{2+}, Ca^{2+}, Mn^{2+}) cations, and is also inhibited in a concentration-dependent, competitive and stereospecific manner by the calcium channel-blocking drugs diltiazem and verapamil (Wade *et al.* 1986), such that a close spatial relationship may exist between PAF binding sites and membrane calcium channels in the human platelet.

Little is known about the structure of the PAF platelet receptor protein. The receptor is heat labile and sensitive to treatment with protease enzymes (Valone, 1984). Two studies in which solubilized platelet membrane preparations have been loaded with [^{3}H]PAF as a marker, and analysed by SDS-PAGE or sucrose density gradient centrifugation, have reported that the receptor is a single protein with M_r estimates of 180 000 and 220 000 respectively (Valone, 1984; Chau & Jii, 1988). Internalization of the receptor and metabolism of PAF, reflected by the presence of a second low affinity site in binding studies at room temperature or 37 °C, but not 4 °C (Figure 2.5), does not appear essential for platelet activation (Kloprogge & Akkerman, 1984; Tuffin & Wade, 1987). In washed human platelet preparations, [^{3}H]PAF receptor occupancy (high affinity binding sites) correlates with shape change and threshold aggregatory responses (Tuffin *et al.* 1985). Exposure of washed, unstirred platelet suspensions to PAF at 37 °C causes a specific and rapid desensitization of the cells to subsequent addition of PAF but not other agonists (Chesney *et al.* 1985), suggesting the occurence of an uncoupling event which parallels that for adrenaline or TXA_2 referred to earlier.

Pharmacological characterization of platelet PAF receptors has awaited the identification of potent, selective antagonists, a number of which, including CV 3988, BN 52021, WEB 2086 and L-659989, have now become available. From

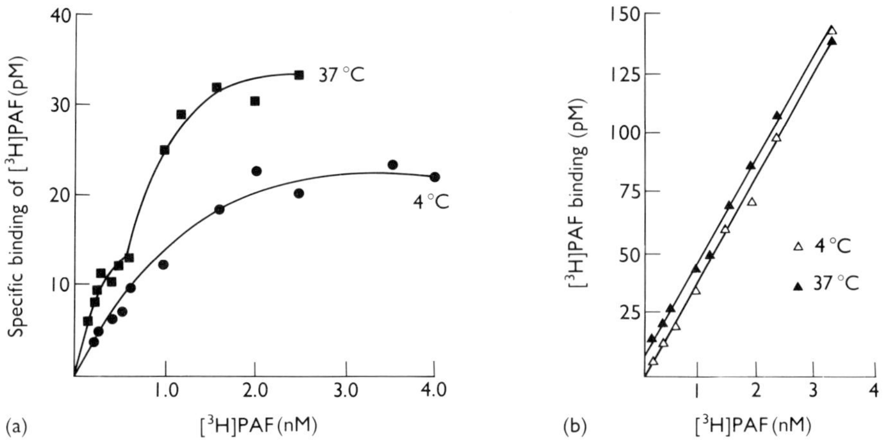

Figure 2.5 Temperature dependent radioligand binding to washed human platelets. (a) In the example shown, $[^3H]C_{18}$-PAF binding demonstrates a two phase isotherm at 37 °C (and in most experiments at room temperature) but exhibits only a single phase at 4 °C. (b) Scatchard analysis for the high affinity site reveals a similar dissociation constant (K_D) and number of sites per platelet (245 ± 30 vs 300 ± 10) at 37 °C and 4 °C respectively (from Tuffin & Wade, 1987). A number of other lipophilic platelet ligands demonstrate similar multicomponent binding isotherms; caution is advised with respect to interpretation (see Zierler, 1989).

the estimation of binding site parameters and the comparison of antagonist rank-order potency in platelets, polymorphonuclear leucocytes and macrophages, considerable evidence has accumulated for the existence of PAF receptor subtypes, with the platelet receptor being initially assigned the notation PAF_1 (Lambrecht & Parnham, 1986; Stewart & Dusting, 1988).

Prostaglandin inhibitory agonists

The prostaglandins E_1 (PGE_1), D_2 (PGD_2) and I_2 (prostacyclin; PGI_2) each demonstrate potent anti-aggregatory activity on human platelets (Ball *et al.* 1970; Smith *et al.* 1974; Moncada *et al.* 1976). Binding of $[^3H]PGD_2$ to washed human platelet preparations is specific, rapid, saturable and reversible (Cooper & Ahern, 1979). Scatchard analysis reveals a single population of several hundred high affinity binding sites per platelet (Table 2.5). The finding that $[^3H]PGD_2$ binding is poorly displaced by PGE_1 or PGI_2 has indicated the presence of a discrete platelet PGD_2 (DP) receptor population (Cooper & Ahern, 1979; Siegl *et al.* 1979a). Studies with $[^3H]PGE_1$ and $[^3H]PGI_2$ not only confirm that these agonists bind to a membrane receptor distinct from that PGD_2, but suggest that both act at the same adenylyl cyclase linked PGI_2 (IP) receptor. Binding with either ligand is again saturable and specific, but in contrast to PGD_2, the presence of two-component binding isotherms reveals a second low affinity binding site (μM) in addition to the high affinity (nM) population (Schafer *et al.* 1979; Siegl *et al.*

1979b). Estimates vary, but in general most investigators have described a population of between 1000 and 3000 high affinity [^{3}H]PGI$_2$ or [^{3}H]PGE$_1$ sites per human platelet (Table 2.5) (Siegl *et al.* 1979b; Eggerman *et al.* 1987). PGI$_2$ competitively displaces [^{3}H]PGE$_1$ whereas PGD$_2$ ia 1000-fold less active, and conversely, PGE$_1$ will displace bound [^{3}H]PGI$_2$ with PGD$_2$ again inactive. Moreover, in aggregation experiments, prior exposure of platelets to PGE$_1$, or PGI$_2$ induces refractoriness of the cells to either of these agonists, but not to PGD$_2$ (Miller & Gorman, 1979).

Most recently, evidence from the study of [^{3}H]PGE$_2$ binding has emerged which suggests that human platelets possess a population of PGE$_2$ (EP) receptors in addition to those of PGI$_2$ and PGD$_2$ (Eggerman *et al.* 1986). Although PGE$_1$ will compete at [^{3}H]PGI$_2$ binding sites with reduced affinity (above), it will reverse [^{3}H]PGE$_2$ binding on an equimolar basis, and high affinity binding of [^{3}H]PGE$_1$ appears to be at least in part explainable by binding to EP rather than IP receptor sites. However, the existence of a physiological role for platelet EP receptors is open to question. Prostaglandin E$_2$ is substantially less active than PGI$_2$ or PGE$_1$ as an inhibitor of aggregatory responses, and at high concentrations has been reported to potentiate ADP-induced aggregation. Despite the presence of EP receptors on the platelet, the anti-aggregatory activity of PGE$_1$ and PGE$_2$ nevertheless correlates closely with IC$_{50}$ values against [^{3}H]PGI$_2$ receptor binding (Eggerman *et al.* 1987).

Solubilization of the platelet PGI$_2$ (IP) receptor in buffer containing Triton X-100, followed by chromatographic purification and analysis using SDS-PAGE indicates a receptor protein with two subunits of approximate M_r' 190 000 (Dutta-Roy & Sinha, 1987). Binding of PGE$_1$ to this purified protein is rapid, specific, saturable and displaced by PGI$_2$. Surprisingly, two binding sites of high (K_D 9.8 nM) and low (K_D 0.7 μM) affinity are reported to be present in the single protein. Furthermore, incubation of the purified receptor protein with platelets previously depleted of the native IP receptor by mild treatment with buffer containing Triton X-100 detergent, significantly restored the ability of both PGI$_2$ and PGE$_1$ to stimulate adenylyl cyclase.

There is some evidence for the heterogeneity of PGI$_2$ (IP) receptors across the animal species in platelets, and between platelets and smooth muscle preparations, although a classification has not been attempted. The anti-aggregatory potency of PGI$_2$ (and PGD$_2$) varies between tissues by up to an order of magnitude. Certain analogues of PGI$_2$ possess antagonist activity at IP receptors on vascular smooth muscle but are agonists on the platelet. Caution is, however, advisable regarding the interpretation of cross tissue potency data in the light of the significant PGE-like stimulatory activity at smooth muscle EP receptors exhibited by some stable PGI$_2$ analogues such as iloprost or 6a-carba PGI$_2$ and additional work is needed to clarify the issue (see Armstrong *et al.* 1989).

Interaction of the platelet with α-thrombin

The precise nature of the interaction of α-thrombin with the platelet remains controversial. Although a polypeptide ligand, α-thrombin-induced platelet responses have much in common with events which follow exposure of platelets to low molecular weight excitatory agonists. For example, binding studies employing washed or gel-filtered platelets and [^{125}I]thrombin have established that association of the ligand is rapid, specific, saturable and reversible (Table 2.4). Multicomponent binding isotherms revealing two, and in some reports, three separate binding sites, have been described. In general, the data indicate the presence of a high affinity binding site ($K_D < 1\,nM$) with estimates of 300–700 sites per platelet (Tollefsen *et al.* 1974; Martin *et al.* 1976). Recent studies with colloidal-gold labelled α-thrombin as a probe lend further support to these estimates (Handley & Chien, 1985). Evidence can be cited, however, which indicates a role for both proteolytic and hormonal (receptor mediated) events, such that a two site coupling mechanism, perhaps involving the catalytic site of α-thrombin and a second exosite has been proposed (McGowan & Detwiler, 1986). Notably, when α-thrombin is chemically inactivated by agents such as diisopropyl fluorophosphate (DFP), it will still bind to platelets but fails to induce activation alone, or to compete with native α-thrombin (Tollefsen *et al.* 1974; Workman *et al.* 1977); γ-thrombin will not bind to high affinity α-thrombin receptors (McGowan & Detwiler, 1986), and a short exposure of washed platelets to chymotrypsin causes a significant delay in the onset of the response to α-thrombin, such that it becomes indistinguishable from that induced by γ-thrombin (Tam *et al.* 1980; McGowan *et al.* 1983a). In addition, the platelet granule secretory response is irreversible following a brief exposure of the cells to α-thrombin, activation of platelets by α-thrombin is also blocked by the potent leech salivary gland anticoagulant polypeptide hirudin (K_i:10^{-10}M), and a platelet surface membrane glycoprotein, GpV, has been identified as a substrate for α-thrombin (McGowan *et al.* 1983b).

Despite the findings described above, new evidence increasingly favours a receptor occupancy-based mechanism. The stimulation of platelets by α-thrombin is rapid, is coupled via a G-protein, and is followed by a cascade of intracellular biochemical events characteristic of many platelet agonists (Brass *et al.* 1986; Rock & Jackowski, 1987). The time course and concentration-response relationship for α-thrombin-induced formation of inositol phosphates and secretion of amine storage granules are closely parallel, and the receptor can be rapidly desensitized (Huang & Detwiler, 1987). The hypothesis that hydrolysis of GpV is involved in the activation of the platelet has also become untenable. A near maximal disappearance of single platelets from washed cell suspensions occurs at 1.0 nM α-thrombin, despite no detectable release of the cleavage product GpV_{FR}. Maximal hydrolysis of platelet surface membrane GpV is not achieved until 30–45 minutes after addition of α-thrombin, chymotrypsin cleaves GpV without inducing aggregation, and a polyclonal antibody raised against a major proteolytic fragment of GpV blocks α-thrombin-induced cleavage of GV_{FR} but not platelet activation (Knupp & White, 1985; Bienz *et al.* 1986; Ruda *et al.* 1988). Finally, caution is advisable in the interpretation of data generated using α-thrombin active-site inhibitors as these agents may induce conformational changes in other parts of the α-thrombin molecule. Certainly, the binding of hirudin to α-thrombin blocks not only the catalytic site, but also sterically interferes with other regions such as the adjacent apolar binding site, the domain responsible for fibrinogen recognition, and also possibly the Tyr–Pro–Pro–Arg sequence since chemotactic activity is compromised (Fenton, 1988).

If platelet aggregation induced by α-thrombin does not require proteolytic activity, and is a function of surface membrane receptor occupancy, it should be possible to identify small peptides or analogues thereof which exhibit agonist or antagonist activity. Interestingly, Ruda *et al.* (1988) have described two such novel modified tripeptide molecules, SC40476 and SC42619, which demonstrate weak partial agonist and antagonist activity at the platelet α-thrombin receptor, but do not interfere significantly with cleavage by α-thrombin of either fibrinogen or the low molecular weight chromogenic substrate S-2238. Despite the presence of partial agonist activity SC40476 fails to cause detectable release of GpV_{FR}. However, it is still necessary to invoke a multicomponent recognition site for α-thrombin on the platelet, a scheme for which is outlined in Fig. 2.6, since pretreatment with chymotrypsin (see above) renders washed platelets significantly more sensitive to the inhibition of α-thrombin-induced aggregation by SC42619 and also by a further analogue SC43583 (Ruda *et al.* 1990).

There is some evidence to suggest that the binding of α-thrombin to platelets may occur at least in part via the GpIbα subunit of the GpIb–IX complex (see Fig. 2.3). Binding of α-thrombin and platelet aggregation is reduced in platelets from patients with Bernard–Soulier syndrome (Jamieson & Okumura, 1978). When [^{125}I]thrombin is covalently crosslinked to platelets and membrane proteins are subsequently analysed by SDS-PAGE and autoradiography, the label is predominantly associated with a M_r 200 000 species which is absent from Bernard–Soulier platelets (Takamatsu *et al.* 1986). This process is prevented by pretreatment with a polyclonal antibody raised to the glycocalicin fragment of GpIbα, but is not blocked by a monoclonal antibody (6D1) specific for the vWF binding region, indicating interaction with a separate domain. Although platelet stimulation by α-thrombin decreases subsequent binding of vWF (George & Torres, 1988), this may be attributable to a steric effect, and currently available information indicates that α-thrombin could interact with a site on GpIbα distinct from that at which vWF binding occurs.

The data remain equivocal, however, since comparative binding studies carried out in the presence of the α-thrombin inhibitors PPACK and TLCK suggest that whilst GpIbα might function as one platelet recognition site for α-thrombin, its

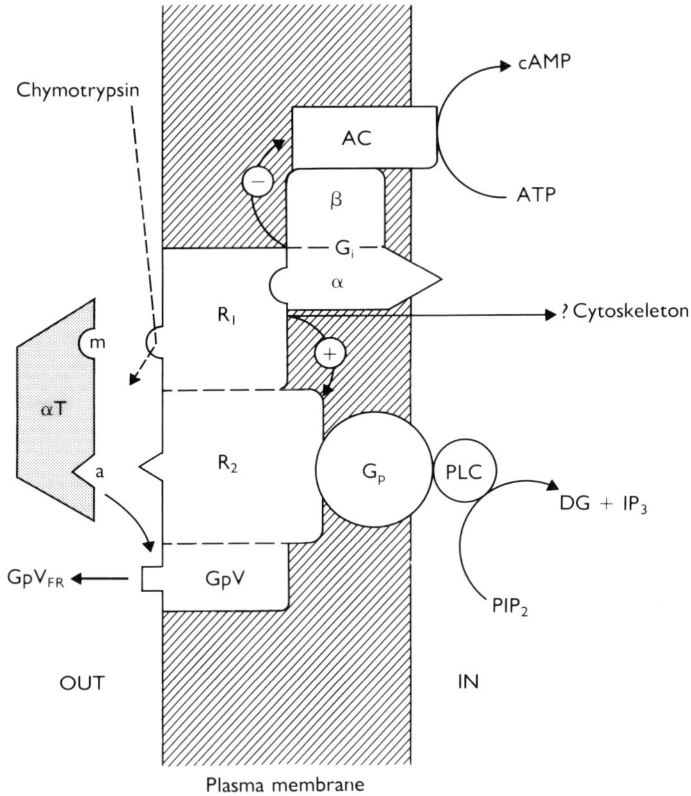

Figure 2.6 Scheme for the multisite interaction of α-thrombin (αT) with the human platelet plasma membrane. The model comprises a macromolecular domain (m) recognizing a high affinity binding site (R_1) negatively coupled via G_i to adenylyl cyclase (AC), and a putative additional active site on α-thrombin (a) interacting with a second membrane component (R_2) perhaps coupled via G_P to phospholipase C (PLC). In this hypothesis, R_1 is the chymotrypsin sensitive binding site, pretreatment with which reveals slower responses through R_2 alone. Cleavage of GpV is included in the scheme, but from recent evidence, appears unlikely to contribute to α-thrombin-induced platelet responses. (Personal communication from E. Ruda.)

removal by protease treatment reveals the presence of a binding site of unknown identity which remains quite capable of supporting platelet aggregation (Harmon & Jamieson, 1986, 1988). In particular, it also remains unclear why relatively few high affinity α-thrombin binding sites are present when specific monoclonal antibody studies indicate the existence of some 25 000 molecules of GpIb per platelet (see earlier), and why the decreased membrane GpIb content in Bernard–Soulier syndrome platelets correlates only poorly with the degree of impairment of the α-thrombin aggregatory response. Accordingly, the likelihood exists that the primary platelet receptor for α-thrombin has yet to be identified, and that binding to GpIbα may either account for low affinity binding, or represent only part of a much larger receptor complex.

Formation and stabilization of platelet aggregates

The fibrinogen receptor: GpIIb–IIIa

Fibrinogen has long been recognized as an essential cofactor for platelet aggregatory responses induced by agonists such as ADP. Patients suffering from congenital afibrinogenaemia possess extended bleeding times and platelet aggregation is severely compromised. Similarly, platelets prepared as washed cell suspensions, or maintained in plasma depleted of fibrinogen, fail to respond normally in the presence of agonists, whilst the addition of fibrinogen restores sensitivity. Monovalent anti-fibrinogen antibody antigen-binding fragments (Fab) inhibit aggregation, and whilst it is accepted that under normal physiological conditions extracellular and membrane associated fibrinogen largely facilitate aggregation, fibrinogen secreted from the platelet protein-storage granules in the presence of a powerful agonist such as thrombin, is also able to support a response even in washed suspensions. It has been shown that fibrinogen associates with the platelet surface on activation (Peerschke *et al.* 1980) and early electron microscopy studies established that fibrinogen acts as a 'bridge' between platelets during the aggregatory process (Shirasawa & Chandler, 1969). However, the interaction of fibrinogen with the platelet appears to be reversible if the release reaction has not occurred (e.g. disaggregation of ADP-stimulated platelets by PGI_2) and drugs such as dipyridamole prevent fibrinogen binding despite the presence of shape change (Harfenist *et al.* 1981).

The availability of purified [^{125}I]fibrinogen as a radioligand enabled the examination of binding parameters with washed or gel filtered platelets in the absence or presence of excitatory agonists (for a comprehensive review see Peerschke, 1985). On the quiescent discoid platelet, the majority of fibrinogen binding sites are unavailable (Marguerie *et al.* 1979). However, when platelets are stimulated by agonists such as α-thrombin, collagen, ADP or adrenaline, specific high affinity fibrinogen receptors are rapidly exposed (DiMinno *et al.* 1983). Under these assay conditions, the binding of [^{125}I]fibrinogen is specific, saturable, pH and divalent cation concentration dependent (i.e. supported by Ca^{2+} or Mg^{2+}; dissociated by EDTA (ethylene diaminetetra-acetate)). Importantly, agonist dose–response relationships can be demonstrated such that fibrinogen receptor occupancy correlates with platelet activation (Marguerie *et al.* 1980; Peerschke *et al.* 1980; Peerschke, 1985). Platelets have been reported to bind from 5000 to upwards of 50 000 molecules of fibrinogen per cell depending on the agonist and stimulatory concentration employed. Over a period of time, however, binding of fibrinogen to the platelet surface is stabilized and becomes irreversible (Marguerie *et al.* 1980).

Opinions have differed with respect to the existence of one or two populations of fibrinogen receptors (Marguerie *et al.* 1979; DiMinno *et al.* 1983), but the possibility has been raised that two component binding isotherms, observed in certain studies at higher ligand concentrations, reflect interaction between receptors or clustering rather than a true second site (Peerschke, 1982). For example, the presence of fibrinogen in plasma at saturating concentrations with respect to its platelet receptor, coupled with the observation that high fibrinogen concentrations can actually decrease aggregation, has prompted speculation that some degree of negative receptor cooperativity, which decreases binding affinity with increasing occupancy may be necessary as an important physiological control mechanism (Peerschke, 1985). Moreover, electron microscopy has provided clear evidence for fibrinogen receptor clustering on α-thrombin stimulated platelets (Loftus & Albrecht, 1984). Recent immunogold-labelling studies have further shown that this is an event driven by receptor occupancy, which may facilitate interaction with the platelet cytoskeleton, rather than being a prerequisite for fibrinogen binding *per se* (Isenberg *et al.* 1987).

The initial evidence to indicate a role for the surface membrane GpIIb and GpIIIa molecules in fibrinogen binding, arose from the study of platelets from patients with Glanzmann's thrombasthenia, which revealed a dramatic decrease in the labelling of these two glycoproteins (Phillips & Agin, 1977; Nurden & Caen, 1979). Platelets from such patients fail to bind fibrinogen, and respond abnormally to a spectrum of agonists including ADP and α-thrombin (Mustard *et al.* 1979). Although GpIIb and GpIIIa migrate as separate proteins on SDS-PAGE (Table 2.1) and are products of separate genes, there is considerable evidence to suggest that they associate on the surface membrane as a complex. A 1:1 stoichiometry is present between GpIIb and GpIIIa in normal platelets (Jennings & Phillips, 1982), and expression of both polypeptides is decreased in Glanzmann's thrombasthenia (Shulman & Karpatkin, 1980). Chemical crosslinking experiments support a specific interaction of fibrinogen with a complex of GpIIb and GpIIIa on the platelet surface membrane. Monoclonal antibodies directed against the GpIIb–IIIa complex recognize the same number of platelet membrane sites as are revealed in fibrinogen binding experiments, block the binding of [^{125}I]fibrinogen, and prevent platelet aggregation induced by collagen, ADP or arachidonic acid (Bennett *et al.* 1982; Coller *et al.* 1983a; DiMinno *et al.* 1983). Indeed, GpIIb and GpIIIa isolated from platelet membranes in Triton X-100 lysates dissociate on addition of EDTA, re-associate on addition of calcium, and bind fibrinogen in the presence of calcium only when complex formation has occurred (Nachman & Leung, 1982; Jennings & Phillips, 1982; Fujimura & Phillips, 1983).

Thus, the two subunit polypeptide GpIIb and the single polypeptide chain of GpIIIa are present in the platelet surface membrane as a non-covalently linked, calcium-dependent heterodimeric complex (Fig. 2.7) which is now recognized to correspond to the α and β-subunits respectively of other members of the integrin superfamily of membrane-adhesion receptors referred to earlier (Table 2.3) (Hynes, 1987; Ginsberg *et al.* 1988). Both GpIIb and GpIIIa have been cloned and sequenced. GpIIb is a 1008 amino acid protein which is synthesized as a single polypeptide chain and then post-translationally cleaved to yield the two subunit chains GpIIbα (871 residues) and GpIIbβ (137 residues) present at the cell surface

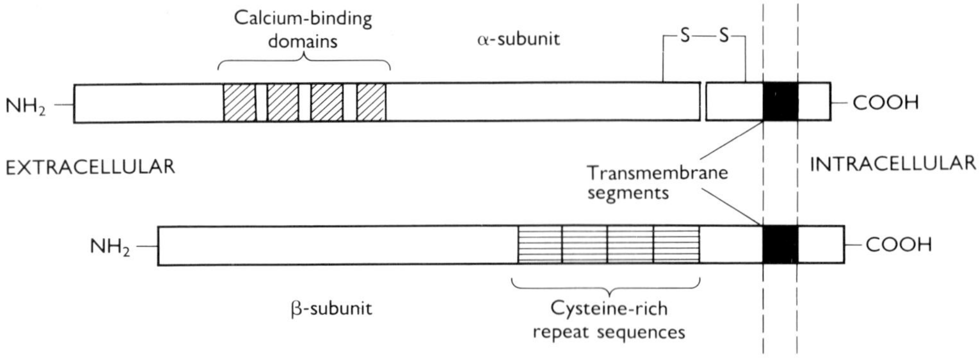

Figure 2.7 Structural model representing the key features of the adhesion receptor or integrin family, as applicable to the fibrinogen receptor of the human platelet (adapted from Phillips *et al.* 1988). Each receptor possesses two subunits (α and β) which form a calcium-dependent noncovalently linked complex. In the case of the fibrinogen receptor, the α-subunit is post-translationally cleaved to give heavy (GpIIbα) and light (GpIIbβ) chains which are linked by disulphide bonding, whereas the β subunit (GpIIIa) is preserved as a single polypeptide. Cytoplasmic domains are short, being only 20 (GpIIbβ) and 41 (GpIIIa) amino acids respectively.

(Fitzgerald *et al.* 1987a; Loftus *et al.* 1987, 1988). A certain degree of homology (36–44%) is present with the α-subunit polypeptides of the related fibroblast fibronectin receptor and the endothelial cell vitronectin receptor. Notably, since GpIIb had previously been shown to bind calcium, four repeated sequences of some 30 amino acids homologous with calcium binding domains on other proteins are present (Fitzgerald *et al.* 1987a). Platelet GpIIIa, a 762 amino acid polypeptide, contains no less than 56 cysteine residues arranged in four cysteine rich tandem repeat sequences, all of which initially appear to be disulphide linked. The protein possesses a short C-terminal cytoplasmic domain, a 29 residue transmembrane segment, and a long N-terminal extracellular domain. A number of potential N-linked glycosylation sites are present. The properties of both the α (GpIIb) and β (GpIIIa) subunits are therefore characteristic of all the surface membrane integrin receptor family so far identified (Fitzgerald *et al.* 1987b). Specifically, on the basis of these data, GpIIIa in the platelet appears identical to the endothelial cell GpIIIa (Fitzgerald *et al.* 1987b). Interestingly, the genes for GpIIb and GpIIIa are both encoded on chromosome 17, and as might be predicted, there is evidence for a close physical linkage (Bray *et al.* 1988).

In addition to fibrinogen, the platelet GpIIb–IIIa complex is able to bind fibronectin and vWF (Plow *et al.* 1984), such that thrombasthenic platelets also bind significantly reduced levels of these polypeptides (Ginsberg *et al.* 1983). Similarly, the binding of fibrinogen, fibronectin and vWF to normal platelets is equally inhibited by monoclonal antibodies directed against the GpIIb–IIIa complex, suggesting the possibility of shared recognition domains (Plow *et al.* 1985b). Since plasma fibrinogen is present in large excess, it seems unlikely that vWF actively binds to GpIIb–IIIa unless locally secreted from platelet protein-storage granules during the aggregatory process. Despite the fact that fibrinogen, fibronectin and vWF are large multimeric proteins, it has become evident that short, discrete peptide recognition sequences are responsible for the interaction of these proteins with GpIIb–IIIa. Three structurally unrelated candidate peptide sets have been identified by inhibition studies, but of these, Gly–Pro–Arg–Pro is now recognized to prevent fibrinogen binding to platelets by binding to fibrinogen itself (Plow *et al.* 1987a).

The Arg–Gly–Asp-containing sequences were first highlighted in cleavage experiments designed to identify the domain in fibronectin which governs its attachment to fibroblasts. Early experiments also demonstrated that proteolytic fragments of fibrinogen, which lack the C-terminal residues of the Aα-fibrinogen chain, support aggregation of platelets less efficiently than the intact fibrinogen molecule (Niewiarowski *et al.* 1977). Isolated intact fibrinogen Aα-chains themselves bind to platelets and induce aggregation (Hawiger *et al.* 1982). Sequence data has revealed that fibrinogen, fibronectin and vWF each possess Arg–Gly–Asp-containing peptide domains; two are present in fibrinogen at positions 95–97 and 572–574 on the Aα-chain. The Arg–Gly–Asp peptides bind directly to platelets and can be chemically crosslinked to both the GpIIbα and GpIIIa subunits in the complex. Such Arg–Gly–Asp-containing tetra or penta peptides inhibit fibrinogen binding to ADP-stimulated platelets and appear to behave as competitive antagonists of adhesive protein binding, since their activity can be reversed by the addition of fibrinogen (Plow *et al.* 1985b; Gartner & Bennett, 1985). This effect is more complex than simply direct competition, however, as variation of the size and sequence of the Arg–Gly–Asp-containing peptide alters the relative potency against the binding of different adhesive proteins. Chemically modified peptides demonstrate further enhanced potency, and binding of human fibrinogen fragment X, which lacks the Aα-chain Arg–Gly–Asp sequence, is also inhibited by Arg–Gly–Asp-containing peptides (Ruggeri *et al.* 1986; Plow *et al.* 1987b). Nevertheless, it is possible to extract GpIIb–IIIa from crude platelet lysates by affinity chromatography using an Arg–Gly–Asp-containing peptide coupled to a CNBr-Sepharose solid support in a column, and to elute the GpIIb–IIIa complex with free peptide (Pytela *et al.* 1986).

Secondly, a decapeptide located at the C-terminus of the fibrinogen γ-chain (γ 402–411) has also been strongly implicated in the interaction of fibrinogen with platelet GpIIb–IIIa (Kloczewiak *et al.* 1984; Plow *et al.* 1984). This peptide actively prevents fibrinogen, fibronectin and vWF binding to platelets, inhibits platelet aggregation and like the Arg–Gly–Asp–Ser tetrapeptide causes the clustering of surface GpIIb–IIIa molecules (Isenberg *et al.* 1987). Fibrinogen with an alternative γ-chain C-terminal sequence binds poorly to platelets (Peerschke *et al* 1986) whereas peptides from the native γ-chain C-terminal region crosslinked to a solid support avidly bind GpIIb–IIIa (Lam *et al.* 1987). Thus, fibrinogen contains at least two peptide sequences on the Aα and γ-chains which are important in the binding of the protein to platelets, and are believed to recognize discrete but interacting domains on the GpIIb–IIIa complex.

Attention is becoming increasingly focused towards achieving a greater understanding of how the GpIIb–IIIa complex functions. Although monodispersed GpIIb–IIIa is present on the surface membrane of resting platelets, activation via intracellular second messengers is necessary to reveal the specific binding site for adhesive proteins, and it is accepted that agonists induce a calcium-dependent conformational change within the complex (Coller, 1985). Peptides based on the Arg–Gly–Asp or fibrinogen γ-chain 402–411 sequences, alter the conformation of affinity chromatography purified GpIIb–IIIa complex, such that its sedimentation coefficient decreases and Stoke's radius increases, consistent with some degree of unfolding of the complex, and allowing GpIIbα to become a substrate for thrombin (Parise *et al.* 1987). Studies with monoclonal antibodies (PAC-1, PMI-1) demonstrate that the conformational change reveals new epitopes in the GPIIb–IIIa complex, and specifically in the C-terminal region of GpIIbα, which are exposed by treatment of platelets with EDTA, stimulation with ADP, or incubation of purified GpIIb–IIIa complex with Arg–Gly–Asp-containing peptides (Shattil *et al.* 1985; Frelinger *et al.* 1988). Interestingly, in crosslinking experiments, whereas the Arg–Gly–Asp–Ser tetrapeptide links to both GpIIb and GpIIIa, the fibrinogen γ-chain labels only GpIIb (Santoro & Lawing, 1987). This lends further support to the supposition that GpIIb is the subunit which confers the receptor specificity of the complex, and either undergoes or dictates the subsequent conformational change. In addition, there is evidence for the presence of GpIIb–IIIa at intracellular locations in the open canalicular system (Woods *et al.* 1986) and protein-storage granules (Wencel-Drake *et al.* 1986), and for increased expression of GpIIb–IIIa at the platelet surface in the presence of strong agonists (e.g. thrombin) such that a newly exposed receptor pool can become available on stimulation (Niiya *et al.* 1987). The clustering of GpIIb–IIIa complexes induced by the binding of fibrinogen or the small peptides (above) is not a phenomenon unique to this receptor, but it is tempting to speculate that it is a critical event, involved either in stabilization of the binding complex (see also thrombospondin below), cytoskeletal rearrangement, or even ion channel modulation (Brass, 1985). Certainly, platelets from thrombasthenic patients are reported to be deficient in α-actinin as well as GpIIb–IIIa. The presence of GpIIb–IIIa in the Triton X-100 insoluble residue of platelet lysates has been described, and data from experiments with cytochalasin B and colchicine support the possibility of increased association of GpIIb–IIIa with the cytoskeleton during platelet aggregation (Peerschke & Zucker, 1980; Painter *et al.* 1985; Wheeler *et al.* 1985). Consequently, clustering of the receptor has been proposed as an event necessary to establish focal areas within the membrane which facilitate cytoskeletal anchoring.

The thrombospondin receptor: GpIV

The observation that thrombin-stimulated platelets secrete a high molecular weight 'thrombin sensitive' protein was first reported by Baenziger *et al.* (1971). This platelet protein-storage granule constituent, termed thrombospondin, is a large multifunctional glycoprotein (M_r 450 000, 3% carbohydrate, pI 4.7) comprised of three disulphide-linked subunit polypeptide chains. Notably, multiple calcium binding domains are present, and the binding of calcium to thrombospondin elicits a conformational change in the tertiary structure of the protein (Lawler & Hines, 1986). Thrombospondin is capable of binding to heparin, forms complexes with fibrinogen, fibronectin, collagen or plasminogen (Silverstein *et al.* 1984), and contains the Arg–Gly–Asp recognition peptide (Lawler & Hines, 1986). Exposure of thrombospondin to proteolytic enzymes induces cleavage of an N-terminal polypeptide which contains the heparin-binding domain (Coligan & Slater, 1984) whereas the fibrinogen binding site is located in a separate M_r 120–140 000 fragment (Dixit *et al.* 1984). Thrombospondin is not a major circulating constituent protein in the plasma, but in addition to its presence in the platelet, is synthesized by mononuclear cells, smooth muscle cells and vascular endothelium. It is, therefore, a possibly significant component of the vessel wall extracellular matrix, with some preliminary data to indicate increased levels in atherosclerotic lesions (Wight *et al.* 1985).

The belief that thrombospondin might play an important role in platelet aggregatory responses gained credence from experiments demonstrating that anti-thrombospondin monovalent (Fab) antibodies partially inhibit thrombin, collagen or ADP-induced aggregation of gel filtered platelet suspensions (Leung, 1984). The antibody caused rapid reversal of primary wave aggregation, abolished the second wave of the response, and also inhibited platelet binding of fibrinogen. Thrombospondin itself demonstrates saturable, specific and calcium-dependent binding to platelets, which is substantially enhanced in thrombin stimulated cells, and reveals some 35 000 sites per platelet with a K_D of 250 nM (Wolff *et al.* 1986). Despite the presence of the Arg–Gly–Asp tripeptide sequence (Leung, 1984), prevention of thrombospondin binding by antibodies to the GpIIb–IIIa complex (Plow *et al.* 1985b) and the observation that bound thrombospondin co-clusters on the platelet surface with GpIIb–IIIa (Asch *et al.* 1985), it has become apparent that thrombospondin binds not to GpIIb–IIIa, but to a closely related membrane site. Briefly, thrombospondin binding is normal in platelets from patients with Glanzmann's thrombasthenia (Aiken *et al.* 1986; Wolff *et al.* 1986); a monoclonal antibody (P8) specific for thrombospondin blocks thrombin-induced aggregation but not fibrinogen binding (Boukerche & McGregor, 1988); and thrombospondin is reported not to bind to an affinity column purified preparation of GpIIb–IIIa complex incorporated into lecithin liposomes which still recognizes fibrinogen or fibronectin (Pytela *et al.* 1986).

Accordingly, attention has increasingly focussed on GpIV as the putative membrane receptor for thrombospondin. This platelet surface glycoprotein is an M_r 88 000 single chain polypeptide which contains a high proportion (28%) of carbohydrate (Table 2.1) and unusually, is resistant to proteolysis by trypsin or chymotrypsin. It has recently been purified to homogeneity by Tsuji & Osawa (1986). An important clue to the identity of GpIV as the thrombospondin receptor arose through studies with another monoclonal antibody, OKM5. This antibody was initially reported to be directed against an unidentified cell surface antigen, also M_r 88 000, and believed to play a fundamental role in malarial parasite (*Plasmodium falciparum*) infected erythrocyte adherence to monocytes or endothelial cells (Barnwell *et al.* 1985). Indeed, thrombospondin contains a highly conserved amino acid sequence homologous not only with properdin (a plasma glycoprotein that stabilizes the C3BnBb enzyme complex of the alternative pathway of complement activation) but also with a protein recently cloned and sequenced which is expressed during the erythrocyte stage of the malaria parasite's life cycle, and referred to as thrombospondin-related anonymous protein or TRAP (Robson *et al.* 1988). Since circulating monocytes and macrophages, like platelets, possess a membrane population of thrombospondin receptors (Silverstein & Nachman, 1987); binding of thrombospondin to the M_r 88 000 protein also appears saturable and specific; and OKM5 is now known to specifically recognize GpIV (Asch *et al.* 1987), it now seems certain that the M_r 88 000 protein and GpIV are synonymous, and moreover, that GpIV is the thrombospondin receptor on a variety of cell types including the platelet.

It is apparent from the above information that one potentially important function of thrombospondin may therefore be to act as a cell–cell bridging molecule (analogous to fibrinogen) which mediates attachment, for example, of platelets to monocytes (Silverstein & Nachman, 1987). Similarly, with respect to platelet aggregation, thrombospondin is clearly a key participant in the development of irreversible aggregates through its ability to co-cluster with the GpIIb–IIIa complex and to stabilize the binding of fibrinogen. Conceivably therefore, a sequence of events occurs whereby stimulation of platelets exposes GpIIb–IIIa binding sites for fibrinogen which, through formation of a macromolecular surface membrane complex with GpIV and thrombospondin, become stabilized and anchored via the platelet cytoskeleton (shown in Fig. 2.8 as proposed by Nachman *et al.* 1987).

New functions for platelet surface glycoproteins

The reader will have gathered from the foregoing information that the present time is one of rapid expansion in the available knowledge base with respect to structure and function of the platelet surface membrane receptor proteins. The conclusion that the platelet is well-equipped to specifically interact with both low molecular weight excitatory or inhibitory agonists, and high molecular weight polypeptide ligands at different levels of affinity and capacity is clearly justified.

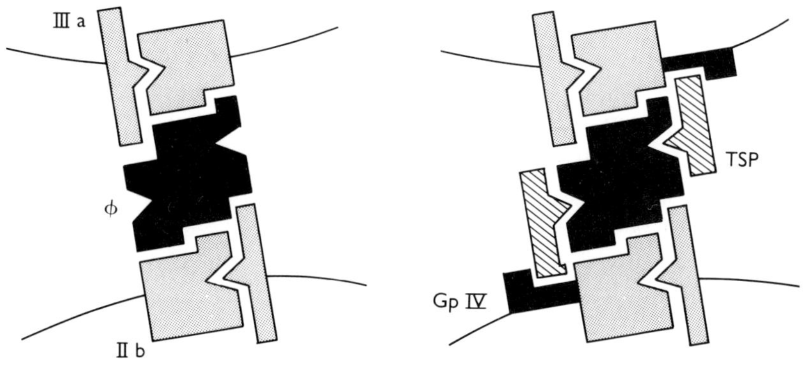

Figure 2.8 Hypothetical model for a two step process in the macromolecular assembly of GpIIb–IIIa, fibrinogen, GpIV and thrombospondin on the surface of an activated platelet. Binding of fibrinogen to its receptor (left) results in a reversible cell–cell interaction (primary aggregation). Following release of thrombospondin (TSP) and co-clustering of GpIV with GpIIb–IIIa, the interaction is stabilized by thrombospondin binding to GpIV and also to fibrinogen at a site discrete from the loci which recognise GpIIb–IIIa. (Reproduced from Nachman *et al.* (1987) with permission.)

However, whilst information continues to accumulate on those receptors involved in haemostatic functions such as the adhesion and formation of aggregates, there is clear evidence that we are only just beginning to comprehend the contribution that circulating blood platelets may make to other physiological processes. Two notable examples, without which this review would be incomplete, are the potential role of the platelet in the acceleration of local fibrinolysis (via receptors for plasminogen) and in immune-based disorders involving immunoglobulin Fc receptors and interaction with the complement system.

Plasminogen binding

This potentially exciting area derives from the initial observation that platelets are able to bind plasminogen in a specific and saturable manner, and with high capacity. Moreover, the 37 000 sites per platelet evident on the resting cell increases by up to an order of magnitude following stimulation by α-thrombin (Miles & Plow, 1985). Plasminogen binding to monocytes, granulocytes, lymphocytes and vascular endothelial cells has also been reported, whilst urokinase can also bind to monocytes or granulocytes (Plow *et al.* 1986), but not platelets. Calculations suggest that at the circulating concentration of plasminogen in plasma (1–2 μM), approximately 1% is likely to be cell-associated (Miles & Plow, 1987). This may, however, underestimate the physiological importance of cell-bound plasminogen in local fibrinolysis. Firstly, plasminogen bound to platelets is significantly more efficiently activated by tissue plasminogen activator than soluble plasminogen (Miles & Plow, 1987). Secondly, α-thrombin-stimulated platelets express increased numbers of binding sites (above). Finally, there is some evidence to suggest that plasmin generated on the cell surface may be protected from inhibitor complex formation with α_2-antiplasmin (Plow *et al.* 1986). Tissue plasminogen activator (tPA), receptors for which have been described on endothelial cells but not platelets, may be similarly protected from inactivation by plasminogen activator inhibitor (PAI-l) under these circumstances.

Plasminogen binding to platelets requires detailed characterization, but has been suggested to occur primarily through two mechanisms: the formation of fibrin on the platelet surface, and via an as yet undefined mechanism involving binding to sites on GpIIb–IIIa distinct from those recognized by adhesive proteins. Evidence for this (reviewed by Miles & Plow, 1988) focuses on the requirement for the putative receptor to be a prominent surface membrane polypeptide, the apparent absence of plasminogen binding to platelets from patients with Glanzmann's thrombasthenia, and the lack of enhanced binding induced by α-thrombin in an afibrinogenaemic patient. Further support is provided by the recognized ability of α-thrombin to cleave fibrinogen to fibrin on the cell surface, and the known high affinity of plasminogen for fibrin(ogen). However, it should also be recalled that α-thrombin stimulation of platelets induces secretion of thrombospondin which, linked via its receptor GpIV, can co-cluster with GpIIb–IIIa on platelet activation (above). Thrombospondin itself binds to plasminogen (Silverstein *et al.* 1984), and will form a ternary complex with tPA and plasminogen on a solid support system *in vitro*, such that a 40-fold decrease in K_m and a similar magnitude of increase in catalytic efficiency has been described for the conversion of plasminogen to plasmin by tPA in this system. Again, it is claimed tht plasmin is protected from inhibition by α_2-antiplasmin under these circumstances (Silverstein *et al.* 1985; Nachman *et al.* 1987). Nevertheless, the position remains equivocal with respect to a primary role for thrombospondin, most notably since although thrombasthenic platelets lack plasminogen binding sites, surface expression of thrombospondin is apparently normal (Aiken *et al.* 1986). Current data does not, however, appear to preclude the possibility that optimum enhancement of local fibrinolysis in α-thrombin-stimulated platelets or endothelial cells might only be achieved through co-clustering of the macromolecular GpIIb–IIIa-fibrinogen/GpIV-thrombospondin complex. More importantly, localization of plasminogen and tPA on the cell surface leading to plasmin generation appears to be an attractive and potentially key mechanism for promoting local fibrinolysis and proteolysis (Fig. 2.9), such that it may well be of importance in both clot lysis and tissue remodelling.

Cytoxicity and allergy

The potential contribution of platelets to primary defence mechanisms such as antibody-dependent cytotoxicity, and via parallel mechanisms, to immune complex disorders, organ transplant rejection, and most recently hypersensitivity reactions including bronchial asthma, has steadily become apparent. Platelets possess a glycoprotein receptor for the third component of complement (C3b) which re-

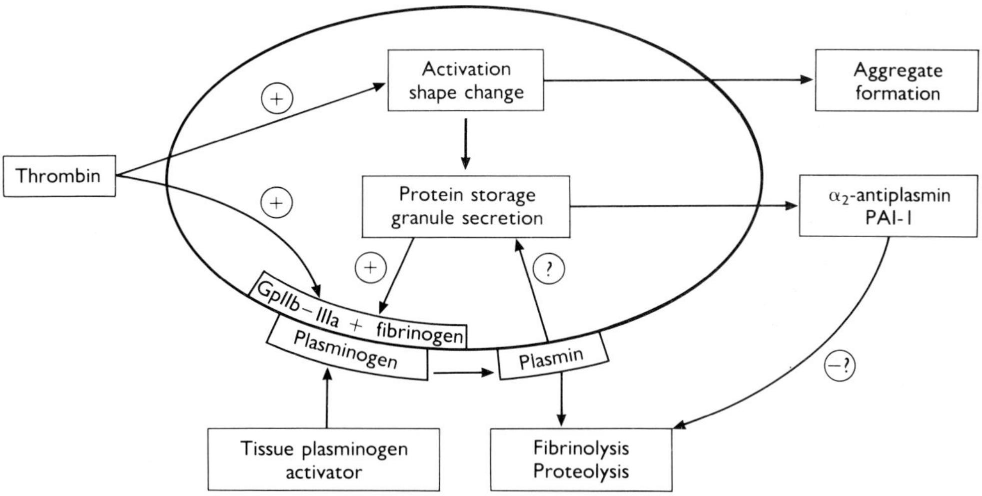

Figure 2.9 Scheme for events which might influence local fibrinolysis on the α-thrombin stimulated platelet surface. GpIIb–IIIa and fibrin(ogen) are currently believed to play key roles in plasminogen binding. Fibrinogen secretion from the protein storage granules may be the mechanism for α-thrombin enhanced plasminogen binding (see text). Plasmin is variously reported to enhance or inhibit platelet activation depending on concentration present. There is some evidence to suggest that plasmin is protected from inactivation by α_2-antiplasmin in this system. A parallel situation may apply to tissue plasminogen activator and plasminogen activator inhibitor (PAI-l) although curiously, *in vitro* the latter appears to be secreted predominantly in a latent form. Similar mechanisms (with the additional presence of utokinase plasminogen activator (UPA) receptors) may operate on the vascular endothelial cell surface.

sembles that on mononuclear cells (Yu *et al.* 1986), and Fc receptors for both IgG and IgE antibodies (Rosenfeld *et al.* 1985; Joseph *et al.* 1986).

Historically, the ability of aggregated immunoglobulins to induce platelet aggregation and secretion of the dense granule constituent 5-HT has been recognized for more than a decade. Specific and saturable radioligand binding of IgG dimers and oligomers to platelets has been described (Karas *et al.* 1982). The platelet IgG receptor, in common with certain lymphocytes and endothelial cells, possesses low affinity for monomeric IgG, but considerable capacity to bind IgG aggregates or IgG-coated particles. Rosenfeld *et al.* (1985) have shown, by a combination of surface labelling studies, immunoprecipitation from platelet lysates and affinity purification on IgG-Sepharose, that the platelet IgG receptor is an M_r 40 000 glycoprotein specifically recognized by a murine monoclonal antibody originally developed against this protein in human monocytes and U937 cells. The same monoclonal antibody inhibits platelet aggregation induced by heat-aggregated IgG, but not by agonists such as thrombin or collagen. Although the antibody fails to induce aggregation directly, addition of a second bridging antibody (goat anti-mouse Ig) results in an ADP-dependent aggregatory response suggesting that the M_r 40 000 component is coupled to secretory mechanisms. Heat-aggregated IgG can also render platelets hyperaggregable, and in some circumstances, may play a role in the formation and stabilization of aggregates (Parbtani *et al.* 1987). The platelet IgG receptor is evidently of the FcγRII type, and there is currently no evidence for the presence of high affinity monomeric IgG (FcγRI) receptors on these cells.

Flow cytofluorometric analysis employing indirect labelling via a mouse monoclonal anti-human IgE and FITC-conjugated rabbit anti-mouse IgG has also recently revealed a sub-population (20%) of human platelets in normal donor samples which possess high affinity Fc receptors for IgE (Joseph *et al.* 1986). Incidence increases (up to 50%) in patients with high levels of circulating IgE such as atopic individuals or those with parasitic infections. Binding of ^{125}I-labelled IgE to normal donor platelets is specific, saturable, and inhibited by a 50-fold excess of unlabelled IgE or by pretreatment with a polyclonal anti-FcεR antibody. Heat-aggregated IgG is without effect. A two component binding isotherm indicates the presence of several hundred high affinity (K_a $3.3 \times 10^7\,M^{-1}$) sites per platelet and a much greater number (up to 60000) low affinity sites (K_a $7.8 \times 10^5\,M^{-1}$). The IgE receptor on the human platelet appears antigenically related to the IgE receptor on other leukocytes since both a monoclonal anti-eosinophil FcεR and a polyclonal anti-lymphocyte FcεR antibody inhibit IgE-dependent platelet activation. The receptor has consequently been designated as of the M_r 45000 FcεRII type, rather than the FcεRI-receptor present on mast cells. The human lymphocyte cDNA for the FcεRII receptor has been cloned, sequenced and expressed in COS-7 cells (Ikuta *et al.* 1987). It is a 321 amino acid polypeptide with a putative 24 residue transmembrane segment close to the N-terminal (i.e. C-terminal is probably extracellular), and potential asparagine-linked glycosylation sites are present. There is significant homology in the C-terminal domain with sugar binding animal lectins such as the asialoglycoprotein receptor which binds galactose, and the chicken-hepatic lectin which recognizes *N*-acetylglucosamine, which may indicate a role for glycosylated residues on IgE in ligand recognition and binding.

Interestingly, the platelet IgE receptor appears not to be associated in any way with the formation of aggregates, but rather with the ability of platelets to mount a reaginic antibody-dependent cytotoxic response against helminth parasites such as *Schistosoma mansoni* through oxidative killing (as demonstrated *in vitro* by chemiluminescence) (Capron *et al.* 1986). Its possible relevance to both this host defence mechanism and a role for IgE-activated platelets in allergic responses are considered in detail elsewhere in this volume.

References

Adelstein, R.S., Pollard, T.D. & Kuehl, W.M. (1971) Isolation and characterization of myosin and two myosin fragments from human blood platelets. *Proc Natl Acad Sci USA* **68**, 2703–2707.

Aiken, M.L., Ginsberg, M.H. & Plow, E.F. (1986) Identification of a new class of inducible receptors in platelets. Thrombospondin interacts with platelets via a GpIIb.-IIIa independent mechanism. *J Clin Invest* **78**, 1713–1716.

Argraves, W.S., Suzuki, S., Arai, H., Thompson, K.,

Pierschbacher, M.D. & Ruoslahti, E. (1987) Amino acid sequence of the human fibronectin receptor. *J Cell Biol* **105**, 1183–1190.

Armstrong, R.A., Jones, R.L. & Wilson, H.H. (1983) Ligand binding to thromboxane receptors on human platelets: correlation with biological activity. *Br J Pharmacol* **79**, 953–964.

Armstrong, R.A., Lawrence, R.A., Jones, R.L., Wilson, N.H. & Collier, A. (1989) Functional and ligand binding studies suggest heterogeneity of prostacyclin receptors. *Br J Pharmacol* **97**, 657–668.

Asch, A.S., Leung, L.L.K., Polley, M. & Nachman, R.L. (1985) Platelet membrane topography: colocalization of thrombospondin and fibrinogen with the glycoprotein IIb–IIIa complex. *Blood* **66**, 926–934.

Asch, A.S., Barnwell, J., Silverstein, A.L. & Nachman, R.L. (1987) Isolation of the thrombospondin membrane receptor. *J Clin Invest* **79**, 1054–1061.

Baenziger, N.L., Brodie, G.N. & Majerus, P.W. (1971) A thrombin sensitive protein of human platelet membranes. *Proc Natl Acad Sci USA* **68**, 240–243.

Ball, G., Brereton, G.G., Fulwood, M., Ireland, D.M. & Yates, P. (1970) Effect of prostaglandin E_1 alone and in combination with theophylline or aspirin on collagen-induced platelet aggregation and on platelet nucleotides including adenosine 3′,5′-cyclic monophosphate. *Biochem J* **120**, 709–718.

Barber, A.J. & Jamieson, G.A. (1970) Isolation and characterization of plasma membranes from human platelets. *J Biol Chem* **245**, 6359–6365.

Barnes, M.J. (1985) Collagens in atherosclerosis. *Coll Relat Res* **5**, 65–97.

Barnett, D.B., Swart, S.S., Nahorski, S.R. & Cook, N. (1985) Characterization of human platelet adrenoceptors. In Westwick, J., Scully, M.F., MacIntyre, D.E. & Kakkar, V.V. (eds) *Mechanisms of Stimulus–Response Coupling in Platelets*, pp. 97–108. Plenum Press, London.

Barnwell, J.W., Ockenhouse, C.F. & Knowles, D.M. (1985) Monoclonal antibody OKM5 inhibits the *in vitro* binding of *Plasmodium falciparum*-infected erythrocytes to monocytes, endothelial, and C32 melanoma cells. *J Immunol* **135**, 3494–3497.

Baumgartner, H.R. (1977) Platelet interaction with collagen fibrils in flowing blood. I. Reaction of human platelets with α-chymotrypsin digested subendothelium. *Thromb haemost* **37**, 1–16.

Bennett, J.S., Colman, R.F. & Colman, R.W. (1978) Identification of adenine nucleotide binding proteins in human platelet membranes by affinity labeling with 5′-p-fluorosulphonylbenzoyl adenosine. *J Biol Chem* **253**, 7346–7354.

Bennett, J.S., Vilaire, G. & Cines, D.B. (1982) Identification of the fibrinogen receptor on human platelets by photoaffinity labelling. *J Biol Chem* **257**, 8049–8054.

Benovic, J.L., Regan, J.W., Matusi, H., Mayor, F., Cotecchia, S., Leeb-Lundberg, L.M.F., Caron, M.G. & Lefkowitz, R.J. (1987) Agonist-dependent phosphorylation of the α_2-adrenergic receptor by the β-adrenergic receptor kinase. *J Biol Chem* **262**, 17251–17253.

Berndt, M.C., Gregory, C., Kabral, A., Zola, H., Fournier, D. & Castaldi, P.A. (1985) Purification and preliminary characterization of the glycoprotein Ib complex in the human platelet membrane. *Eur J Biochem* **151**, 637–649.

Bhagwat, S.S., Hamann, P.R. & Still, W.C. (1985a) Synthesis of thromboxane A_2. *J Am Chem* Soc **107**, 6372–6376.

Bhagwat, S.S., Hamann, P.R., Still, W.C., Bunting, S. & Fitzpatrick, F.A. (1985b) Synthesis and structure of the platelet aggregation factor thromboxane A_2. *Nature* **315**, 511–513.

Bienz, D., Schnippering, W. & Clementson, K.J. (1986) Glycoprotein V is not the thrombin activation receptor on human blood platelets. *Blood* **68**, 720–725.

Boon, N.A., Elliott, J.M., Grahame-Smith, D.G., St John-Green, T. & Stump, K. (1983) A comparison of α-adrenoceptor binding characteristics of intact human platelets identified by [^{3}H]yohimbine and [^{3}H]dihydroergocryptine. *J Auton Pharmacol* **3**, 89–95.

Boukerche, H. & McGregor, J.L. (1988) Characterization of an anti-thrombospondin monoclonal antibody P8 that inhibits human blood platelet functions: normal binding of P8 to thrombin-activated Glanszmann thrombasthenic platelets. *Eur J Biochem* **171**, 383–392.

Boyles, J., Fox, J.E.B., Phillips, D.R. & Sternberg, D.E. (1985) Organization of the cytoskeleton in resting, discoid platelets: preservation of actin filaments by a modified fixation that prevents osmium damage. *J Cell Biol* **101**, 1463–1472.

Brass, L.F. (1985) Ca^{2+} transport across the platelet plasma membrane. A role for membrane glycoproteins IIb and IIIa. *J Biol Chem* **260**, 2231–2236.

Brass, L.F., Laposata, M., Banga, H.S. & Rittenhouse, S.E. (1986) Regulation of the phosphoinositide hydrolysis pathway in thrombin-stimulated platelets by a pertussis toxin-sensitive guanine nucleotide-binding protein. Evaluation of its contribution to platelet activation and comparisons with the adenylate cyclase inhibitory protein, G_i. *J Biol Chem* **261**, 16838–16847.

Bray, P.F., Barsh, G., Rosa, J-P., Luo, X.Y., Magenis, E. & Shuman, M.A. (1988) Physical linkage of the genes for platelet membrane glycoproteins IIb and IIIa. *Proc Natl Acad Sci USA* **85**, 8683–8687.

Bunting, S., Buchanan, L.V., Holzgrefe, H.H. & Fitzpatrick, F.A. (1987) Pharmacology of synthetic thromboxane A_2. *Adv Prostaglandin Thromboxane Leukotriene Res* **17**, 192–197.

Burch, R., Mais, D., Pepkowitz, S. & Halushka, P.V. (1985) Hydrodynamic properties of a thromboxane A_2 prostaglandin H_2 antagonist binding site solubilized from human platelets. *Biochem Biophys Res Commun* **132**, 961–968.

Burke, S.E., Lefer, A.M., Nicolaou, K.C., Smith, G.M. & Smith, J.B. (1983) Responsiveness of platelets and coronary arteries from different species to synthetic thromboxane and prostaglandin endoperoxide analogues. *Br J Pharmacol* **78**, 287–292.

Burnstock, G., Cusack, N.J., Hills, J.M., Mackenzie, I. & Meghji, P. (1983) Studies on the stereo-selectivity of the P_2-purinoceptor. *Br J Pharmacol* **79**, 907–913.

Bylund, D.B., Ray-Prenger, C. & Murphy, T.J. (1988) Alpha-2A and alpha-2B adrenergic receptor subtypes: antagonist binding in tissues and cell lines containing only one subtype. *J Pharmacol Exp Ther* **245**, 600–607.

Capron, A., Dessaint, J.P., Capron, M., Joseph, M., Ameisen, J.C. & Tonnel, A.B. (1986) From parasites to allergy: a second receptor for IgE. *Immunology Today* **7**, 15–18.

Chau, L.Y. & Jii, Y.J. (1988) Characterization of tritium-labelled platelet activating factor receptor complex solubilized from rabbit platelet membranes. *Biochim Biophys Acta* **970**, 103–112.

Cheresh, D.A., Pytela, R., Pierschbacher, M.D., Klier, F.G., Ruoslahtl, E. & Reisfeld, R.A. (1987) An Arg–Gly–Asp-directed receptor on the surface of human melanoma cells exists in a divalent cation-dependent functional complex with the disialoganglioside GD2. *J Cell Biol* **105**, 1163–1173.

Chesney, C.M., Pifer, D.D. & Huch, K.M. (1985) Densitization of human platelets by platelet-activating factor. *Biochem Biophys Res Commun* **127**, 24–30.

Chiang, T.M. & Kang, A.H. (1982) Isolation and purification of collagen α_1(I) receptor from human platelet membrane. *J Biol Chem* **257**, 7581–7586.

Chiang, T.M., Jin, A. & Kang, A.H. (1987) Platelet-collagen interaction. Inhibition by a monoclonal antibody raised against collagen receptor. *J Immunol* **139**, 887–892.

Clemetson, K.J., McGregor, J.L., James, E., Dechavanne, M. & Luscher, E.F. (1982) Characterization of the platelet membrane glycoprotein abnormalities in Bernard–Soulier syndrome and comparison with normal by surface-labeling techniques and high-resolution two-dimensional gel electrophoresis. *J Clin Invest* **70**, 304–311.

Coligan, J.E. & Slater, H.S. (1984) Structure of thrombospondin. *J Biol Chem* **259**, 3944–3948.

Coller, B.S. (1981) Inhibition of von Willebrand factor-dependent platelet function by increased platelet cyclic AMP and its prevention by cytoskeleton-disrupting agents. *Blood* **57**, 846–855.

Coller, B.S. (1985) A new murine monoclonal antibody reports an activation-dependent change in the conformation and/or microenvironment of the platelet glycoprotein IIb-IIIa complex. *J Clin Invest* **76**, 101–108.

Coller, B.S., Peerschke, E.I., Scudder, L.E. & Sullivan, C.A. (1983a) A murine monoclonal antibody that completely blocks the binding of fibrinogen to platelets produces a thrombasthenic-like state in normal platelets and binds GpIIb and GpIIIa. *J Clin Invest* **72**, 325–338.

Coller, B.S., Peerscheke, E.I., Scudder, L.E. & Sullivan, C.A. (1983b) Studies with a murine monoclonal antibody that abolishes ristocetin-induced binding of von Willebrand factor to platelets: additional evidence in support of GpIb as a platelet receptor for von Willebrand factor. *Blood* **61**, 99–110.

Collier, N.C. & Wang, K. (1982) Purification and properties of human platelet P235. A high molecular weight protein substrate of endogenous calcium-activated proteases. *J Biol Chem* **257**, 6937–6943.

Colman, R.W. & Figures, W.R. (1984) Characteristics of an ADP receptor mediating platelet activation. *Mol Cell Biochem* **59**, 101–111.

Cooper, B. & Ahern, D. (1979) Characterization of the platelet PGD_2 receptor. Loss of PGD_2 receptors in platelets of patients with myeloproliferative disorders. *J Clin Invest* **64**, 586–590.

Cooper, B., Handin, R.I., Young, L.H. & Alexander, R.W. (1978) Agonist regulation of the human platelet α-adrenergic receptor. *Nature* **274**, 703–706.

Cote, G., Lewis, W.G. & Smillie, L.B. (1978) Non-polymerizability of platelet tropomyosin and its NH_2- and COOH-terminal sequences. *FEBS Lett* **91**, 237–241.

Demushkin, V.P., Fomenko, A.M., Plyashkevich, Y.G., Shchurin, M.R. & Brusov, O.S. (1987) High and low-affinity tritiated imipramine binding sites on human platelets: separate determination and involvement of sulphur-containing bonds. *Eur J Biochem* **140**, 171–178.

DiMinno, G., Thiagarajan, P., Perussia, B., Martinez, J., Shapiro, S., Trinchieri, G. & Murphy, S. (1983) Exposure of platelet fibrinogen-binding sites by collagen, arachidonic acid and ADP: Inhibition by a monoclonal antibody to the GpIIb.IIIa complex. *Blood* **61**, 140–148.

Dixit, V.M., Grant, G.A., Frazier, W.A. & Santoro, S.A. (1984) Isolation of the fibrinogen binding region of platelet thrombospondin. *Biochem Biophys Res Commun* **119**, 1075–1081.

Dohlman, H.G., Caron, M.G. & Lefkowitz, R.J. (1987) A family of receptors coupled to guanine nucleotide regulatory proteins. *Biochemistry* **26**, 2657–2664.

Du, X., Beutier, L., Ruan, C., Castaldi, P.A. & Berndt, M.C. (1987) Glycoprotein Ib and glycoprotein IX are fully complexed in the intact platelet membrane. *Blood* **69**, 1524–1527.

Dutta-Roy, A.K. & Sinha, A.K. (1987) Purification and properties of prostaglandin E_1-prostacyclin receptor of human blood platelets. *J Biol Chem* **262**, 12685–12691.

Eggerman, T.L., Anderson, N.H. & Robertson, R.P. (1986) Separate receptors for prostacyclin and prostaglandin E_2 on human gel-filtered platelets. *J Pharmacol Exp Ther* **236**, 568–573.

Eggerman, T.L., Hartzell, C.J., Selfe, S. & Anderson, N.H. (1987) The single prostacyclin receptor of gel-filtered platelets provides a correlation with anti-aggregatory potency of PGI_2 mimics. *Thromb Res* **45**,

645–660.

Elliott, J.M. & Grahame-Smith, D.G. (1982) The binding characteristics of [^{3}H]dihydroergocryptine on intact human platelets. *Br J Pharmac* **76**, 121–130.

Fenton, J.W. (1988) Regulation of thrombin generation and functions. *Semin Thromb Hemost* **14**, 234–240.

Figures, W.R., Scearce, L.M., Defeo, P., Stewart, G., Zhou, G., Chen, J., Daniel, J., Colman, R.F. & Colman, R.W. (1987) Direct evidence for the interaction of the nucleotide affinity analog 5'-P-fluorosulphonylbenzoyladenosine with a platelet ADP receptor. *Blood* **70**, 796–803.

Fitzgerald, L.A., Poncz, M., Steiner, B., Rall, S.C., Bennett, J.S. & Phillips, D.R. (1987a) Comparison of cDNA-derived protein sequences of the human fibronectin and vitronectin receptor α-subunits and platelet glycoprotein IIb. *Biochemistry* **26**, 8158–8165.

Fitzgerald, L.A., Steiner, B., Rall, S.C., Lo, S. & Phillips, D.R. (1987b) Protein sequence of endothelial glycoprotein IIIa derived from a cDNA clone. Identity with platelet glycoprotein IIIa and similarity to Integrin. *J Biol Chem* **262**, 3936–3939.

Fitzsimmons, C.M., Cawston, T.E. & Barnes, M.J. (1986) The platelet reactivity of collagen type I: evidence for multiple platelet-reactive sites in the type I collagen molecule. *Thromb Haemost* **56**, 95–99.

Fox, J.E.B. (1985a) Identification of actin-binding protein as the protein linking the membrane skeleton to glycoproteins on platelet plasma membranes. *J Biol Chem* **260**, 11970–11977.

Fox, J.E.B. (1985b) Linkage of a membrane skeleton to integral membrane glycoproteins in human platelets. Identification of one of the glycoproteins as glycoprotein Ib. *J Clin Invest* **76**, 1673–1683.

Fox, J.E.B. (1987) The platelet cytoskeleton. In Verstraete, M., Vermylen, J., Lijen, R. & Arnout, J. (eds) *Thrombosis and Haemostasis*, pp. 175–225. Leuven University Press, Belgium.

Fox, J.E.B. & Boyles, J.K. (1988) The membrane skeleton — a distinct structure that regulates the function of cells. *Bioessays* **8**, 14–18.

Fox, J.E.P., Boyles, J.K., Reynolds, C.C. & Phillips, D.R. (1984) Actin filament content and organization in unstimulated platelets. *J Cell Biol* **98**, 1985–1991.

Fox, J.E.B., Reynolds, C.C. & Johnson, M.M. (1987a) Identification of glycoprotein Ibβ as one of the major proteins phosphorylated during exposure of intact platelets to agent that activate cyclic AMP-dependent protein kinase. *J Biol Chem* **262**, 12627–12631.

Fox, J.E.B., Reynolds, C.C., Morrow, J.S. & Phillips, D.R. (1987b) Spectrin is associated with membrane-bound actin filaments in platelets and is hydrolyzed by the Ca^{2+}-dependent protease during platelet activation. *Blotoid* **69**, 537–545.

Fox, J.E.B., Aggerbeck, L.P. & Berndt, M.C. (1988a) Structure of the glycoprotein Ib.IX complex from platelet membranes. *J Biol Chem* **263**, 4882–4890.

Fox, J.E.B., Boyles, J.K., Berndt, M.C., Steffen, P.K. & Anderson, L.K. (1988b) Identification of a membrane skeleton in platelets. *J Cell Biol* **106**, 1525–1538.

Frelinger, A.L., Lam, S.C-T., Plow, E.F., Smith, M.A., Loftus, J.C. & Ginsberg, M.H. (1988) Occupancy of an adhesive glycoprotein receptor modulates expression of an antigenic site involved in cell adhesion. *J Biol Chem* **263**, 12397–12402.

Frielle, T., Collins, S., Daniel, K.W., Caron, M.G., Lefkowitz, R.J. & Kobilka, B.K. (1987) Cloning of the cDNA for the human β_1-adrenergic receptor. *Proc Natl Acad Sci USA* **84**, 7920–7924.

Fujimura, K. & Phillips, D.R. (1983) Calcium cation regulation of glycoprotein IIb–IIIa complex formation in platelet plasma membranes. *J Biol Chem* **258**, 10247–10252.

Gartner, T.K. & Bennett, J.S. (1985) The tetrapeptide analogue of the cell attachment site of fibronectin inhibits platelet aggregation and fibrinogen binding to activated platelets. *J Biol Chem* **260**, 11891–11894.

George, J.N. (1978) Studies on platelet plasma membranes. IV. Quantitative analysis of platelet membrane glycoproteins by (^{125}I)-diazotized duodosulfanilic acid labelling and SDS-polyacrylamide gel electrophoresis. *J. Lab. Clin. Med.* **92**, 430–446.

George, J.N. & Torres, M.M. (1988) Thrombin decreases von Willebrand factor binding to platelet glycoprotein Ib. *Blood* **71**, 1253–1259.

George, J.N., Nurden, A.T. & Phillips, D.R. (1984) Molecular defects in interactions of platelets with the vessel wall. *New Engl J Med* **311**, 1084–1098.

George, J.N., Nurden, A.T. & Phillips, D.R. (1985) *Platelet Membrane Glycoproteins*. Plenum Press, New York-London.

Giancotti, F.G., Comoglio, P.M. & Tarone, G. (1986) A 135 000 molecular weight plasma membrane glycoprotein involved in fibronectin-mediated cell adhesion: Immunofluorescence localization in normal and RSV-transformed fibroblasts. *Exp Cell Res* **163**, 47–54.

Giancotti, F.G., Languino, L.R., Zanetti, A., Peri, G., Tarone, G. & Dejana, E. (1987) Platelets express a membrane protein complex immunologically related to the fibroblast fibronectin receptor and distinct from GpIIb–IIIa. *Blood* **69**, 1535–1538.

Giancotti, F.G., Comoglio, P.M. & Tarone, G. (1988) Interaction of fibroblasts, haemopoietic cells and platelets with extracellular matrix; characterization and role of a common cell surface glycoprotein. *Ann NY Acad Sci* **511**, 65–76.

Ginsberg, M.H., Forsyth, J., Lightsey, A., Chediak, J. & Plow, E.F. (1983) Reduced surface expression and binding of fibronectin by thrombin-stimulated thrombasthenic platelets. *J Clin Invest* **71**, 619–624.

Ginsberg, M.H., Loftus, J.C. & Plow, E.F. (1988) Cytoadhesins, integrins and platelets. *Thromb Haemost* **59**, 1–6.

Gonella, P.A. & Nachmias, V.T. (1981) Platelet activation and microfilament bundling. *J Cell Biol* **89**, 146–151.

Grant, J.A. & Scrutton, M.C. (1980) Interaction of selective α-adrenoceptor agonists and antagonists with human and rabbit blood platelets. *Br J Pharmac* **71**, 121–134.

Hack, N. & Crawford, N. (1984) Two-dimensional polyacrylamide-gel electrophoresis of the proteins and glycoproteins of purified human platelet surface and intracellular membranes. *Biochem J* **222**, 235–246.

Handa, M., Titani, K., Holland, L.Z., Roberts, J.R. & Ruggeri, Z.M. (1986) The von Willebrand factor-binding domain of platelet membrane glycoprotein Ib. Characterization by monoclonal antibodies and partial amino acid sequence analysis of proteolytic fragments. *J Biol Chem* **261**, 12579–12585.

Handley, D.A. & Chien, S. (1985) Ultrastructure studies of endothelial and platelet receptor binding of thrombin-colloidal gold probes. *Eur J Cell Biol* **39**, 391–398.

Harden, T.K. (1983) Agonist-induced desensitization of the β-adrenergic receptor-linked to adenylate cyclase. *Pharmacol Rev* **35**, 5–32.

Harfenist, E.J., Packham, M.A., Kinlough-Rathbone, R.L. & Mustard, J.F. (1981) Inhibitors of ADP-induced platelet aggregation prevent fibrinogen binding to rabbit platelets and cause rapid deaggration and dissociation of bound fibrinogen. *J Lab Clin Med* **97**, 680–688.

Harmon, J.T. & Jamieson, G.A. (1986) Activation of platelets by α-thrombin is a receptor-mediated event. *J Biol Chem* **261**, 15928–15933.

Harmon, J.T. & Jamieson, G.A. (1988) Platelet activation by thrombin in the absence of the high-affinity thrombin receptor. *Biochemistry* **27**, 2151–2157.

Hartig, P.R. (1989) Molecular biology of 5-HT receptors. *TIPS* **10**, 64–69.

Haslam, R.J. & Cusack, N.J. (1981) Blood platelet receptors for ADP and for adenosine. In Burnstock, G. (ed) *Receptors and Recognition*, vol **B12**, pp. 223–285. Chapman & Hall, London.

Haslam, R.J. & Rosson, G.M. (1972) Effect of vasopressin on human blood platelets. *J Physiol (Lond)* **219**, 36p–38p.

Haslam, R.J., Davidson, M.M.L. & Desjardins, J.V. (1978) Inhibition of adenylate cyclase by adenosine analogues in preparations of broken and intact human platelets. Evidence for the unidirectional control of platelet function by cyclic AMP. *Biochem J* **176**, 83–95.

Hawiger, J., Timmons, S., Kloczewiak, M., Strong, D.D. & Doolittle, R.F. (1982) Gamma and alpha chains of human fibrinogen possess sites reactive with human platelet receptors. *Proc Natl Acad Sci USA* **79**, 2068–2071.

Hemler, M.E., Huang, C. & Schwarz, L. (1987) The VLA protein family. Characterization of five distinct cell surface heterodimers each with a common 130 000 molecular weight β-subunit. *J Biol Chem* **262**, 3300–3309.

Hemler, M.E., Crouse, C., Takada, Y. & Sonnenberg, A. (1988) Multiple very late antigen (VLA) heterodimers on platelets. Evidence for distinct VLA-2, VLA-5 (fibronectin receptor) and VLA-6 structures. *J Biol Chem* **263**, 7660–7665.

Houdijk, W.P.M. & Sixma, J.J. (1985) Fibronectin in artery subendothelium is important for platelet adhesion. *Blood* **65**, 598–603.

Hsu, C.Y., Knapp, D.R. & Halushka, P.V. (1979) The effects of α-adrenergic agents on human platelet aggregation. *J Pharmacol Exp Ther* **208**, 366–370.

Huang, E.M. & Detwiler, T.C. (1987) Thrombin-induced phosphoinsitide hydrolysis in platelets: receptor occupancy and densensitization. *Biochem J* **242**, 11–18.

Hynes, R.O. (1986) Integrins: a family of cell surface receptors. *Cell* **48**, 549–554.

Ikuta, K., Takami, M., Kim, C.W., Honjo, T., Miyoshi, T., Tagaya, Y., Kawake, T. & Yodoi, J. (1987) Human lymphocyte Fc receptor for IgE: sequence homology of its cloned cDNA with animal lectins. *Proc Natl Acad Sci USA* **84**, 819–823.

Ill, C.R., Engvall, E. & Ruoslahti, E.J. (1984) Adhesion of platelets to laminin in the absence of activation. *J Cell Biol* **99**, 2140–2145.

Isenberg, W.M., McEver, R.P., Phillips, D.R., Shuman, M.A. & Bainton, D.F. (1987) The platelet fibringen receptor: an immunogold-surface replica study of agonist-induced ligand binding and receptor clustering. *J Cell Biol* **104**, 1655–1663.

Jakobs, K.H., Saur, W., & Schultz, G. (1978) Characterization of α and β-adrenergic receptors linked to human platelet adenylate cyclase. *N S Arch Pharmacol* **302**, 285–291.

Jamieson, G.A. & Okumura, T. (1978) Reduced thrombin binding and aggregation in Bernard–Soulier platelets. *J Clin Invest* **61**, 861–864.

Jennings, L.K. & Phillips, D.R. (1982) Purification of GpIIb and III from human platelet plasma membranes and characterization of a calcium dependent GpIIb–III complex. *J Biol Chem* **257**, 10458–10466.

Jones, R.L., Wilson, N.H., Armstrong, R.A. & Tymkewycz, P.M. (1987) Developments in the characterization of prostaglandin endoperoxide/thromboxane receptors. In Lagarde, M. (ed) *Biology of Icosanoids*, Colloque INSERM Vol **152**, 335–344. Inserm, Paris.

Joseph, M., Capron, A., Ameisen, J-C., Capron, M., Vorng, H., Pancre, V., Kusnierz, J-P. & Auriault, C. (1986) The receptor for IgE on blood platelets. *Eur J Immunol* **16**, 306–312.

Karas, S.P., Rosse, W.F. & Kurlander, R.J. (1982) Characterization of the IgG-Fc receptor on human platelets. *Blood* **60**, 1272–1282.

Karliner, J.S., Motulsky, H.J. & Insel, P.A. (1982) Apparent 'down-regulation' of human platelet α_2-adrenergic receptors is due to retained agonist. *Mol Pharmacol* **21**, 36–43.

Kaulen, H.D. & Gross, R. (1973) Metabolic properties of human platelet membranes. I. Characterization of platelet membranes prepared by sucrose and Ficoll density gradients. *Thromb Diath Haemorr* **30**, 199–214.

Kerry, R. & Scrutton, M.C. (1983) Platelet β-adrenoceptors. *Br J Pharmacol* **79**, 681–691.

Kerry, R., Scrutton, M.C. & Wallis, R.B. (1984) Mammalian platelet adrenoceptors. *Br J Pharmacol* **81**, 91–102.

Kim, B.K., Steiner, M. & Baldini, M.G. (1980) Serotonin binding sites of human blood platelets. *Anal Biochem* **106**, 92–98.

Kinoshita, T., Nachman, R.L. & Minick, R. (1979) Isolation of human platelet plasma membranes with polylysine beads. *J Cell Biol* **82**, 688–696.

Kloczewiak, M., Timmons, S., Lukas, T.J. & Hawiger, J. (1984) Platelet receptor recognition sites on human fibrinogen. Synthesis and structure-function relationship of peptides corresponding to the carboxy-terminal segment of the γ-chain. *Biochemistry* **23**, 1767–1774.

Kloprogge, E. & Akkerman, J.W.N. (1984) Binding kinetics of PAF-acether (1-0-alkyl-2-acetyl-sn-glycero-3-phosphocholine) to intact human platelets. *Biochem J* **223**, 901–909.

Knupp, C.L. & White, G.C. (1985) Effect of active site-modified thrombins on the hydrolysis of platelet-associated glycoprotein V by native thrombin. *Blood* **65**, 578–583.

Kobilka, B.K., Matsui, H., Kobilka, T.S., Yang-Feng, T.L., Francke, U., Caron, M.G., Lefkowitz, R.J. & Regan, J.W. (1987a) Cloning, sequencing and expression of the gene coding for the human platelet α-adrenergic receptor. *Science* **238**, 650–656.

Kobilka, B.K., Dixon, R.A.F., Frielle, T., Dohlman, H.G., Bolanowski, M.A., Sigal, I.S., Yang-Feng, T.L., Francke, U., Caron, M.G. & Lefkowitz, R.J. (1987b) cDNA for the human β_2-adrenergic receptor: a protein with multiple membrane-spanning domains and encoded by a gene whose chromosomal location is shared with that of the receptor for platelet-derived growth factor. *Proc Natl Acad Sci USA* **84**, 46–50.

Kobilka, B.K., Kobilka, T.S., Daniel, K., Regan, J.W., Caron, M.G. & Lefkowitz, R.J. (1988) Chimeric α_2-, β_2-adrenergic receptors: delineation of domains involved in effector coupling and ligand binding specificity. *Science* **240**, 1310–1316.

Koteliansky, V.E., Gneushev, G.N., Glukhova, M.A., Venyaminov, S.Y. & Muszbek, L. (1984) Identification and isolation of vinculin from platelets. *FEBS Lett* **165**, 26–30.

Kramer, R.M., Patton, G.M., Pritzker, C.R. & Deykin, D. (1984) Metabolism of platelet-activating factor in human platelets. *J Biol Chem* **259**, 13316–13320.

Kunicki, T.J., Nugent, D.J., Staats, S.J., Orchekowski, R.P., Wayner, E.A. & Carter, W.G. (1988) The human fibroblast class II extracellular matrix receptor mediates platelet adhesion to collagen and is identical to the platelet glycoprotein Ia–IIa complex. *J Biol Chem* **263**, 4516–4519.

Lagarde, M., Guichardant, M., Menashi, S. & Crawford, N. (1982) The phospholipid and fatty acid composition of human platelet surface and intracellular membranes isolated by high voltage free flow electrophoresis. *J Biol Chem* **257**, 3100–3104.

Lam, S.C-T., Plow, E.F., Smith, M.A., Andrieux, A., Ryckwaert, J.J., Marguerie, G.A. & Ginsberg, M.H. (1987) Evidence that arginyl-glycyl-aspartate peptides and fibrinogen gamma chain peptides share a common binding site on platelets. *J Biol Chem* **262**, 947–950.

Lambrecht, G. & Parnham, M.J. (1986) Kadsurenone distinguishes between different platelet activating factor receptor subtypes on macrophages and polymorphonuclear leucocytes. *Br J Pharmacol* **87**, 287–289.

Landon, F. & Olomucki, A. (1983) Isolation and physico-chemical properties of blood platelet α-actinin. *Biochim Biophys Acta* **742**, 129–134.

Landon, F., Huc, C., Thome, F., Oriol, C. & Olomucki, A. (1977) Human platelet actin. Evidence of β and γ forms and similarity of properties with sarcomeric actin. *Eur J Biochem* **81**, 571–577.

Langer, S.Z. & Raisman, R. (1983) Binding of [^{3}H]imipramine and [^{3}H]desimipramine as biochemical tools for studies in depression. *Neuropharmacology* **22**, 407–413.

Lawler, J.W. & Hines, R.O. (1986) The structure of human thrombospondin, an adhesive glycoprotein with multiple calcium binding sites and homologies with several different proteins. *J Cell Biol* **103**, 1635–1648.

Leung, L.L.K. (1984) Role of thrombospondin in platelet aggregation. *J Clin Invest*, **74**, 1764–1772.

Leysen, J.E., Awouters, F., Kennis, L., Laduron, P.M., Vandenberk, J. & Janssen, P.A.J. (1981) Receptor binding profile of R41468, a novel antagonist at 5-HT_2 receptors. *Life Sci* **28**, 1015–1022.

Lind, S.E., Yin, H.I. & Stossel, T.P. (1982) Human platelets contain gelsolin. A regulator of actin filament length. *J Clin Invest* **69**, 1384–1387.

Loftus, J.C. & Albrecht, R.M. (1984) Redistribution of the fibrinogen receptor of human platelets following surface activation. *J Biol Chem* **99**, 822–829.

Loftus, J.C., Plow, E.F., Frelinger, A.L., D'Souza, S.E., Dixon, D., Lacy, J., Sorge, J. & Ginsberg, M.H. (1987) Molecular cloning and chemical synthesis of a region of platelet glycoprotein IIb involved in adhesive function. *Proc Natl Acad Sci USA* **84**, 7114–7118.

Loftus, J.C., Plow, E.F., Jennings, L.K. & Ginsberg, M.H. (1988) Alternative proteolytic processing of platelet membrane glycoprotein IIb. *J Biol Chem* **263**, 11025–11028.

Lopez, J.A., Chung, D.W., Fujikawa, K., Hagen, F.S., Papayannopoulou, T. & Roth, G.J. (1987) Cloning of the α-chain of human platelet glycoprotein Ib: a transmembrane protein with homology to leucine-rich α_2-glycoprotein. *Proc Natl Acad Sci USA* **84**, 5615–5619.

MacFarlane, D.E., Srivastava, P.C. & Mills, D.C.B. (1983) 2-methylthioadenosine [β-^{32}P]diphosphate. An agonist and radioligand for the receptor that inhibits the accumulation of cyclic AMP in intact blood platelets. *J Clin Invest* **71**, 420–428.

Mais, D.E., Burch, R.M., Saussy, D.L., Kochel, P.J. & Halushka, P.V. (1985) Binding of a thromboxane A_2

prostaglandin H_2 receptor antagonist to washed human platelets. *J Pharmacol Exp Ther* **235**, 729–734.

Mais, D.E., DeHoll, D., Sightler, H. & Halushka, P.V. (1988) Different pharmacologic activities for [3-azapinane thromboxane A_2 analogs in platelets and blood vessels. *Eur J Pharmacol* **148**, 309–315.

Majerus, P.W., Tollefsen, D.M. & Shuman, M.A. (1976) The interaction of platelets with thrombin. In Gordon, J.L. (ed) *Platelets in Biology and Pathology*, pp. 241–260. Elsevier/North Holland, Amsterdam.

Marguerie, G.A., Plow, E.G. & Edgington, T.S. (1979) Human platelets possess an inducible and saturable receptor specific for fibrinogen. *J Biol Chem* **254**, 5357–5663.

Marguerie, G.A., Edgington, T.S. & Plow, E.F. (1980) Interaction of fibrinogen with its platelet receptor as part of a multistep reaction in ADP-induced platelet aggregation. *J Biol Chem* **255**, 154–161.

Markey, F., Persson, T. & Lindberg, U. (1981) Characterisation of platelet extracts before and after stimulation with respect to the possible role of profilactin as microfilament precursor. *Cell* **23**, 145–153.

Martin, B.M., Wasiewski, W.W., Fenton, J.W. & Detwiler, T.C. (1976) Equilibrium binding of thrombin to platelets. *Biochemistry* **15**, 4886–4893.

McBride, P.A., Mann, J.J., Polley, M.J., Wiley, A.J. & Sweeney, J.A. (1987) Assessment of binding indices and physiological responsiveness of the 5-HT_2 receptor on human platelets. *Life Sci* **40**, 1799–1809.

McGowan, E.B. & Detwiler, T.C. (1986) Modified platelet responses to thrombin. Evidence for two types of receptors or coupling mechanisms. *J Biol Chem* **261**, 739–746.

McGowan, E.B., Yeo, K.T. & Detwiler, T.C. (1983a) The action of calcium-dependent protease on platelet surface glycoproteins. *Arch Biochem Biophys* **227**, 287–301.

McGowan, E.B., Duig, A. & Detwiler, T.C. (1983b) Correlation of thrombin-induced glycoprotein V hydrolysis and platelet activation. *J Biol Chem* **258**, 11243–11248.

Menashi, S., Weintroub, H. & Crawford, N. (1981) Characterization of human platelet surface and intracellular membranes isolated by free flow electrophoresis. *J Biol Chem* **256**, 4095–4101.

Miles, L.A. & Plow, E.F. (1985) Binding and activation of plasminogen on the platelet surface. *J Biol Chem* **260**, 4303–4311.

Miles, L.A. & Plow, E.F. (1987) Receptor mediated binding of the fibrinolytic components, plasminogen and urokinase, to peripheral blood cells. *Thromb Haemost* **58**, 936–942.

Miles, L.A. & Plow, E.F. (1988) Plasminogen receptors: ubiquitous sites for cellular regulation of fibrinolysis. *Fibrinolysis* **2**, 61–71.

Miller, O.V. & Gorman, R.R. (1979) Evidence for distinct prostaglandin I_2 and D_2 receptors in human platelets. *J Pharm Exp Ther* **210**, 134–140.

Mills, D.C.B. & Smith, J.B. (1972) The control of platelet responsiveness by agents that influence cyclic AMP metabolism. *Ann NY Acad Sci* **201**, 391–399.

Moncada, S., Gryglewski, R.J., Bunting, S. & Vane, J.R. (1976) An enzyme isolated from arteries transforms prostaglandin endoperoxides to an unstable substance that inhibits platelet aggregation. *Nature* **263**, 663–665.

Morton, L.F., Fitzsimmons, C.M., Rauterberg, J. & Barnes, M.J. (1987) Platelet reactive sites in collagen. Collagens I and III possess different aggregatory sites. *Biochem J* **248**, 483–487.

Motulsky, H.J. & Insel, P.A. (1982a) [^{3}H]-Dihydroergocryptine binding to α-adrenergic receptors of human platelets: a reassessment using the selective radioligands [^{3}H]prazosin, [^{3}H]yohimbine and [^{3}H]rauwolscine. *Biochem Pharmacol* **31**, 2591–2597.

Motulsky, H.J. & Insel, P.A. (1982b) Adrenergic receptors in man. Direct identification, physiologic regulation, and clinical alteration. *New Engl J Med* **307**, 18–29.

Motulsky, H.J., Shattil, S.J., Ferry, N., Rozansky, D. & Insel, P.A. (1986) Desensitization of epinephrine-initiated platelet aggregation does not alter binding to the α-adrenergic receptor or receptor coupling to adenylate cyclase. *Mol Pharmacol* **29**, 1–6.

Murray, R. & Fitzgerald, G.A. (1989) Regulation of thromboxane receptor activation in human platelets. *Proc Natl Acad Sci USA* **86**, 124–128.

Mustard, J.F., Kinlough-Rathbone, R.L., Packham, M.A., Perry, D.W., Harfenist, E.J. & Pai, K.R. (1979) Comparison of fibrinogen association with normal and thrombasthenic platelets on exposure to ADP or chymotrypsin. *Blood* **545**, 987–993.

Nachman, R.L. & Leung, L.L.K. (1982) Complex formation of platelet membrane glycoprotein IIb and IIIa with fibrinogen. *J Clin Invest* **69**, 263–269.

Nachman, R.L., Silverstein, R.L. & Asch, A.S. (1987) Thrombospondin: cell biology of an adhesive glycoprotein. In Verstraete, M., Vermylen, J., Lijnen, R. & Arnout, J. (eds) *Thrombosis and Haemostasis*, pp. 81–91, Leuven University Press, Leuven.

Nachmias, V.T., Sullender, J.S. & Fallon, J.R. (1979) Effects of local anaesthetics on human platelets: filopodial suppression and endogenous proteolysis. *Blood* **53**, 63–72.

Narumiya, S., Okuma, M. & Ushikubi, F. (1985) Binding of radioiodinated 13-azapinane thromboxane antagonist to platelets: correlation with antiaggregatory activity in different species. *Br J Pharmacol* **88**, 323–331.

Nieuwenhuis, H.K., Akkerman, J.W.N., Houdijk, W.P.M. & Sixma, J.J. (1985) Human blood platelets showing no response to collagen fail to express surface glycoprotein Ia. *Nature* **318**, 470–472.

Niewiarowski, S., Budzynski, A.Z. & Lipinske, B. (1977) Significance of the intact polypeptide chains of human fibrinogen in ADP-induced platelet aggregation. *Blood* **49**, 635–644.

Niiya, K., Hodson, E., Bader, R., Byers-Ward, V., Kozid, J.A., Plow, E.F. & Ruggeri, Z.M. (1987) Increased surface expression of the membrane glycoprotein IIb.IIIa complex induced by platelet activation. Relationship to the binding of fibrinogen and platelet aggregation. *Blood* **70**, 475–483.

Nurden, A.T. (1987) Platelet membrane glycoproteins and their clinical aspects. In Verstraete, M., Vermylen, J., Lijnen, H.R. & Arnout, J. (eds) *Thrombosis and Haemostasis*, pp. 93–125. Leuven University Press, Leuven.

Nurden, A.T. & Caen, J.P. (1978) Membrane glycoproteins and human platelet function. *Br J Haematol* **38**, 155–160.

Okita, J.R., Pidard, D., Newman, P.J., Montgomery, R.R. & Kunicki, T.J. (1985) On the association of glycoprotein Ib and actin-binding protein in human platelets. *J Cell Biol* **100**, 317–321.

Painter, R.G. & Ginsberg, M.H. (1984) Centripetal myosin redistribution in thrombin stimulated platelets, relationship to platelet factor 4 secretion. *Exp Cell Res* **155**, 198–212.

Painter, R.G., Prodouz, K.N. & Gaarde, W. (1985) Isolation of a subpopulation of glycoprotein IIb–III from platelet membranes that is bound to membrane actin. *J Cell Biol* **100**, 652–657.

Parbtani, A., Clark, W.F., Caveney, A. & Reid, B. (1987) Binding of aggregated immunoglobulins to the human platelet Fc receptors: a mechanism of platelet to platelet bridging. *Thromb Haemost* **58**, 966–970.

Parise, L.V., Helgerson, S.L., Steiner, B., Nannizzi, L. & Phillips, D.R. (1987) Synthetic peptides derived from fibrinogen and fibronectin change the conformation of purified glycoprotein IIb–IIIa. *J Biol Chem* **262**, 12597–12602.

Peerschke, E.I.B. (1982) Evidence for interaction between fibrinogen receptors. *Blood* **60**, 973–977.

Peerschke, E.I.B. (1985) The platelet fibrinogen receptor. *Semin Haematol* **22**, 241–259.

Peerschke, E.I.B. & Zucker, M.B. (1980) Relationship of ADP-induced fibrinogen binding to platelet shape change and aggregation elucidated by use of colchicine and cytochalasin B. *Thromb Haemost* **43**, 58–60.

Peerschke, E.I.B., Zucker, M.B., Grant, R.A., Egan, J.J. & Johnson, M.M. (1980) Correlation between fibrinogen binding to human platelets and platelet aggregability. *Blood* **55**, 841–847.

Peters, J.R. & Grahame-Smith, D.G. (1980) Human platelet 5-HT receptors: characterization and functional association. *Eur J Biochem* **68**, 243–256.

Phillips, D.R. & Agin, P.P. (1977) Platelet plasma membrane glycoproteins. Evidence for the presence of non equivalent disulphide bonds using non-reduced–reduced two-dimensional gel electrophoresis. *J Biol Chem* **252**, 2121–2126.

Phillips, D.R. & Baughan, A.K. (1983) Fibrinogen binding to human platelet plasma membranes. Identification of two steps requiring divalent cations. *J Biol Chem* **258**, 10240–10246.

Phillips, D.R., Jenkins, C.S.P., Luscher, E.F. & Larrieu, M.J. (1975) Molecular differences of exposed surface proteins on thrombasthenic platelet plasma membranes. *Nature* **257**, 599–600.

Phillips, D.R., Charo, I.F., Parise, L.V. & Fitzgerald, L.A. (1988) The platelet membrane glycoprotein IIb–IIIa complex. *Blood* **71**, 831–843.

Pho, D.B., Desbruyeres, E., Der Terrossian, E. & Olomucki, A. (1986) Cytoskeletons of ADP and thrombin-stimulated blood platelets. Presence of a caldesmon-like protein, α-actinin and gelsolin at different steps of the stimulation. *FEBS Lett* **202**, 117–121.

Pischel, K.D., Hemler, M.E., Huang, C., Bluestein, H.G. & Woods, V.L. (1987a) Use of the monoclonal antibody 12F1 to characterize the differentiation antigen VLA-2. *J Immunol* **138**, 226–233.

Pischel, K.D., Bluestein, H.G. & Woods, V.L. (1987b) Platelet glycoprotein Ia, Ic and IIa are physiochemically indistinguishable from the very late activation antigens adhesion-related proteins of lymphocytes and other cell types. *J Clin Invest* **81**, 505–513.

Plow, E.F., Srouji, A.H., Meyer, D., Marguerie, G. & Ginsberg, M.H. (1984) Evidence that three adhesive proteins interact with a common recognition site on activated platelets. *J Biol Chem* **259**, 5388–5391.

Plow, E.F., Marguerie, G.A. & Ginsberg, M.H. (1985a) Fibronectin binding to thrombin-stimulated platelets: evidence for fibrin(ogen) independent and dependent pathways. *Blood* **66**, 26–32.

Plow, E.F., McEver, R.P., Coller, B.S., Woods, V.L., Marguerie, G.A. & Ginsberg, M.H. (1985b) Related binding mechanisms for fibrinogen, fibronectin, von Willebrand factor, and thrombospondin on thrombin-stimulated human platelets. *Blood* **66**, 724–727.

Plow, E.F., Freaney, D.E., Plescia, J. & Miles, L.A. (1986) The plasminogen system and cell surfaces: evidence for plasminogen and urokinase receptors on the same cell type. *J Cell Biol* **103**, 2411–2420.

Plow, E.F., Marguerie, G.A. & Ginsberg, M.H. (1987a) Fibrinogen, fibrinogen receptors, and the peptides that inhibit these interactions. *Biochem Pharmacol* **36**, 4035–4040.

Plow, E.F., Pierschbacher, M.D., Ruoslahti, E., Marguerie, G.A. & Ginsberg, M.H. (1987b) Arginyl–Glycyl–Aspartic acid sequences and fibrinogen binding to platelets. *Blood* **70**, 110–115.

Pollard, T.D., Fujiwara, K., Handin, R. & Weiss, G. (1977) Contractile proteins in platelet activation and contraction. *Ann NY Acad Sci* **283**, 218–236.

Pritchett, D.B., Bach, A.W.J., Wozny, M., Taleb, O., Dal Toso, R., Shih, J.C. & Seeburg P.H. (1988) Structure and functional expression of cloned rat serotonin 5-HT_2 receptor. *EMBO J* **7**, 4135–4140.

Pytela, R., Pierschbacher, M.D., Plow, E.F. & Ruoslahti, E. (1985) Identification and isolation of a 140 kd cell surface glycoprotein with properties expected of a fibronectin receptor. *Cell* **40**, 191–198.

Pytela, R., Pierschbacher, M.D., Ginsberg, M.H., Plow, E.F. & Ruoslahti, E. (1986) Platelet membrane glycoprotein IIb–IIIa: member of a family of Arg–Gly–Asp–specific adhesion receptors. *Science* **231**, 1559–1562.

Regan, J.W., Kobilka, T.S., Yang-Feng, T.L., Caron, M.G., Lefkowitz, R.J. & Kobilka, B.K. (1988) Cloning and expression of a human kidney cDNA for an α_2-adrenergic receptor subtype. *Proc Natl Acad Sci USA* **85**, 6301–6305.

Robson, K.J.H., Hall, J.R.S., Jennings, M.W., Harris, T.J.R., Marsh, K., Newbold, C.I., Tate, V.E. & Weatherall, D.J. (1988) A highly conserved amino-acid sequence in thrombospondin, properdin, and in proteins from sporozoites and blood stages of a human malaria parasite. *Nature* **335**, 79–82.

Rock, C.O. & Jackowski, S. (1987) Thrombin and nucleotide-activated phosphatidylinositol 4,5-bisphosphate phospholipase C in human platelet membranes. *J Biol Chem* **262**, 5492–5498.

Rosenberg, S., Stracher, A. & Lucas, R.C. (1981a) Isolation and characterization of actin and actin-binding protein from human platelets. *J Cell Biol* **91**, 201–211.

Rosenberg, S., Stracher, A. & Burridge, K. (1981b) Isolation and characterization of a calcium-sensitive α-actinin-like protein from human platelet cytoskeletons. *J Biol Chem* **256**, 12986–12991.

Rosenfeld, S.J., Looney, R.J., Leddy, J.P., Phipps, D.C., Abraham, G.N. & Anderson, C.L. (1985) Human platelet Fc receptor for Immunoglobulin G. *J Clin Invest* **76**, 2317–2322.

Ruda, E.M., Petty, A., Scrutton, M.C., Tuffin, D.P. & Manley, P.W. (1988) Identification of small peptide analogues having agonist and antagonist activity at the platelet thrombin receptor. *Biochem Pharmacol* **37**, 2417–2426.

Ruda, E.M., Scrutton, M.C., Manley, P.W. & Tuffin, D.P. (1990) Thrombin receptor antagonists: structure-activity relationships for the platelet thrombin receptor and effects on prostacyclin synthesis by human umbilical vein endothelial cells. *Biochem Pharmacol* **39**, 373–381.

Ruggeri, Z.M., De Marco, L., Gatti, L., Bader, R. & Montgomery, R.R. (1983) Platelets have more than one binding site for von Willebrand factor. *J Clin Invest* **72**, 1–12.

Ruggeri, Z.M., Houghton, R.A., Russell, S.R. & Zimmerman, T.S. (1986) Inhibition of platelet function with synthetic peptides designed to be high-affinity antagonists of fibrinogen binding to platelets. *Proc Natl Acad Sci USA* **83**, 5708–5712.

Sakariassen, K.S., Bolhuis, P.A. & Sixma, J.J. (1979) Human blood platelet adhesion to artery subendothelium is mediated by factor VIII-von Willebrand factor bound to the subendothelium. *Nature* **279**, 636–638.

Sakariassen, K.S., Nievelstein, P.F.E.M., Coller, B.S. & Sixma, J.J. (1986) The role of platelet membrane glycoproteins Ib and IIb–IIIa in platelet adherence to human artery subendothelium. *Br J Haematol* **63**, 681–691.

Santoro, S.A. (1986) Identification of a 160 000 dalton platelet membrane protein that mediates the initial divalent cation-dependent adhesion of platelets to collagen. *Cell* **46**, 913–920.

Santoro, S.A. & Lawing, W.J. (1987) Competition for related but non-identical binding sites on the glycoprotein IIb.IIIa complex by peptides derived from platelet adhesive proteins. *Cell* **48**, 867–873.

Santoro, S.A., Rajpara, S.M., Staatz, W.D. & Woods, V.L. (1988) Isolation and characterization of a platelet surface collagen binding complex related to VLA-2. *Biochem Biophys Res Commun* **153**, 217–223.

Schafer, A.I., Cooper, D., O'Hara, O. & Handin, R.I. (1979) Identification of platelet receptors for prostaglandins I_2 and D_2. *J Biol Chem* **254**, 2914–2917.

Schollmeyer, J.V., Rao, G.H.R. & White, J.G. (1978) An actin binding protein in human platelets: interactions with α-actinin on gelation of actin and the influence of cytochalasin B. *Am J Pathol* **93**, 433–441.

Scrutton, M.C., Thompson, N.T. & Hallam, T.J. (1986) Vasopressin. In Holmsen H. (ed) *Platelet Function and Metabolism*, Vol. II, pp. 69–82 CRC Press, Boca Raton.

Shadle, P.J. & Barondes, S.H. (1982) Adhesion of human platelets to immobilized trimeric collagen. *J Cell Biol* **95**, 361–365.

Shattil, S.J. & Cooper, R.A. (1976) Membrane microviscosity and human platelet function. *Biochemistry* **15**, 4832–4837.

Shattil, S.J. & Cooper, R.A. (1978) Role of membrane lipid composition, organization, and fluidity in human platelet function. *Prog Haemost Thromb* **4**, 59–86.

Shattil, S.J., Hoxie, J.A., Cunningham, M. & Brass, L.F. (1985) Changes in the platelet membrane glycoprotein IIb–IIIa complex during platelet activation. *J Biol Chem* **260**, 11107–11114.

Shirasawa, K. & Chandler, A.B. (1969) Fine structure of the bond between platelets in thrombi and platelet aggregates induced by adenosine diphosphate. *Am J Pathol* **57**, 127–154.

Shulman, S. & Karpatkin, S. (1980) Crossed immunoelectrophoresis of human platelet membranes. Diminution of major antigens in Glanzmann's thrombasthenia and Bernard–Soulier syndrome. *J Biol Chem* **255**, 4320–4327.

Sibley, D.R. & Lefkowitz, R.J. (1985) Molecular mechanisms of receptor desensitization using the β-adrenergic receptor-coupled adenylate cyclase system as a model. *Nature* **317**, 124–129.

Siegl, A.M., Smith, J.B. & Silver, M.J. (1979a) Specific binding sites for prostaglandin D_2 on human platelets. *Biochem Biophys Res Commun* **90**, 291–296.

Siegl, A.M., Smith, J.B., Silver, M.J., Nicolaou, K.C.

& Ahern, D. (1979b) Selective binding sites for [^{3}H]prostacyclin on platelets. *J Clin Invest* **63**, 215–220.

Silverstein, R.L. & Nachman, R.L. (1987) Thrombospondin binds to monocytes-macrophages and mediates platelet-monocyte adhesion. *J Clin Invest* **79**, 867–874.

Silverstein, R.L., Leung, L.L.K., Harpel, P.C. & Nachman, R.L. (1984) Complex formation of platelet thrombospondin with plasminogen. *J Clin Invest* **74**, 1625–1633.

Silverstein, R.L., Nachman, R.L., Leung, L.L.K. & Harpel, P.C. (1985) Activation of immobilized plasminogen by tissue plasminogen activator: multimolecular complex formation. *J Biol Chem* **260**, 10346–10352.

Sixma, J.J. & Molenaar, I. (1966) Microtubules and microfibrils in human platelets. *Thromb Diath Haemorr* **16**, 153–162.

Smith, J.B., Silver, M.J., Ingerman, C.M. & Kocsis, J.J. (1974) Prostaglandin D_2 inhibits the aggregation of human platelets. *Thromb Res* **5**, 291–299.

Solum, N.O. & Olsen, T.M. (1984) Glycoprotein Ib in the Triton-insoluble (cytoskeletal) fraction of blood platelets. *Biochim Biophys Acta* **799**, 209–220.

Sonnenberg, A., Janssen, H., Hogervorst, F., Calafat, J. & Hilgers, J. (1987) A complex of platelet glycoproteins Ic and IIa identified by a rat monoclonal antibody. *J Biol Chem* **262**, 10376–10383.

Sonnenberg, A., Modderman, P.W. & Hilgers, J. (1988) Laminin receptor on platelets is the integrin VLA-6. *Nature* **336**, 487–489.

Stel, H.V., Sakariassen, K.S., de Groog, P.G., van Mourik, J.A. & Sixma, J.J. (1985) Von Willebrand factor in the vessel wall mediates platelet adherence. *Blood* **65**, 85–92.

Stewart, A.G. & Dusting, G.J. (1988) Characterization of receptors for platelet-activating factor on platelets, polymorphonuclear leukocytes and macrophages. *Br J Pharmacol* **94**, 1225–1233.

Strader, C.D., Sigal, I.S., Blake, A.D., Cheung, A.H., Register, R.B., Rands, E., Zemick, B.A., Candelore, M.R. & Dixon, R.A.F. (1987) The carboxyl terminus of the hamster β-adrenergic receptor expressed in mouse L cells is not required for receptor sequestration. *Cell* **49**, 855–863.

Strasser, R.H., Benovic, J.L., Caron, M.G. & Lefkowitz, R.J. (1986) β-agonist and prostaglandin E_1-induced translocation of the β-adrenergic receptor kinase: evidence that the kinase may act on multiple adenylate cyclase coupled recetors. *Proc Natl Acad Sci USA* **83**, 6362–6366.

Takada, Y., Huang, C. & Hemler, M.E. (1987) Fibronectin receptor structures in the VLA family of heterodimers. *Nature* **326**, 607–609.

Takamatsu, J., Horne, M.K. & Granick, H.R. (1986) Identification of the thrombin receptor on human platelets by chemical crosslinking. *J Clin Invest* **77**, 362–368.

Tam, S.W., Fenton, J.W. & Detwiler, T.C. (1980) Platelet thrombin receptor: binding of α-thrombin is coupled to signal generation by a chymotrypsin sensitive mechanism. *J Biol Chem* **255**, 6626–6632.

Tao, R.V.P., Sweeley, C.C. & Jamieson, G.A. (1973) Sphingolipid composition of human platelets. *J Lipid Res* **14**, 16–25.

Titani, K., Takio, K., Handa, M. & Ruggeri, Z.M. (1987) Amino acid sequence of the von Willebrand factor-binding domain of platelet membrane glycoprotein Ib. *Proc Natl Acad Sci USA* **84**, 5610–5614.

Tollefsen, D.M., Feagler, J.R. & Majerus, P.W. (1974) The binding of thrombin to the surface of human platelets. *J Biol Chem* **249**, 2646–2651.

Touqui, L., Jacquemin, C., Dumarey, C. & Vargaftig, B.B. (1985) 1-O-alkyl-2-acyl-sn-glycero-3-phosphorylcholine is the precursor of plateletactivating factor in stimulated rabbit platelets. Evidence for an alkylacetyl-glycero-phosphorylcholine cycle. *Biochim Biophys Acta* **833**, 111–118.

Tsuji, T. & Osawa, T. (1986) Purification and chemical characterization of platelet membrane glycoprotein IV. *J Biochem (Tokyo)* **100**, 1077–1085.

Tsuji, T., Tsunehisa, S., Watanabe, Y., Yamamoto, K., Tohyama, H. & Osawa, T. (1983) The carbohydrate structure of human platelet glycocalicin: the structure of the major Ser/Thr-linked chain. *J Biol Chem* **258**, 6335–6339.

Tuffin, D.P. & Wade, P.J. (1987) Interaction of PAF-acether with the human platelet: receptor binding and pharmacology. In Reid, E., Cook, G.M.W. & Luzio, J.P. (eds) *Cells, Membranes and Disease*, pp. 171–183. Plenum, New York.

Tuffin, D.P., Davey, P., Dyer, R.L., Lunt, D.O. & Wade, P.J. (1985) Specific binding of [^{3}H]1-O-octadecyl PAF-acether to washed human platelets. In Westwick, J., Scully, M.F., MacIntyre, D.E. & Kakkar, V.V. (eds) *Mechanisms of Stimulus–Response Coupling in Platelets*, pp. 83–96. Plenum Press, New York.

Turitto, V.T., Weis, H.J., Zimmerman, T.S. & Sussman, I. (1985) Factor VIII — von Willebrand factor in subendothelium mediates platelet adhesion. *Blood* **65**, 823–830.

Valone, F.H. (1984) Isolation of a platelet membrane protein which binds the platelet-activating factor. *Immunology* **52**, 169–174.

Wade, P.J., Lunt, D.O., Lad, N., Tuffin, D.P. & McCullagh, K.G. (1986) Effect of calcium and calcium antagonists on [^{3}H]PAF-acether binding to washed human platelets. *Thromb Res* **41**, 251–262.

Wayne, E.A. & Carter, W.G. (1987) Identification of multiple cell adhesion receptors for collagen and fibronectin in human fibrosarcoma cells. *J Cell Biol* **105**, 1873–1884.

Wencel-Drake, J.D., Plow, E.F., Kunicki, T.J., Woods, V.L., Keller, D.M. & Ginsberg, M.H. (1986) Localization of internal pools of membrane glycoproteins involved in platelet adhesive responses. *Am J Pathol* **124**, 324–334.

Wheeler, M.E., Gerrard, J.M. & Carroll, R.C. (1985) Reciprocal transmembranous receptor-cytoskeleton interactions in concanavalin A activated platelets. *J Cell Biol* **101**, 993–1000.

White, J.G. (1974) Electron microscopic studies of platelet secretion in the electron microscope. *Prog Haemost Thromb* **2**, 49–98.

White, J.G. (1984) Arrangements of actin filaments in the cytoskeleton of human platelets. *Am J Pathol* **117**, 207–217.

White, J.G. (1987a) Platelet ultrastructure. In Bloom, A.L. & Thomas, D.P. (eds) *Haemostasis and Thrombosis*, 2nd edn, pp. 20–46. Churchill Livingstone, U.K.

White, J.G. (1987b) Views of the platelet cytoskeleton at rest and at work. *Ann NY Acad Sci* **509**, 156–176.

White, J.G. & Rao, G.H.R. (1983) Influence of a microtubule stabilizing agent on platelet structural physiology. *Am J Path* **112**, 207–217.

White, J.G. & Sauk, J.J. (1984) Microtubule coils in spread blood platelets. *Blood* **64**, 470–478.

White, J.G., Burris, S.M., Hasegawa, D. & Johnson, M. (1984) Micropipette aspiration of human blood platelets: a defect in Bernard–Souliere syndrome. *Blood* **63**, 1249–1252.

Wight, T.N., Raugi, G.J., Mumby, S.M. & Bornstein, P. (1985) Light microscopic immunolocation of thrombospondin in human tissues. *J Histochem Cytochem* **33**, 291–302.

Wolff, R., Plow, E.F. & Ginsberg, M.H. (1986) Interaction of thrombospondin with resting and stimulated human platelets. *J Biol Chem* **261**, 6840–6846.

Woods, V.L., Wolff, L.E. & Keller, D.M. (1986) Resting platelets contain a substantial centrally located pool of glycoprotein IIB–IIIa complex which may be accessible to some but not other extracellular proteins. *J Biol Chem* **261**, 15242–15251.

Workman, E.F., White, G.C. & Lundlad, R.L. (1977) Structure function relationship in the interaction of α-thrombin with platelets. *J Biol Chem* **252**, 7118–7123.

Wyler, B., Bienz, D., Clemetson, K.J. & Luscher, E.F. (1986) Glycoprotein Ib is the only phosphorylated major membrane glycoprotein in human platelets. *Biochem J* **234**, 373–379.

Yu, G-H., Holers, M., Seya, T., Ballard, L. & Atkinson, J.P. (1986) Identification of a third component of complement-binding glycoprotein of human platelets. *J Clin Invest* **78**, 494–501.

Zierler, K. (1989) Misuse of nonlinear Scatchard Plots. *TIBS* **14**, 314–317.

3: The Biochemical Basis for the Regulation of Platelet Responsiveness

Michael C. Scrutton and Christopher M. Athayde

Introduction

Blood platelets play a central role in the maintenance of vascular integrity. They are involved in initiating haemostatic plug formation at a site of vascular injury by promoting coagulation and subsequent wound healing. Activation of platelets at such sites results from their interaction with coagulation factors (e.g. thrombin), hormones (e.g. vasopressin), autocoids (e.g. adenosine diphosphate (ADP), thromboxane A_2) or non-platelet surfaces (e.g. collagen) (adhesion).

A number of responses to stimulation are required if the platelet is to fulfil its haemostatic role. The nature of these responses, and the order in which they occur, is dependent on the nature of the stimulus. For example, adhesion to newly exposed collagen fibrils in a damaged area of a blood vessel causes spreading of the platelets on this surface followed by thromboxane A_2 synthesis, secretion and phosphatidylserine exposure. Aggregation of other platelets on the adherent monolayer then occurs as a consequence of their stimulation by the released autocoids. The increase in the phosphatidylserine content of the outer leaflet of the plasma membrane enhances the activation of Factor X and the conversion of prothrombin to thrombin, and thus promotes fibrin deposition in the damaged area.

Stimulation by a soluble agonist such as thrombin typically causes shape change in which platelets are rapidly converted from the discoid morphology of the quiescent cell to a sphere possessing multiple pseudopodia. This response is associated with a general rearrangement of the cytoskeleton and is accompanied by centralization of the secretory granules tightly encircled by a microtubular ring which had previously been located just below the plasma membrane (Carrol *et al.* 1982). Shape change induced by soluble agonists is generally followed by aggregation and secretion but phosphatidylserine exposure is not increased. The aggregation response can often be resolved into two phases — primary and secondary aggregation. The primary response involves the formation of a relatively unstable aggregate and is associated with the appearance of fibrinogen receptors on the platelet surface since fibrinogen, as well as Ca^{2+}, is necessary to obtain platelet–platelet interaction (Fujimura & Phillips, 1983; Phillips & Baughan, 1983). Without further stimulation platelets will dissociate from this loose aggregate thus producing a reversible response. Secondary, or irreversible, aggregation occurs as a consequence of further stimulation, or exposure to a more potent initial stimulus, and involves consolidation of the aggregate associated with secretion. The contents of the amine and protein storage granules contribute to aggregate consolidation by providing, respectively, autocoids (ADP, 5-hydroxytryptamine 5-HT), which recruit further platelets, and proteins (fibrinogen, thrombospondin) which enhance aggregate stability (Nachmann *et al.* 1987). Other proteins released as a consequence of protein storage granule secretion promote wound-healing (platelet-derived growth factor) and leukocyte chemotaxis. Under some conditions lysosomal secretion can also occur but the physiological role (if any) of lysosomal enzyme release in haemostasis is unclear. For some agonists (ADP, adrenaline) at all concentrations and at suboptimal concentrations of others (collagen, platelet activating factor (PAF) vasopressin), secretion and secondary aggregation are dependent on arachidonate mobilization from membrane phospholipids and conversion of this fatty acid to thromboxane A_2 via the cyclooxygenase pathway. Receptors for this cyclooxygenase metabolite, as well as for other prostaglandins which are produced in much smaller quantities, are present on the platelet plasma membrane (Crawford & Scrutton, 1987). Arachidonate is also metabolized in platelets via the 12-lipoxygenase pathway but the physiological importance of lipoxygenase pathway products is much less clear. They may have a role as mediators of chemotaxis (Lagarde, 1987).

In the platelet as in other cells responses to changes in the environment are obtained by sensing these changes using plasma membrane receptors. The occupancy of such receptors by suitable agonists is transduced into appropriate responses via elaborate and interacting intracellular signalling (or signal transduction) mechanisms. Both the nature of the mechanisms present in a given cell and the way in which they interact differ widely. In the platelet it is accepted that most, if not all, conventional excitatory agonists cause cellular activation by increasing cytosolic Ca^{2+} and plasma membrane 1,2-diacylglycerol concentrations. Such activation is opposed by increases in intracellular cyclic adenosine monophosphate (cAMP) and cyclic guanosine monophosphate (cGMP) concentrations. These latter responses result, respectively, from occupancy of plasma membrane receptors for inhibitory agonists which are linked to adenylyl cyclase and from activation of the cytosolic guanylyl cyclase. In the terminology proposed by Rasmussen (1981) the platelet is therefore an example of a cell in which there is an antagonistic relationship between Ca^{2+} and cAMP (or cGMP) as the intracellular second messengers.

We will outline briefly the nature of these signal transduction mechanisms and the manner in which they may interact in a cell such as the platelet. We will then consider in more detail the nature of platelet responses and the way in which these responses are mediated by particular elements of the signal transduction pathways. Unless specifically stated otherwise the discussion relates to human platelets on which most of the studies have been performed. Although platelets obtained from other mammals possess similar signal transduction pathways some differences of detail have been described. These differences are, however, much less marked than the spectrum of excitatory and inhibitory agonists to which this cell responds in different mammalian species (Dodds, 1978).

A number of recent reviews have covered this area including those by Haslam (1987) and Siess (1989).

Signal transduction pathways and their interactions

Ca^{2+}

Cytosolic [Ca^{2+}] in the resting platelet is estimated as 0.05–0.1 μM using the fluorescent probes Fura2 or Quin2. Most excitatory agonists induce an increase in cytosolic [Ca^{2+}] from this resting level as measured using these probes (Table 3.1), although the approximate extent of the observed increase ranges from two-fold for 5-HT to 20-fold for thrombin (MacIntyre *et al.* 1985c). In the absence of extracellular Ca^{2+}, cytosolic [Ca^{2+}] returns to its resting level within 1–2 minutes after addition of agonist (Pollock *et al.* 1986). In the presence of millimolar extracellular Ca^{2+} the magnitude of the initial increase in cytosolic [Ca^{2+}] is not markedly enhanced but the time course of the increase is prolonged due to the opening of plasma membrane divalent cation channels (Hallam & Rink, 1985b). The extent to which the increase in cytosolic [Ca^{2+}] is prolonged varies with the agonist used. It is particularly marked on stimulation by thrombin when cytosolic [Ca^{2+}] remains elevated for a considerable time after addition of this agonist (Rink *et al.* 1982).

When Fura2 or Quin2 are used as the probe, neither collagen nor adrenaline cause a detectable increase in cytosolic [Ca^{2+}] provided that secretion and thromboxane A_2 synthesis are prevented (Table 3.1) (Thompson & Scrutton, 1985 Pollock *et al.* 1986). Contrasting results are obtained when intracelluar [Ca^{2+}] is measured using the chemiluminescent photoprotein aequorin. In this latter system, resting platelet [Ca^{2+}] is estimated as 0.3 μM and ten to 30-fold increases in this parameter are detected as a result of stimulation by all excitatory agonists tested thus far, including collagen and adrenaline (Table 3.1). Such increases in intracellular [Ca^{2+}] are also observed on the addition of activators of protein kinase C such as 12-O-tetradecanoylphorbol-13-acetate (TPA) and 1-oleoyl-2-acetyl glycerol (OAG) (Ware *et al.* 1985; Ware *et al.* 1986; Ware *et al.* 1988). The reason for the difference in the results obtained when the fluorescent probes and the photoprotein are used to measure intracellular [Ca^{2+}] is still unclear. The explanation may reside either in the procedures required to introduce the photoprotein into the cytosol or in properties inherent to the probe itself. Factors which may be important are discussed below.

1 Loading procedures — Quin2 and Fura2 are loaded into cells as their membrane-permeant acetoxymethyl esters followed by hydrolysis by cytosolic esterases to

Table 3.1 Responses and effects on signal transduction pathways induced by different excitatory agonists and other agents
(a) Responses

Excitatory agonist (agent)	Shape change	Aggregation	Thromboxane A_2 synthesis	Secretion from: Amine storage granule	Protein storage granule	Lysosome	Phosphatidyl serine exposure
Collagen	+(?)	+	+	+	+	+	+
Thrombin	+	+	+	+	+	+	–
PAF	+	+	+	+	+	±	–
Vasopressin	+	+	+	+	+	±	–
Thromboxane A_2	+	+	+	+	+	–	–
ADP	+	+	±	–	–	–	–
5-HT	+	+	±(?)	–†	–†	–	–
Adrenaline	–	±*	±*	–	–	–	–
A23187/ Ionomycin	+	+	+	+	+	+(?)	+

(b) Signal transduction mechanisms

Excitatory agonist (agent)	Increase in intracellular $[Ca^{2+}]$ detected by: Fura2	Aequorin	Increase in [1,2-diacyl glycerol]‡	Increase in inositol $trisPO_4$	Decrease in elevated [cAMP]	Increase in [cGMP]**
Collagen	−	+	+	+	?	+
Thrombin	+	+	+	+	+(high conc.)	+
PAF	+	+	+	+	−	+
Vasopressin	+	?	+	+	−	+
Thromboxane A_2	+	+	+	+	−	+
ADP	+	+	±	±(?)	+	+
5-HT	+	?	±	?	+	+
Adrenaline	−	+	−	−	?	+
A23187/	+	+	−	−	+	+
Ionomycin					?	

The symbols represent: (+) moderate/strong response; (−) no response, (±) weak response; (?) uncertain.

* Marked variability is observed in the extent of the response in different humans. Adrenaline does not cause these responses in platelets obtained from subprimate mammals.

† Except on an inconsistent basis in a minority of humans. It is not clear whether such secretion is directly dependent on occupancy of the $5\text{-}HT_2$ receptor or is a secondary consequence of thromboxane A_2 synthesis.

‡ Usually measured as enhanced incorporation of $[^{32}P]$ into phosphatidate in platelets prelabelled with $[^{32}P]^{\dagger}$ phosphate.

§ In some cases the increase has been shown to occur in inositol-1,4,5-trisphosphate.

△ Most agonists possess the capacity to inhibit adenylate cyclase in membrane preparations but this capacity is less widely expressed in the intact platelet.

** The increases in cGMP are not a direct consequence of receptor occupancy but result from platelet−platelet (aggregation) or platelet-matrix (adhesion) contact (Edgecombe & Scrutton, 1987).

Collagen induces aggregation as a secondary consequence of its ability to induce secretion and thromboxane A_2 synthesis.

The pattern of responses indicated (a) is based on Table 7 of Crawford and Scrutton (1987). The nature of the signal transduction mechanisms (b) is drawn from references cited in the text except for PAF (Hallam *et al.* 1984a; Shulka, 1985) and for vasopressin (Hallam *et al.* 1984b) yield the membrane-impermeant free acid (Tsien, 1981). In contrast aequorin is loaded by treating the cells either with ethylene glycol tetra acetic acid (EGTA) + ATP^{4-} or with graded doses of dimethylsulfoxide (Johnson *el at.* 1985; Yamaguchi *et al.* 1986). Both these latter methods presumably cause extensive damage to the plasma membrane in order to permit uptake of a protein of molecular mass 21 kDa. It is, therefore, most surprising that no leakage of cytosolic proteins or adenine nucleotides accompanies aequorin uptake when this probe is loaded using the EGTA/ATP^{4-} method (Johnson *et al.* 1985).

2 Intracellular probe concentrations and buffering capacity — the absolute increase in fluoresence caused by binding of Ca^{2+} to Quin2 is relatively small and necessitates loading of this probe to near millimolar levels in the cytosol. At such levels transient increases in cytosolic [Ca^{2+}] are suppressed and some decrease in cellular responsiveness is observed due to the marked increase in the cytosolic buffering capacity for Ca^{2+} (Tsien *et al.* 1982; Pollock & Rink, 1986). A considerably greater absolute increase in fluorescence occurs on formation of the Ca^{2+}–Fura2 complex and adequate sensitivity can be achieved with this probe at an intracellular concentration of 20–30 μM (Pollock & Rink, 1986). At this level the addition to the physiological buffering capacity is minimal. There is little evidence that either Ca^{2+} transients or physiological responses are suppressed in Fura2-loaded platelets provided that an acceptable protocol is followed. Aequorin is typically loaded to a final concentration of 1–10 nM and therefore causes no increase in cytosolic Ca^{2+} buffering (Cobbold & Rink, 1987).

3 Detection range and sensitivity — both Quin2 and Fura2 follow a classical saturation curve with K_D values for the Ca^{2+} complex of 0.11 μM (Quin2) or 0.22 μM (Fura2). Increases in cytosolic [Ca^{2+}] over the physiological range therefore cause a three- to six-fold increase in fluorescence with little further increase occurring when [Ca^{2+}] rises above 2–3 μM (Cobbold & Rink, 1987). These probes cannot, therefore, be used to determine whether cytosolic [Ca^{2+}] increases into the 5–10 μM range, a point which is important in the context of responses, such as phosphatidylserine exposure, which may involve Ca^{2+}-dependent cytoskeletal protein degradation (see later). In contrast aequorin, which binds 3 moles of Ca^{2+} per mole of protein with a K_D of 1–2 μM and a 10^5-fold increase in luminescence, provides better potential for detection of increases in [Ca^{2+}] in this upper concentration range. Furthermore, because of the marked increase in luminesence aequorin would be likely to highlight localized elevations in [Ca^{2+}] which might be insufficient to be reflected in a significant increase in average cytosolic [Ca^{2+}] (Cobbold & Rink, 1987).

This latter difference in probe properties provides the currently favoured explanation for the difference in the results obtained when intracellular [Ca^{2+}] is measured using either Quin2/Fura2 or aequorin (Table 3.1) (Johnson *et al.* 1985). However it is pertinent to note that the properties of aequorin also make this probe an effective detector of a small percentage of dying cells in the preparation. Given the nature of the loading protocols employed, preparations containing aequorin might be expected to contain such dead or dying cells which are unable to maintain normal Ca^{2+} homeostasis and hence show markedly elevated cytosolic [Ca^{2+}] (El-Mofty *et al.* 1975). Notably single cell imaging analysis using Fura2 has failed to detect significant intra- or interplatelet Ca^2+ heterogeneity (Hallam *et al.* 1986).

Increases in platelet cytosolic [Ca^{2+}] could result from operation of a range of mechanisms which allow cells to increase their Ca^{2+} levels in response to stimulation. Some of these mechanisms are described below.

1 Ca^{2+} influx from the extracellular medium via voltage-operated channels.

2 Ca^{2+} influx from the extracellular medium via receptor-operated channels.

3 Ca^{2+} mobilization from an intracellular store which is now generally accepted as being a specialized region (or regions) of the smooth endoplasmic reticulum. In the platelet this organelle is often described as the dense tubular system. Ca^{2+} release from this store is mediated by an increase in the cytosolic concentration of inositol-1,4,5-trisphosphate (I(1,4,5,)P_3) resulting from agonist-induced activation of phosphoinositide phosphodiesterase (phospholipase C) (see later).

4 Ca^{2+} influx from the extracellular medium via a plasma membrane Na^+/Ca^{2+} antiport.

5 Ca^{2+} influx from the extracellular medium via channels which open as a consequence of physical disturbance to the plasma membrane, e.g. the 'stretch-activated' Ca^{2+} channels of endothelial cells (Lansman *et al.* 1987).

Of these, platelets have clearly been shown to possess mechanism **3** since addition of I(1,4,5)P_3 to permeabilized preparations causes Ca^{2+} release (Authi & Crawford, 1985) as in many other cells; and to lack mechanism **1** since stimulation by agonists which increase cytosolic [Ca^{2+}] does not cause a significant change in membrane potential (MacIntyre & Rink, 1982; Sage & Rink, 1986). The status of the contribution of the other mechanisms to an increase in platelet cytosolic [Ca^{2+}] is, however, less clear.

In contrast to voltage-operated Ca^{2+} channels which are now clearly defined molecular entities (Seagar *et al.* 1988) the evidence supporting the existence of discrete receptor-operated Ca^{2+} channels is fragmentary. Few, if any, compounds acting selectively on such channels have yet been described and patch-clamp analysis has thus far failed to provide convincing evidence supporting the existence of such channels in most cell types which have been examined (Hallam & Rink, 1989). It has, therefore, been postulated that agonist-induced Ca^{2+} influx is not a direct event as shown in Fig. 3.1(c) but rather arises as an indirect consequence either of polyphosphoinositide breakdown (Irvine & Moor, 1986; Morris *et al.* 1987) (Fig. 3.1b) or of intracellular Ca^{2+} mobilization (Putney, 1986) (Fig. 3.1a). A close coupling of Ca^{2+} influx to intracellular Ca^{2+} mobilization (Fig. 3.1a) is indicated in some cells, e.g. parotid acinar cells, since depleted intracellular Ca^{2+} stores can be refilled by Ca^{2+} present in the extracellular fluid without any detectable increase in average cytosolic [Ca^{2+}] (Putney, 1986). However in other cells, e.g. endothelial cells, in which depletion of intracellular Ca^{2+} stores causes

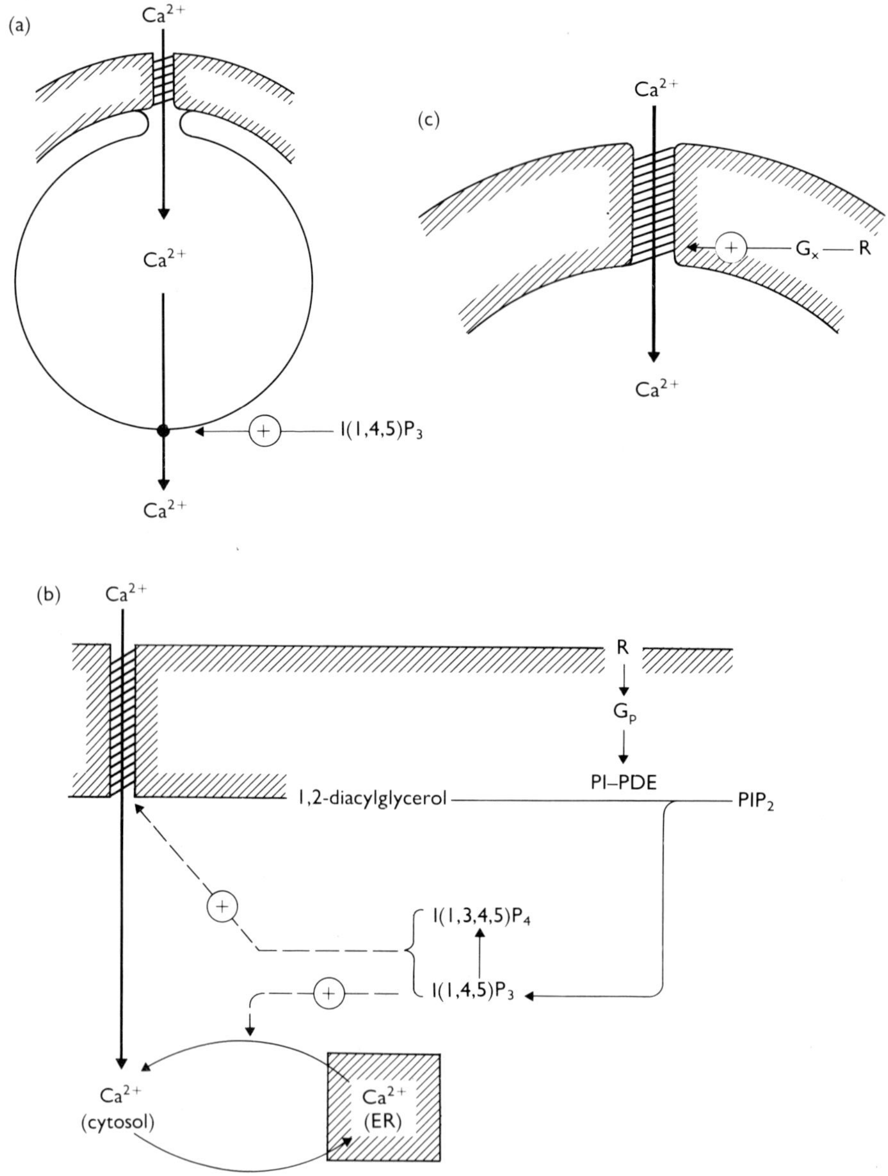

Figure 3.1 Proposed mechanisms to explain receptor-operated Ca^{2+} influx. (a) The capacitance model proposed by Putney (1986) in which direct Ca^{2+} influx into a specific intracellular pool is regulated by Ca^{2+} mobilization from this pool controlled by $I(1,4,5)P_3$ and hence related to agonist-induced activation of phosphoinositide phosphodiesterase (PI-PDE) with consequent breakdown of phosphatidyl inositol-4,5-bisphosphate (PIP_2). (b) The $I(1,3,4,5)P_4$ model as proposed by Irvine and Moor (1986) in which Ca^{2+} influx is regulated directly by $I(1,3,4,5)P_4$ in combination with $I(1,4,5)P_3$ presumptively by activation of the plasma membrane Ca^{2+} channel. (ER = endoplasmic reticulum.) (c) Direct control of Ca^{2+} influx in which the receptor (R) is coupled directly to the Ca^{2+} channel possibly via a G-protein (G_X).

agonist-independent divalent cation influx (Hallam *et al.* 1989) and agonist-induced Mn^{2+} influx is clearly initiated *after* intracellular Ca^{2+} mobilization (Hallam *et al.* 1988), an increase in average cytosolic $[Ca^{2+}]$ *does* occur during refilling of the depleted Ca^{2+} stores (Hallam *et al.* 1989). Hence the relationship between cytosolic Ca^{2+} and the mechanism by which depleted intracellular Ca^{2+} stores are refilled is unclear.

Platelet studies using stopped-flow fluorimetry have shown that Ca^{2+} and Mn^{2+} influx induced by agonists such as thrombin occurs only after a significant delay which is slightly, but significantly, shorter than that which characterizes the initiation of intracellular Ca^{2+} mobilization by such agonists (Sage & Rink, 1987; Sage *et al.* 1989). These data are not easily reconciled with the postulate that Ca^{2+} influx is controlled by indirect mechanisms of the type shown in Fig. 3.1 (a and b). They appear more consistent with Ca^{2+} influx via a receptor-operated channel which is activated independently of the mechanisms responsible for initiating intracellular Ca^{2+} mobilization. Such an entity has recently been demonstrated by patch-clamp analysis of thrombin-stimulated platelet membrane vesicles enriched in plasma membrane which were inserted into a planar phospholipid bilayer (Zschauer *et al.* 1988). The agonist-induced Ca^{2+} current observed in these latter studies is unlikely to be explained on the basis of the mechanism shown in Fig. 3.1(b) since the Ca^{2+}-activated kinase responsible for inositol-1,3,4,5-tetrakisphosphate ($I(1,3,4,5)P_4$) formation is a cytosolic enzyme in other cells (Biden & Wolheim, 1986). The mechanism shown in Fig. 3.1(a) could still be operative in this preparation since the purity of the membrane fractions was not clearly established and structures such as that shown in Fig. 3.1(a) might in any case be isolated as part of a plasma membrane fraction. If such structures are present they might provide an explanation for the repeated reports of 'plasma-membrane-associated Ca^{2+}' in various cells.

A receptor-operated Ca^{2+} channel is particularly likely to be responsible for ADP-induced Ca^{2+} influx into platelets. This agonist has little, if any, capacity to induce phosphoinositide breakdown or to increase the levels of $I(1,4,5)P_3$ in human platelets (Fisher *et al.* 1985; Daniel *et al.* 1986), but at high concentration activates entry of Ca^{2+} or Mn^{2+} without measurable delay (Sage & Rink, 1987; Sage *et al.* 1989). The operation of such an ADP-gated Ca^{2+} channel has been directly demonstrated in very recent patch-clamp studies on intact platelets (Mayhaut-Smith *et al.* 1990). Neither the difference in the time courses of the increase in cytosolic $[Ca^{2+}]$ induced by ADP and thrombin nor the initiation of Ca^{2+} influx before intracellular Ca^{2+} mobilization seen in the stopped-flow studies are observed in a continuous-flow system (Jones & Gear, 1988). However the time resolution of this latter system does not appear adequate to resolve events occurring prior to 500 milliseconds and hence the earlier processes detected in the stopped-flow analysis cannot be seen using this method.

Agonists such as ADP have been shown to cause an *increase* in $^{23}Na^{+}$ uptake into platelets (Feinberg *et al.* 1977). This effect is however likely to result from activation of Na^+/H^+ exchange (see 1,2-diacylglycerol, inositol-1,4,5-trisphosphate ($I(1,4,5)P_3$) and other inositol phosphates) rather than from any effect on a putative Na^+/Ca^{2+} antiport (Brass, 1984). Hence mechanism (**4**) is unlikely to contribute to elevation of cytosolic [Ca^{2+}]. The effects of physical distortion (mechanism **5**) on Ca^{2+} influx into platelets have not been well characterized although cellular activation resulting from close cell contact, e.g. by centrifugation, might be caused in this way.

Elevation of cytosolic [Ca^{2+}] might also in principle result from inhibition of the mechanisms responsible for removal of Ca^{2+} from the cytosol. However, in the platelet control of these mechanisms appears to be directed to depression of cellular responsiveness by enhancement of the removal of Ca^{2+} from the cytosol (see Cyclic-3,5-AMP).

1,2-diacylglycerol, inositol-1,4,5-trisphosphate ($I(1,4,5)P_3$) and other inositol phosphates

Elevations in intracellular [1,2-diacylglycerol] and (I-1,4,5-P_3] are typically associated with agonist-induced increases in cytosolic [Ca^{2+}] where these increases are not caused by plasma membrane depolarization. It is also generally accepted that in such systems 1,2-diacylglycerol and $I(1,4,5)P_3$ are formed as a result of breakdown of phosphatidylinositol-4,5-bisphosphate by a plasma-membrane-bound phosphoinositide phosphodiesterase (phospholipase C) (Berridge, 1987). Agonist-induced activation of this enzyme is postulated to involve coupling to the receptor via a putative guanine nucleotide binding (G)-protein (G_P) (Berridge, 1987) in a scheme analogous to that which is well established for receptor-mediated control of adenylate cyclase (Gilman, 1987) (Fig. 3.2) (see also Brass, 1988).

There is adequate evidence to suggest that such events occur in the platelet as a consequence of interaction with excitatory agonists such as thrombin, vasopressin, PAF and thromboxane A_2 (Table 3.1). For example both agonists, e.g. thrombin in the presence of guanosine triphosphate and metabolically stable GTP analogues such as guanosine-5′-*O*-(3-thiotriphosphate) (GTPγS) activate phosphoinositide phosphodiesterase in platelet membrane fractions (Hrbolich *et al.* 1987) and cause both 1,2-diacylglycerol and inositol trisphosphate formation in permeabilized platelets (Haslam & Davidson, 1984a; Culty *et al.* 1988). As in other cells, the molecular nature of the G_P protein(s) responsible for receptor-phosphoinositide phosphodiesterase coupling has yet to be defined. However, more than one such protein appears to be involved. Phosphoinositide hydrolysis induced by thrombin or the stable thromboxane A_2 analogue U46619 in permeabilized platelets is GTP-dependent and is inhibited by addition of the metabolically stable guanosine diphosphate (GDP) analogue GDPβS. Although GDPβS has been reported to inhibit agonist-induced responses in intact platelets (Krishnamurthi *et al.* 1988) the status of this effect is uncertain since inhibition of agonist-stimulated polyphosphoinositide hydrolysis by GDPβS occurs only in permeabilized platelets and therefore is dependent on access to an intracellular site (Kucera & Rittenhouse, 1988).

However, only phosphoinositide hydrolysis induced by thrombin is inhibited by pretreatment of the preparation with pertussis toxin (Brass *et al.* 1987). The ability of pertussis toxin to inhibit G_i, the (G)-protein responsible for inhibitory coupling of receptors to adenylate cyclase, is well established and is associated with incorporation of ADP-ribose into the α-subunit of this protein (Milligan, 1988). Pretreatment of platelets with this toxin causes ADP-ribosylation of a polypeptide having a molecular mass (41 kDa) very similar to that of the α-subunit of G_i (Banga *et al.* 1986). Although the identity of G_i with the pertussis-sensitive form of G_P has been suggested for platelets (Brass *et al.* 1988) this postulate is unlikely to be correct since there is little correlation between the ability of different agonists to activate phosphoinositide phosphodiesterase and to inhibit adenylate cyclase. For example, adrenaline causes effective inhibition of adenylate cyclase but is unable to induce polyphosphoinositide hydrolysis (Jakobs *et al.* 1976; Banga *et al.* 1986) while the converse is true for agonists such as vasopressin, PAF and stable analogues of thromboxane A_2 (Haslam, 1987; Brass *et al.* 1986). Furthermore, the relationship between the extents of ADP-ribose incorporation into the 41 kDa polypeptide and of reduction in the thrombin-induced response differ markedly for inhibition of adenylate cyclase and for activation of phosphoinositide phosphodiesterase (Banga *et al.* 1988).

Recently the 41 kDa substrate which is ADP-ribosylated by pertussis toxin has been resolved into two polypeptides having very similar properties and possibly corresponding to two isoenzymes of G_i (Brass *et al.* 1988). It is conceivable that these two pertussis toxin substrates may differ in their sensitivity to ADP-ribosylation and may be differentially coupled to adenylate cyclase and to phosphoinositide phosphodiesterase, respectively. Such an organization would explain the differential sensitivity of the thrombin-induced responses to pertussis toxin treatment observed by Banga *et al.* (1988).

There are, however, some difficulties in accepting a scheme such as that shown in Fig. 3.2 as the complete explanation for agonist-induced phosphoinositide hydrolysis in the platelet.

1 In both permeabilized platelets and in platelet membrane fractions thrombin causes significant phosphoinositide phosphodiesterase activation and production of 1,2,-diacylglycerol and inositol trisphosphate in the absence of GTP, although these responses are stimulated by addition of exogenous GTP (Rock & Jackowski, 1987; Hrbolich *et al.* 1987). These findings, together with earlier observations, have led to the postulate of guanine nucleotide-dependent and -independent routes for activation of phosphoinositide phosphodiesterase (Haslam & Davidson, 1984a) although the apparent existence of a GTP-independent response may in fact result from the presence of tightly bound GTP in the preparations (Knight & Scrutton, 1986a).

2 In the platelet phosphoinositide phosphodiesterase is predominantly a cytosolic enzyme although some membrane-bound activity is also detected. Both forms of

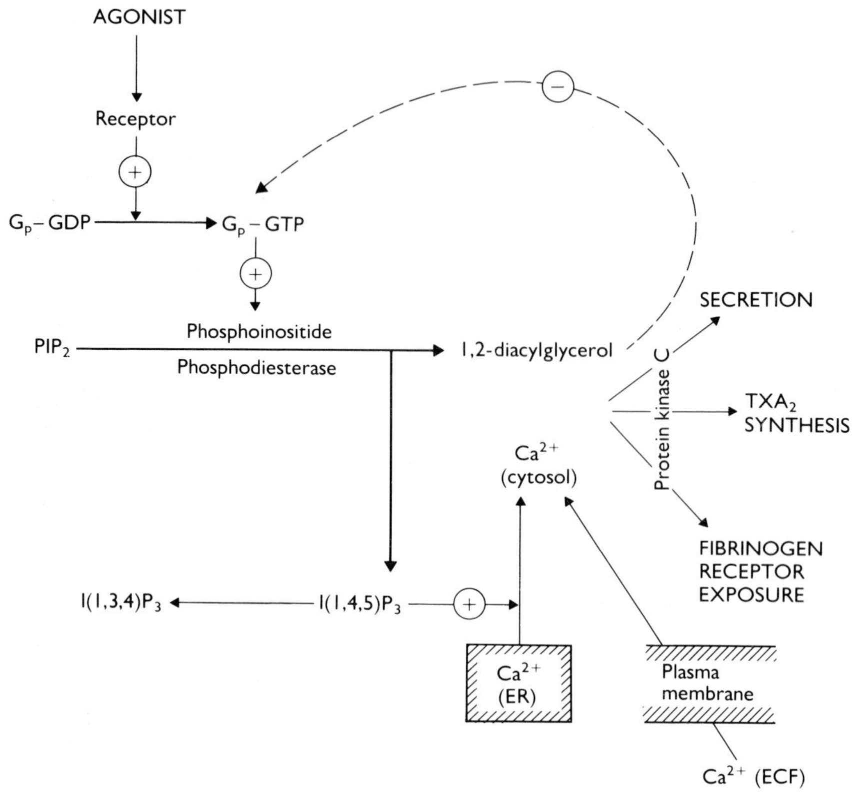

Figure 3.2 Processes in the platelet which may be regulated by Ca^{2+} and 1,2-diacylglycerol via activation of protein kinase C. (ECF = extracellular fluid.)

the enzyme are apparently subject to activation by GTP (Baldassare & Fisher, 1986; Deckmyn *et al.* 1986) although this effect is not specific and can also be observed on addition of other nucleotides or even of ethylene diaminetetra-acetic acid (EDTA) (Rock & Jackowski, 1987). The relationship between the cytosolic and membrane-bound forms of phosphoinositide phosphodiesterase and the mechanisms by which these two isoenzymes are regulated is, therefore, far from clear. It is possible, for example, that phosphoinositide phosphodiesterase undergoes a cytosol–plasma-membrane translocation as a consequence of agonist stimulation comparable to that which is well documented for protein kinase C (Hirota *et al.* 1985).

3 The cytosolic and membrane-bound forms of phosphoinositide phosphodiesterase may differ in their ability to hydrolyse the different phosphoinositides. However, the data suggesting such a difference are derived primarily from *in vitro* studies using purified phospholipids, and in some cases non-physiological Ca^{2+} concentrations. Hence their application to the physiological environment is unclear (Rock & Jackowski, 1987). In more intact systems such as electropermeabilized human platelets (Culty *et al.* 1988) both phosphatidylinositol-4,5-bisphoshate *and phosphatidylinositol-4-phosphate* (but not phosphatidylinositol) are hydrolysed as a consequence of stimulation of phosphoinositide phosphodiesterase by thrombin or GTPγS at a Ca^{2+} concentration (0.1 μM) characteristic of the resting platelet. The predominant substrate hydrolysed under these conditions is phosphatidylinositol-4-phosphate although enough phosphatidylinositol-4,5-bisphosphate is also degraded to achieve the intracellular [I(1,4,5)P_3] required to mobilize intracellular Ca^{2+} stores (Culty *et al.* 1988). If there is variability in the mix of the polyphosphoinositides hydrolysed by phosphoinositide phosphodiesterase in the intact platelet depending on the agonist employed, the observed differences in efficacy for production of 1,2-diacylglycerol and I(1,4,5)P_3 might be explained (Table 3.1). Activation of intact platelets by most, but not all, excitatory agonists causes increases in 1,2-diacylglycerol (usually detected as [^{32}P]-phosphatidate) and in inositol trisphosphates (Table 3.1). Although the increase in inositol trisphosphate is small, as in other cells, it precedes the much larger increase observed in inositol monophosphates (Vickers *et al.* 1984). The relationship between the time courses of formation of inositol bis- and trisphosphates following agonist stimulation is less clear. In most studies both accumulate together (Vickers *et al.* 1984; Watson *et al.* 1985; Siess & Binder, 1985) although Agranoff *et al.* (1983) found that accumulation of inositol trisphosphate preceded that of inositol bisphosphate.

The interpretation of these studies has been complicated by more recent analyses which have shown that most of the inositol trisphosphate detected in stimulated platelets is the 1,3,4-isomer, except at very early times after agonist addition (Culty *et al.*, 1988; King & Rittenhouse, 1989). Accumulation of I(1,3,4,5) P_4 has also been observed under these conditions with a time course similar to that for I(1,4,5)P_3 (King & Rittenhouse, 1989). However, the role(s) of I(1,3,4)P_3 and I(1,3,4,5)P_4 in the platelet is as obscure as in other cells in which these metabolites have been detected.

As noted above a role for I(1,3,4,5,)P_4 together with I(1,4,5)P_3 in inducing Ca^{2+} influx as proposed by Irvine & Moor (1986) appears to be excluded in the platelet since such influx in this cell clearly precedes intracellular mobilization (Sage & Rink, 1986; Sage, 1987). It has recently been shown in permeabilized hepatocytes that I(1,3,4,5)P_4 activates Ca^{2+} sequestration into the endoplasmic reticulum (Hill *et al.* 1988). In this way I(1,3,4,5)P_4 might contribute to the transient nature of the increase in cytosolic [Ca^{2+}] which characterizes the mobilization of this cation from platelet intracellular stores (Pollock & Rink, 1986). Activation of I(1,4,5)P_3 kinase by Ca^{2+} (Biden & Wolheim, 1986) may also regulate the level of I(1,4,5)P_3 and hence indirectly allow control by Ca^{2+} of its own mobilization from intracellular stores.

The increase in [1,2-diacylglycerol] is believed, in part as a consequence of its ability to modulate the response to Ca^{2+}, to have very wide-ranging effects on the initiation and control of platelet responsiveness. These effects, some of which are shown in Fig. 3.2, are proposed to result from activation of protein kinase C.

While a central role for 1,2-diacylglycerol and protein kinase C in co-ordination and modulation of the Ca^{2+} signal is an attractive concept, most of the data cited in support of this postulate are of uncertain validity when applied to the physiological situation. In the intact cell the 1,2-diacylglycerol signal is transient since 1-stearoyl-2-arachidonylglycerol generated by phosphoinositide breakdown (Mauco *et al.* 1984) is rapidly phosphorylated to yield the corresponding phosphatidate (Rittenhouse-Simmons, 1979). Direct evidence for an elevation in [1,2-diacylglycerol] has only been obtained on stimulation by high concentrations of collagen or thrombin (Rittenhouse-Simmons, 1979). For all other agonists the increase in this metabolite can only be detected as an enhanced labelling of phosphatidate in [^{32}P]-loaded platelets (see Table 3.1, footnote). Agonist-stimulated 1,2-diacylglycerol formation is probably localized, both to, and within, the plasma membrane since polyphosphoinositides are exclusively present in this membrane (Mauco *et al.* 1987) and the sites of degradation are likely to be restricted. Hence no realistic estimates can be made of the concentrations achieved in these areas. The natural 1,2-diacylglycerol is too lipophilic to permit its use in intact or permeabilized cell studies. Hence the role of this compound in signal transduction mechanisms is typically probed using more hydrophilic analogues such as OAG or 1,2-dioctanoyl glycerol (diC_8) at relatively high concentration (10–100 μM). Such analogues are effective activators of protein kinase C and are rapidly phosphorylated (Bishop & Bell, 1986; Brass & Laposta, 1987) thus generating a transient signal. However, their effects on general platelet membrane structure, and hence possibly on the localization and activation of protein kinase C, are likely to differ considerably from those consequential on localized generation of 1-stearoyl-2-arachidonylglycerol in the plasma membrane.

The situation is even less satisfactory when metabolically stable activators of protein kinase C such as phorbol esters are employed since, although such compounds are usually used at nanomolar concentrations, the transience of the natural signal is not mimicked. Effects such as inhibition of agonist-induced phosphoinositide breakdown and of Ca^{2+} mobilization which are only observed after preincubation with phorbol esters (MacIntyre *et al.* 1985a; Zavoico *et al.* 1985) are, therefore, of questionable relevance to normal cellular physiology.

In support of this interpretation, the addition of compounds which inhibit protein kinase C, e.g. staurosporine, fails to enhance phosphatidate synthesis induced by thrombin even when phosphorylation of the 47-kDa major platelet protein substrate of this enzyme is completely abolished (Watson *et al.* 1988). Bidirectional control of platelet responsiveness by the 1,2-diacylglycerol/protein kinase C system (Fig. 3.2) is not, however, completely excluded since under appropriate conditions addition of staurosporine enhances thrombin-induced accumulations of $I(1,3,4)P_3$, $I(1,4,5)P_3$, and $I(1,3,4,5)P_4$ (King & Rittenhouse, 1989). This finding may indicate that activation of inositol trisphosphate-5-monoesterase by protein kinase C (Connolly *et al.* 1986) does occur under physiological conditions. However such data, as well as those showing inhibition of thrombin-induced secretion and aggregation by staurosporine, are uncertain indicators of a role for protein kinase C in these responses since this compound like other less potent inhibitors of the enzyme is far from selective (Watson *et al.* 1988).

Cyclic-3,5-AMP

Stimulation of platelets with inhibitory agonists such as PGI_2, PGD_2 and adenosine causes an increase in intracellular [cAMP] as a consequence of activation of the plasma-membrane-bound adenylyl cyclase. This system resembles that present in other cells since in membrane preparations activation of the enzyme by these agonists is dependent on the addition of GTP thus indicating the involvement of the guanine nucleotide-binding protein (G_s) in receptor–adenylyl-cyclase coupling (Mills, 1982). Conversely, many excitatory agonists have the capacity to cause GTP-dependent inhibition of adenylyl cyclase in platelet membrane fractions (Haslam *et al.* 1985a,b). Such inhibition is mediated via the guanine nucleotide binding protein, G_i, since treatment of membrane fractions or of permeabilized platelets with pertussis toxin abolishes agonist-induced inhibition of adenylyl cyclase (Brass *et al.* 1986). However, only a few agonists e.g. ADP, adrenaline, and α-thrombin (at high concentration) are able to express their capacity for adenylyl cyclase inhibition in the intact cell by limiting the ability of inhibitory agonists to increase intracellular cyclic AMP levels (Table 3.1) (Haslam *et al.* 1985b). The explanation for this discrepancy is unclear at present. Phosphorylation of G_i by protein kinase C with consequent uncoupling of excitatory agonist receptors from adenylyl cyclase as proposed by Jakobs *et al.* (1985) is unlikely to provide an explanation. There is no correlation between the ability of different agonists to activate protein kinase C (as measured by 47-kDa polypeptide phosphorylation) and to express inhibition of adenylyl cyclase in intact platelets (Williams *et al.* 1987). Differential coupling of the receptor to G_p or G_i depending on the lêvel of receptor occupancy has also been proposed (Williams *et al.* 1987) but is not easily reconciled with the observation that proteolytic modification of platelets with chymotrypsin selectively abolishes α-thrombin-induced inactivation of adenylyl cyclase (McGowan & Detwiler, 1986).

There is abundant evidence to support the postulate that an increase in intracellular [cAMP] depresses platelet aggregation and secretion and thereby mediates many of the effects of inhibitory agonists on this cell (Crawford & Scrutton, 1987). The dose/response curve describing inhibition of platelet aggregation and secretion by such agonists, however, lies well to the left of that which characterizes agonist-induced cAMP accumulation although this shift is much less marked for other responses e.g shape change, elevation of average cytosolic [Ca^{2+}], phosphatidate formation. Hence only a small fraction of the total capacity for increasing cAMP levels is required to express some of the inhibitory responses in the absence of an excitatory agonist such as ADP which is capable of depressing adenylyl cyclase activity in the intact cell (Haslam, 1975; Bushfield *et al.* 1985).

The mechanisms by which an increase in [cAMP] acting presumably via protein kinase A depresses platelet responsiveness are less well defined. Some possibilities are shown in Fig. 3.3. Enhancement by cAMP of Ca^{2+} efflux and intracellular sequestration is well documented in other cells in which these two signal transduction mechanisms have an antagonistic relationship e.g. smooth muscle (Rasmussen, 1981). Plasma membrane Ca^{2+}, Mg^{2+}-ATPase activity has never been convincingly demonstrated in the platelet but this activity is prominent in an intracellular membrane fraction which appears to be derived from the endoplasmic reticulum (Hack *et al.* 1986). It is unclear whether an increase in [cAMP] enhances Ca^{2+} sequestration in the platelet since intracellular membrane Ca^{2+}, Mg^{2+}-ATPase activity has been reported either to be (Kaser-Glanzmann *et al.* 1977; Adunyah & Dean, 1987), or not to be (Le Peuch *et al.* 1983; O'Rourke *et al.* 1989), enhanced by addition of this cyclic nucleotide. In any case such an effect is unlikely to provide the primary explanation for depression of platelet responsiveness by cAMP since in the presence of inhibitory agonists or of other agents which activate adenylyl cyclase, e.g. forskolin, the increase in cytosolic [Ca^{2+}] induced by thrombin and PAF is abolished rather than attenuated (Rink & Sanchez, 1984; MacIntyre *et al.* 1985b). This, together with other evidence (Knight & Scrutton, 1987), suggests that an increase in [cAMP] impairs the ability of excitatory agonists to activate phosphoinositide phosphodiesterase thus interfering with both Ca^{2+} mobilization and generation of 1,2-diacylglycerol. It is most likely that G_P is the target for cAMP-dependent phosphorylation and that such phosphorylation enhances the GTPase activity of this protein hence decreasing the lifetime of the activated state. This postulate is supported by the finding that in electropermeabilized platelets addition of cAMP inhibits 5-HT secretion induced by GTP in the presence of non-saturating [Ca^{2+}] but has little effect on this response when induced by the metabolically stable GTP analogue, GTPγS (Knight & Scrutton, 1987). The enhancement by cAMP of agonist-stimulated GTPase activity which is predicted by this model has not yet, however, been demonstrated. In addition Moos and Goldberg (1988) have recently shown that cAMP inhibits Ca^{2+} release from the endoplasmic reticulum induced by $I(1,4,5)P_3$.

Effects of cAMP on G_P, and possibly on Ca^{2+} sequestration by the endoplasmic reticulum, do not, however, provide a full explanation of the inhibitory action of this cyclic nucleotide. For example, they do not readily explain the following features.

1 ATP secretion induced by collagen in the presence of cyclooxygenase blockade is not markedly inhibited by forskolin or PGI_2 (Rink & Sanchez, 1984) although generation of 1,2-diacylglycerol does occur under these conditions (Table 3.1). This finding may be related to the well-established failure of PGI_2 to act as an effective inhibitor of adhesion of platelets to collagen (Higgs *et al.* 1978) and to the mobilization of 1,2-diacylglycerol from phospholipids other than the phosphoinositides (Pollock *et al.* 1986).

2 Elevation of [cAMP] inhibits aggregation induced by adrenaline although this

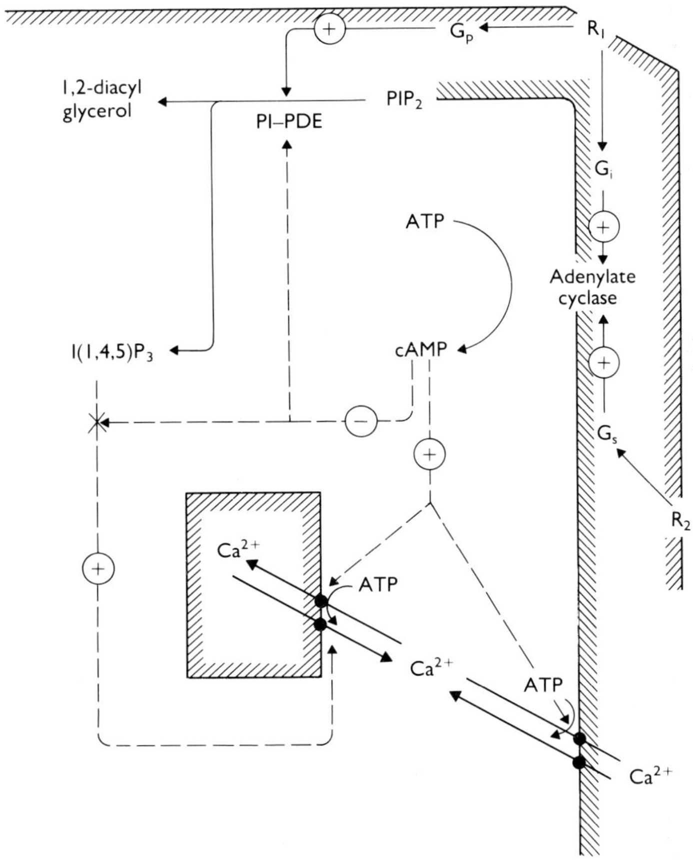

Figure 3.3 Possible sites for regulation of Ca^{2+} sequestration, efflux and mobilization by cyclic AMP (cAMP) in a cell such as the platelet in which Ca^{2+} and cAMP act as antagonistic second messengers.

agonist does not activate phosphoinositide phosphodiesterase, increase average cytosolic [Ca^{2+}] or raise [1,2-diacylglycerol] (Table 3.1).

3 As noted above aggregation and secretion are inhibited at lower cyclic AMP concentrations than responses more directly related to phosphoinositide breakdown (Bushfield *et al.* 1985). This finding probably indicates that cAMP also acts at a site distal to Ca^{2+} in the signal transduction pathways for these responses although such an effect is not seen for Ca^{2+}-driven 5-HT secretion in the electropermeabilized platelet (Knight & Scrutton, 1987).

Interaction between the Ca^{2+}/1,2-diacylglycerol and cAMP signal transduction pathways may also be bidirectional since treatment of platelets with TPA or 1,2-didecanoylglycerol reduces the ability of inhibitory agonists and of forskolin to stimulate adenylyl cyclase, as well as impairing inhibition of this enzyme by excitatory agonists such as adrenaline (Williams *et al.* 1987). It has not been shown that these effects occur as a consequence of physiological 1,2-diacylglycerol generation.

Cyclic-3,5-GMP

Signal transduction pathways involving cGMP are generally less well characterized than those dependent on changes in intracellular [Ca^{2+}] or [cAMP]. Recent studies have shown that cells may contain either a membrane-bound guanylyl cyclase which responds to stimulation by peptide agonists e.g. atrial natiuretic peptide and/or a cytosolic guanylyl cyclase which is activated by free radicals (Waldman & Murad, 1987). It is well established that cGMP mediates inhibitory signal transduction in the platelet and that nitrovasodilators such as sodium nitroprusside inhibit aggregation and secretion as a consequence of activation of a cytosolic guanylyl cyclase and hence of elevation of intracellular [cGMP]. Such compounds have little, if any, ability to increase intracellular [cAMP] (Haslam *et al.* 1980].

Addition of excitatory agonists or of other agents which induce platelet aggregation or agglutination (e.g. divalent cation ionophores, ristocetin) also causes an increase in intracellular [cGMP]. This latter response is not a direct consequence of receptor occupancy but rather results from prolonged contact of the platelet either with other platelets or with a matrix such as a collagen fibril (Haslam, 1975; Edgecombe & Scrutton, 1987). This increase in [cGMP] presumably also results from activation of cytosolic guanylyl cyclase since there is no evidence for the presence of significant membrane-bound activity in the platelet.

Interest in the cGMP/guanylyl cyclase transduction system in the platelet has increased recently with the demonstration that NO released by many types of endothelial cell decreases platelet responsiveness, as well as relaxing vascular smooth muscle, by causing elevation of [cGMP] (Palmer *et al.* 1987; Radomski *et al.* 1987). The effects of the synthetic nitrovasodilators on these two systems are, therefore, now believed to depend on the ability of these compounds to generate NO either within, or near to, the target cell (Moncada *et al.* 1987). This autocoid then activates guanylyl cyclase by interacting with the iron atom in the bound haem of this enzyme (Ignarro *et al.* 1986) and hence an increase in [cGMP] occurs. The mechanism by which platelet–platelet or platelet–matrix contact increases [cGMP] is stil obscure. These increases are small as compared to those induced by the nitrovasodilators and are blocked by redox dyes, e.g. nitroblue tetrazolium, which fail to inhibit activation of guanylyl cyclase induced by sodium nitroprusside. Recently, however, Radomski *et al.* (1990) have shown that contact-induced elevation of [cGMP] results from generation of a low level of NO. The use of the inhibitors may suggest that contact-induced cGMP generation may not cause feedback inhibition of aggregation as suggested by Haslam *et al.* (1980) (Edgecombe & Scrutton, 1988) but has thrown no light on the physiological role of this phenomenon.

The mechanism(s) by which an increase in [cGMP] causes inhibition of platelet responses is equally obscure. Most studies have failed to detect clear-cut differences between the effects of elevation of cAMP and cGMP on signal transduction pathways such as agonist-induced increases in [1,2-diacylglycerol] or cytosolic [Ca^{2+}] (Takai *et al.* 1981; MacIntyre *et al.* 1985b; Henderson *et al.* 1987). Furthermore, in permeabilized platelets cGMP mimics the effect of cAMP on thrombin-induced secretion but is only active at higher concentrations (Haslam *et al.* 1985a). Differences in the interactions of cAMP and cGMP with the excitatory signal transduction mechanisms must, however, exist at some level, since these inhibitory systems exhibit response selectivity. For example, NO is a far more effective inhibitor of the adhesion of platelets to collagen than PGI_2, thus indicating that cGMP has a particular role in regulating this response (Radomski *et al.* 1987). Some differences in the patterns of protein phosphorylation caused by elevation of platelet [cAMP] and [cGMP] have been shown even at the relatively crude level of analysis used thus far in these studies (Haslam *et al.* 1985b). However, since the cellular functions of the phosphorylated polypeptides have not yet been established it is not possible at present to use such data to dissect the system further.

Na^+/H^+ exchange

Stimulation of platelets with certain excitatory agonists (e.g. ADP) has been known for many years to cause Na^+ uptake (Feinberg *et al.* 1977). More recently, this response has been shown to result from enhancement of the activity of a Na^+/H^+ exchange process and to accompany an increase in cytosolic pH (Horne *et al.* 1981). This response is well known in other cells where it is usually associated with induction of cellular proliferation by growth factors (Pouyssegur, 1985), a role which clearly cannot exist in the platelet. The evidence now available suggests rather that Na^+/H^+ exchange may be involved in modulating the aggregation response. For certain agonists, notably adrenaline, aggregation as measured by an increase in light transmittance is markedly reduced in the absence of extracellular Na^+ or in the presence of inhibitors of Na^+/H^+ exchange such as amiloride or its more potent analogues (Horne & Simons, 1978; Connolly & Limbird, 1983). Other agonists (e.g. thrombin) exhibit such effects only when non-saturating agonist concentrations are used to induce the response (Horne *et al.* 1981; Simpson & Rink, 1987).

The role of Na^+/H^+ exchange in platelet signal transduction is far from clear but the proposal that such exchange is an *obligatory* step in agonist-induced Ca^{2+} mobilization (Siffert & Akkerman, 1987) is clearly not correct. Thus, for example:

1 The increase in cytosolic [Ca^{2+}] induced by agonists such as thrombin and PAF precedes the increase in cytosolic pH regardless of the agonist concentration employed (Zavoico & Cragoe, 1988; Sanchez *et al.* 1988);

2 Ca^{2+} mobilization induced by low concentrations of thrombin occurs in platelets

in which the cytosol has been artificially acidified (Zavoico & Cragoe, 1988);
3 Aggregation induced by ADP which is dependent on an increase in cytosolic [Ca^{2+}] is not inhibited by removal of extracellular Na^+ or by addition of inhibitors of Na^+/H^+ exchange at concentrations where this exchange is completely suppressed. At higher inhibitor concentrations aggregation is reduced but this effect is presumably not related to inhibition of Na^+/H^+ exchange (Funder *et al.* 1988).

The suggestion that the increase in cytosolic [Ca^{2+}] is better correlated with an initial transient cytosolic acidification (Sanchez *et al.* 1988) has been shown to be an artefact of transmittance changes associated with shape change (Siffert *et al.* 1989).

Artificial cytosolic alkalization or activation of Na^+/H^+ exchange can, however, *enhance* the increase in cytosolic [Ca^{2+}] and the aggregation and secretion responses induced by non-saturating concentrations of most excitatory agonists (Nakano *et al.* 1987; Sanchez *et al.* 1988). It is still unclear how these latter effects operate, although they may be explained most satisfactorily if Na^+/H^+ exchange and/or cytosolic alkalization enhances agonist-induced arachidonate mobilization (Sweatt *et al.* 1986). As a consequence the extent of aggregation and secretion at low agonist concentration would be enhanced by activation of the amplification loop dependent on thromboxane A_2 synthesis (Connolly & Limbird, 1983). Such an explanation might even accommodate an apparent absolute requirement for Na^+/H^+ exchange in aggregation induced by adrenaline since, as conventionally measured, this response is largely, and often appears entirely, dependent on thromboxane A_2 synthesis (Scrutton & Wallis, 1981). Activation of Na^+/H^+ exchange by protein kinase C (Siffert *et al.* 1987) may then contribute to the mechanism by which agonists such as thrombin enhance Ca^{2+}-driven arachidonate mobilization, although other effects must also be involved since such enhancement can be observed in permeabilized preparations (Halenda & Rehm, 1987) (see Ca^{2+} driven responses). Enhancement of Ca^{2+} mobilization by cytosolic alkalization due to Na^+/H^+ exchange may also contribute to the initial thromboxane A_2-independent aggregation response at low agonist concentration (Siffert & Akkerman, 1988).

Other signal transduction mechanisms

No other well-characterized signal transduction mechanisms have been described in the platelet but a number of unexplained observations suggest that such mechanisms may exist.
1 Thrombin and PAF enhance Ca^{2+}-driven myosin light chain phosphorylation by a mechanism which appears not to depend on activation of protein kinase C or generation of $I(1,4,5)P_3$ (Hallam *et al.* 1985).
2 The stable analogue of thromboxane A_2, U46619, induces platelet shape change over a concentration range well below that required to increase cytosolic [Ca^{2+}] as measured using Fura2 (Simpson *et al.* 1986).

3 Thrombin is able to cause aggregation despite inhibition of protein phosphorylation by treatment of the platelets with staurosporine (Watson & Hambleton, 1989).
4 No satisfactory explanation exists to explain how interaction of platelets with molecules such as IgE enables this cell to participate in cytocidal responses (see Chapter 5).
5 Reports of phagocytosis (Dejesus *et al.* 1972) and of free radical production (Marcus, 1979) by platelets are not readily explained on the basis of our current understanding of its signal transduction pathways.

Signal transduction mechanisms and responses

Cellular signal transduction mechanisms can also be analysed by the use of permeabilized cell preparations to establish the quantitative relationship between the concentration of a given effector and the magnitude of the induced response. With this approach cells may either be selectively permeabilized, e.g. to Ca^{2+} using an appropriate ionophore (Halenda & Rehm, 1987) or more generally permeabilized to allow access and leakage of molecules of increasing size using high voltage discharge, toxins or detergents (Knight & Scrutton, 1986b; Scrutton & Knight, 1987). Although the latter preparations are more extensively damaged — and hence less physiological — they offer the advantage that greater control can be exerted over the signal transduction pathways. It is important to remember, however, that the unrestricted ability to manipulate the concentrations of intracellular metabolites in fully permeabilized cell preparations can be misused to produce responses having no relevance to normal cellular physiology [see, for example, exposure of permeabilized platelets to mM Ca^{2+} (Lapetina *et al.* 1985).

Although generally permeabilized preparations can be used to control the concentration of any cytosolic metabolite and establish its relationship to a given response this approach has been used thus far in the platelet primarily to characterize Ca^{2+}-driven responses.

Ca^{2+}-driven responses

Many platelet responses including shape change (Hallam & Rink, 1985a), secretion (Haslam & Davidson, 1984b; Knight *et al.* 1984; Peltola & Scrutton, 1989, unpublished work), arachidonate mobilization (Halenda & Rehm, 1987) and phosphatidylserine exposure (Verhallen *et al.* 1987) have been shown to be induced directly by Ca^{2+} using permeabilized preparations. In Fig. 3.4 the threshold Ca^{2+} concentration required to induce these, and some other, responses when the permeabilized preparation is challenged with Ca^{2+} in the presence of $MgATP^{2-}$ is compared with the maximal extent to which selected agonists can induce an increase in average cytosolic $[Ca^{2+}]$ as measured using Fura2 (left panel). All the latter data were selected from studies performed at Fura2 loading levels which

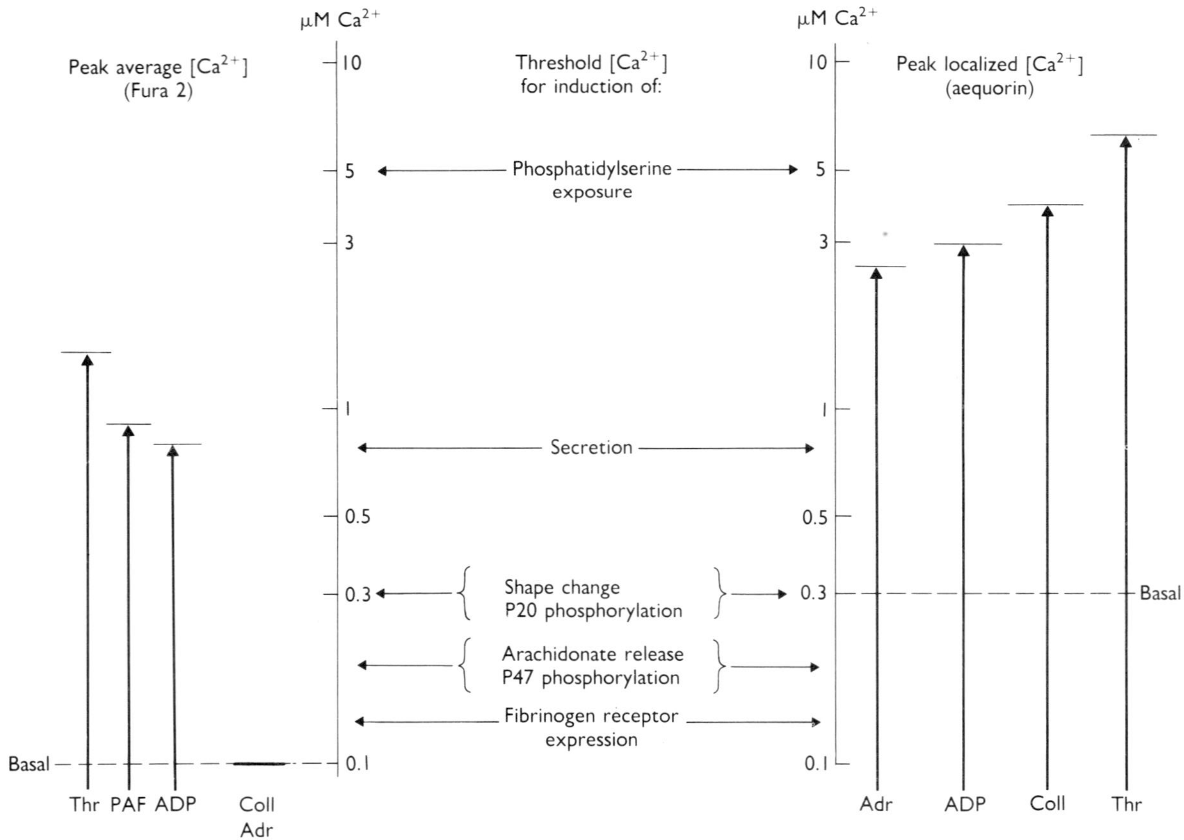

Figure 3.4 Comparison of the maximal extents to which selected excitatory agonists can increase average cytosolic [Ca^{2+}] or localized intracellular [Ca^{2+}] in intact platelets with the threshold [Ca^{2+}] determined for Ca^{2+}-driven responses in permeabilized platelets in the absence of additions other than $MgATP^{2-}$. The values shown for maximal [Ca^{2+}] levels are taken from Pollock and Rink (1986), Pollock *et al.* (1986) and Lanza *et al.* (1987) (Fura2) and from Ware *et al.* (1986) (aequorin). The values for Ca^{2+} thresholds are taken from Knight *et al.* (1984), Verhallen *et al.* (1987), Halenda and Rehm (1987), Haslam and Davidson (1984b), Shattil and Brass (1987), Peltola and Scrutton (1989, unpublished data) and Hallam *et al.* (1985) as well as from our unpublished data. Thr = thrombin; PAF = platelet activating factor; ADP = adenosine diphosphate; Coll = collagen; Adr = adrenaline.

would cause no significant increase in intracellular Ca^{2+}-buffering. In the right panel the comparison is based on measurement of the maximal extent of increase in intracellular [Ca^{2+}] in aequorin-loaded platelets. This latter response appears to reflect the ability of these agonists to induce a localized increase in [Ca^{2+}] (see Ca^{2+}) in a region which may, or may not, be relevant to induction of the response. Comparisons such as those shown in Fig. 3.4 then allow a semi-quantative assessment of the ability of a given agonist to induce a particular response based solely on the effect of this agonist on average cytosolic, or on localized, Ca^{2+} concentration. The comparison also indicates whether the observed extent of the increase in [Ca^{2+}] predicts a capacity to induce a response which is not actually observed. In this analysis we assume that the permeabilized platelet suffers no significant loss of responsiveness to Ca^{2+} as a consequence of the permeabilization procedure. This assumption has been validated for secretory responses in electropermeabilized platelets (Knight *et al.* 1982) but it is less clear whether a similar situation pertains for preparations permeabilized using saponin, digitonin or Streptolysin O. In other cell types, preparations made using these agents are known to suffer a rapid loss of responsiveness (Howell & Gomperts, 1987).

The ability of thrombin to induce shape change, arachidonate mobilization, secretion from all three granules and phosphorylation of P20 and P47, as well as its inability to induce significant phosphatidylserine exposure, (Table 3.1; Lyons *et al.* 1975) can all be explained simply on the basis of the maximal level to which thrombin increases average cytosolic [Ca^{2+}] (Fig. 3.4). A similar conclusion can be drawn for PAF, although the comparison in Fig. 3.4 suggests that the ability of this agonist to induce secretion is barely explained if based solely on its capacity to increase average cytosolic [Ca^{2+}]. However, for several of these responses, addition of thrombin or PAF to the permeabilized preparation either increases the maximal extent of the Ca^{2+}-driven response and/or decreases the threshold [Ca^{2+}] required for its induction (Knight & Scrutton, 1985; Halenda & Rehm, 1987). Such effects clearly enhance the ability of Ca^{2+} to induce these responses and in some cases, e.g. PAF and 5-HT secretion, may be critical to induction of a significant level of response. On the other hand the maximal level to which localized intracellular [Ca^{2+}] is increased in platelets stimulated by thrombin (Fig. 3.4) predicts that this agonist should markedly increase phosphatidylserine exposure, and hence prothrombinase activation. Such a response is not significantly observed when platelets are stimulated with thrombin alone (Table 3.1).

The pattern of responses induced by ADP (Table 3.1) is also predicted correctly on the basis of the level to which this agonist can increase average cytosolic [Ca^{2+}] (Fig. 3.4) except for its apparent inability to induce P47 phosphorylation (Haslam & Lynham, 1977). The inability of adrenaline to increase average cytosolic [Ca^{2+}] also predicts the response pattern observed for this agonist except, apparently, for its weak ability to mobilize arachidonate and hence induce thromboxane A_2 synthesis (Table 3.1). However, it is not clear whether this latter response is a direct consequence of occupancy of the α_2-adrenoceptor rather than being the secondary result of platelet–platelet contact resulting from stimulation by adrenaline. In contrast, if the comparison is based on the maximal levels to which ADP and adrenaline can increase localized intracellular [Ca^{2+}] (Fig. 3.4) we would predict *incorrectly* (Table 3.1) that two agonists should be able directly to induce all the secretory responses and, for ADP, also possibly phosphatidylserine exposure. It would seem, therefore, that the localized increases in intracellular [Ca^{2+}] observed in aequorin-loaded platelets stimulated by ADP, adrenaline and thrombin do not occur at a site which is relevant for Ca^{2+}-driven secretion or phosphatidylserine exposure.

For collagen the situation is less clear. This agonist has the capacity to induce all the responses shown in Fig. 3.4 (Table 3.1) (Lyons *et al.* 1975) but fails to increase average cytosolic [Ca^{2+}]. However, in the presence of this agonist the threshold [Ca^{2+}] for arachidonate mobilization is markedly decreased such that this response occurs at the average cytosolic [Ca^{2+}] (0.1 μM) typical of the resting platelet (Fig. 3.4) (Pollock *et al.* 1986). The effect of collagen on the Ca^{2+}-dependency of other responses has not been examined. If a similar enhancement of sensitivity occurs, the discrepancy highlighted by comparison of Table 3.1 and Fig. 3.4 could be explained. In contrast no such additional factor(s) needs to be invoked if the comparison is based on data obtained using aequorin as the probe (Fig. 3.4) since the maximal level to which collagen increases localized intracellular [Ca^{2+}] is adequate to explain the pattern of responses observed (Table 3.1). For secretion and phosphatidylserine exposure this conclusion does not accord with that reached above on the basis of the data for ADP, adrenaline and thrombin. This further discrepancy can only be explained if we assume that collagen induces a localized increase in intracellular [Ca^{2+}] at a different, and physiologically more relevant, site than the other agonists. Such a postulate is not necessarily unreasonable since the increase in [1,2-diacylglycerol] observed in platelets stimulated by collagen results primarily from hydrolysis of phosphatidylcholine (Pollock *et al.* 1986) whereas agonists such as thrombin and PAF increase [1,2-diacylglycerol] as a consequence of enhanced phosphoinositide breakdown (MacIntyre *et al.* 1985c) (see 1,2-diacylglycerol, inositol-1,4,5-trisphosphate ($I(1,4,5)P_3$) and other inositol phosphates).

The analysis developed thus far has taken no account of the ability of agonists to induce aggregation. The dependence of the aggregation response on intracellular [Ca^{2+}] is not readily studied in permeabilized platelets since binding of fibrinogen to its receptor requires the presence of micromolar Ca^{2+} (Peerschke, 1985). However fibrinogen receptor expression, which is a prerequisite for aggregation, does not require extracellular Ca^{2+} and hence can be examined in permeabilized preparations using a monoclonal antibody such as PAC-1 which binds selectively to the active receptor (Shattil *et al.* 1985). Such studies have shown that Ca^{2+} has no *direct* capacity to induce fibrinogen receptor expression and increases PAC-1 binding only indirectly as a consequence of enhanced thromboxane A_2 synthesis

(Shattil & Brass, 1987). Notably agonists such as thrombin and 11,9-epoxymethano-prostaglandin H_2(U46619) as well as metabolically stable analogues of GTP such as 5′-guanylylimidodiphosphate (GppNHp) do markedly increase PAC-1 binding. This increased response is, at least for GppNHp, largely Ca^{2+}-dependent with a threshold at approximately 0.15 μM (Shattil & Brass, 1987). It is not at present clear how these findings relate to the known ability of divalent cation ionophores (e.g. A23187, ionomycin) to induce aggregation in intact platelets with an average cytosolic Ca^{2+} threshold of approximately 1 μM (Rink *et al.* 1982).

It is pertinent to note in this context that resting platelet intracellular [Ca^{2+}] as estimated using aequorin (0.3 μM) would be adequate, if present at the appropriate site, to induce shape change, P20 and P47 phosphorylation and possibly fibrinogen receptor expression. This is not the case when estimates of average cytosolic [Ca^{2+}] (0.1 μM) in the resting state resulting from studies using Fura2 are used (Fig. 3.4).

Factors which may modulate Ca^{2+}-driven responses

1,2-diacylglycerol/protein kinase C

Many platelet excitatory agonists induce 1,2-diacylglycerol formation as a consequence of activation of phosphoinositide phosphodiesterase (Table 3.1) (see 1,2-diacylglycerol, inositol-1,4,5-trisphosphate ($I(1,4,5)P_3$) and other inositol phosphates) while synthetic 1,2-diacylglycerols are known to decrease the Ca^{2+} concentration required to achieve activation of protein kinase C (Kishimoto *et al.* 1980; Kaibuchi *et al.* 1981; Nishizuka, 1984). Hence it is reasonable to propose that the 1,2-diacyl-glycerol/protein kinase C system is responsible for the enhancement of sensitivity to Ca^{2+} and/or of the maximal extent of response observed when permeabilized platelets are stimulated with Ca^{2+} in the presence of an excitatory agonist such as thrombin. Support for this postulate is provided by two observations.

1 For a range of excitatory agonists there is a reasonable correlation between their capacity to activate phosphoinositide phosphodiesterase in the intact platelet and to decrease the Ca^{2+} requirement for 5-HT secretion in the electropermeabilized platelet (Knight & Scrutton, 1985).

2 Synthetic 1,2-diacylglycerols, as well as other activators of protein kinase C such as TPA, reduce the Ca^{2+} requirement for 5-HT secretion (Knight *et al.* 1984) and arachidonate mobilization (Halenda & Rehm, 1987), and also induce fibrinogen receptor expression at 0.1 μM Ca^{2+} (Shattil & Brass, 1987).

Unfortunately direct evidence for participation of a protein kinase C substrate in any of these Ca^{2+}-driven responses has still not been obtained. The amino acid sequence of the major platelet protein kinase C substrate (P47) has now been deduced from analysis of the nucleotide sequence of the gene which encodes this protein (Tyers *et al.* 1988) but this analysis has failed to throw any light on the biological function of P47. The proposed identification of this protein as $I(1,4,5)P_3$ phosphomonoesterase (Connolly *et al.* 1986) or lipocortin (Touqui *et al.* 1986) has been shown not to be correct (Haslam, 1987).

GTP/guanine nucleotide binding (G) proteins

In many cells GTP and its metabolically stable analogues modulate Ca^{2+}-driven responses indirectly as a consequence of G_P-dependent activation of phosphoinositide phosphodiesterase and resultant 1,2-diacyl-glycerol formation (see 1,2-diacylglycerol, inositol-1,4,5-trisphosphate ($I(1,4,5)P_3$) and other inositol phosphates). In addition GTP and G-proteins have been implicated in direct modulation of Ca^{2+}-driven responses. Such a role was first recognized for lysosomal secretion in neutrophils by Barrowman *et al.* (1986) and is distinguished in permeabilized cell preparations by the following characteristics.

1 In the presence of a metabolically stable GTP analogue, e.g. GTPγS, the response either totally or partially loses its dependence on $[Ca^{2+}]$.

2 Metabolically stable analogues of GDP, e.g. GDPβS, inhibit the Ca^{2+}-driven response in the absence of added GTP or of GTP analogues.

3 GTPγS-stimulated 1,2-diacylglycerol or $I(1,4,5)P_3$ formation can be inhibited, e.g. by the addition of neomycin, without causing a corresponding inhibition of the GTPγS-driven response.

4 Synthetic 1,2-diacylglycerols are not effective in inducing the response when tested at subnanomolar $[Ca^{2+}]$.

The evidence for participation of a modulatory G-protein (G_X) in the platelet responses studied thus far (Table 3.2) is incomplete and does not in any case permit a definitive conclusion. The evidence is most convincing for arachidonate mobilization where Nakashima *et al.* (1987) have shown that neomycin inhibits GTPγS-induced 1,2-diacylglycerol formation at concentrations which have little effect on GTPγS-driven [^{3}H]arachidonate release (see also Fuse & Tai, 1987). Direct transmembrane receptor-phospholipase A_2 coupling cannot, however, occur in the platelet since this enzyme is localized in the endoplasmic reticulum (Lagarde *et al.* 1981). Hence if such coupling exists it must depend on movement of G_X-GTP or of GTP bound to a subunit of G_X from the plasma membrane to the endoplasmic reticulum.

The concept of direct transmembrane coupling involving a G_X protein is most attractive for fibrinogen receptor expression where participation of such a G_X protein would permit direct GTP-dependent communication between the receptor and the plasma membrane glycoprotein IIb–IIIa complex which acts as the fibrinogen receptor (see Chapter 2). The very marked induction of Ca^{2+}-dependent PAC-1 binding by GppNHp is in accord with this postulate although the failure of GDPβS to inhibit PAC-1 binding induced by high [thrombin] suggests that an additional GTP-independent route exists for such receptor–glycoprotein IIb–IIIa complex coupling (Shattil & Brass, 1987).

Table 3.2 Evidence for a role for a modulatory G protein (G_x) in various platelet responses

Response	Ca^{2+}-dependence at saturating [GTPγS] or [GppNHp]	Inhibition of Ca^{2+}-driven response by GDPβS	Differential inhibition of GTPγS-driven response and GTPγS-driven phosphoinositide phosphodiesterase	Induction of response by synthetic 1,2-diacylglycerol at low [Ca^{2+}]	References
Amine storage granule secretion	Complete*	None	n.d.	No[§]	Athayde & Scrutton (1989) (for both amine storage granule secretion and lysosomal secretion)
Lysosomal secretion	Partial[†]	None	n.d.	Small but significant	
Protein storage granule secretion	Complete*	None	n.d.	n.d.	Peltola & Scrutton (1989) (unpublished work)
Arachidonate mobilization	Partial	n.d.	Yes (neomycin)	n.d.	Nakashima *et al.* (1987)
Fibrinogen receptor expression	Partial	None[‡]	n.d.	?**	Shattil & Brass (1987)

* At a calculated [Ca^{2+}] of <0.1 nM.
[†] At a calculated [Ca^{2+}] of approximately 1 nM.
[‡] For the TPA-driven response.
[§] TPA induces a response under these conditions. TPA is also, and more, effective.
** TPA induces a response at 0.1 μM Ca^{2+}.
n.d. = no data.

For the secretory responses the evidence is confusing since some parts of the data support the involvement of such a modulatory G protein, which is usually designated as G_E, while other parts do not (Table 3.2). Selective involvement of a putative G_E protein in platelet lysosomal secretion could have explained the observation that only certain agonists are effective in inducing this response (Table 3.1). However, the data obtained thus far (Table 3.2) do not suggest any marked differences between the effects of the guanine nucleotides on these secretory responses (Athayde & Scrutton, 1989; Peltola & Scrutton, 1989, unpublished data). The agonist selectivity observed for amine storage granule and lysosomal secretion (Table 3.1) appears to arise from the differing effects of 1,2-diacylglycerol on the Ca^{2+}-driven responses (Knight *et al.* 1984).

Phosphatidylserine exposure (prothrombinase activation)

In addition to inducing responses such as shape change and secretion (see Ca^{2+}-driven responses) an increase in cytosolic [Ca^{2+}] into the micromolar range is also one mechanism responsible for increasing phosphatidylserine exposure on the platelet surface and hence enhancing prothrombinase activity (Bevers *et al.* 1983). However, features of this latter response suggest that the underlying mechanism by which an increase in [Ca^{2+}] induces phosphatidylserine exposure may differ qualitatively from that involved in other Ca^{2+}-driven responses. An increase in cytosolic [Ca^{2+}] mediates these latter responses by enhancing Ca^{2+}-dependent protein phosphorylation (see Ca^{2+}-driven responses) whereas Ca^{2+}-driven phosphatidylserine exposure is proposed to be at least in part a consequence of Ca^{2+}-dependent degradation of cytoskeletal proteins such as talin and filamin. The resultant disorganization of the cytoskeleton may remove constraints which localize phosphatidylserine to the inner leaflet of the plasma membrane in the resting platelet and hence permit expression of this phospholipid on the platelet surface (Verhallen *et al.* 1987). This postulate is supported by several lines of evidence.

1 The similar time courses for prothrombinase activation and cytoskeletal degradation observed when platelets are exposed to a range of agents such as divalent cation ionophores, local anaesthetics, F^- and collagen, which induce these responses over time-spans ranging from 20 seconds to 40–50 minutes (Verhallen *et al.* 1987, 1988). Some of these agents, e.g. local anaesthetics, inhibit, rather than enhance other Ca^{2+}-driven responses (Feinstein *et al.* 1976).

2 The similar dependence of prothrombinase activation and cytoskeletal degradation on Ca^{2+} concentration as measured in platelets permeabilized selectively to this cation using a divalent cation ionophore (Verhallen *et al.* 1987).

3 The effect of inhibitors of Ca^{2+}-dependent neutral protease (calpain) such as leupeptin which, when they are active, block both cytoskeletal degradation and prothrombinase activation (Verhallen *et al.* 1988). Such compounds do not cause agonist non-selective inhibition of other Ca^{2+}-driven responses although they do block these responses when induced by thrombin as a consequence of their action as seryl protease inhibitors (Ruda & Scrutton, 1987).

It is, however, unlikely that an acute increase in cytosolic [Ca^{2+}] is the only, or even physiologically the most important, element in the signal transduction mechanism which mediates agonist-induced phosphatidylserine exposure. As noted above (Ca^{2+}-driven responses) there is no correlation between the ability of a series of agonists to induce phosphatidylserine exposure and the extent to which these agonists increase intraplatelet [Ca^{2+}]. This lack of correlation exists whether the comparison is based on measurement of average cytosolic [Ca^{2+}] using Fura2 or of localized intracellular [Ca^{2+}] using aequorin (Fig. 3.4). The increase in plasma membrane [1,2-diacylglycerol] which occurs as a consequence of stimulation with collagen (Rittenhouse-Simmons, 1984) might provide an alternative mechanism for enhancing phosphatidylserine exposure on the platelet surface since localized generation of 1,2-diacylglycerol is known to form non-bilayer structures and hence to facilitate transbilayer movement of phospholipids (Quinn & Chapman, 1980). However, other agonists such as thrombin and PAF which increase platelet 1,2-diacylglycerol levels (Table 3.1) fail to increase phosphatidylserine exposure significantly unless, in the case of thrombin, they are added together with collagen (Bevers *et al.* 1983).

The extent of *net* phosphatidylserine exposure on the platelet surface depends, however, not only on movement of this phospholipid from the inner to the outer leaflet of the plasma membrane, but also on its movement from the outer to the inner leaflet catalysed by ATP-dependent amino-phospholipid translocase (Sune *et al.* 1987; Bevers *et al.* 1989) (Fig. 3.5). Increased phosphatidylserine exposure may, therefore, be induced by inhibition of aminophospholipid translocase as well as by enhanced cytoskeletal degradation. Translocase activity is decreased by a fall in the sulphydryl:disulphide ratio caused by addition of -SH oxidizing agents such as diamide (Connor & Schroit, 1988). This effect may explain the ability of diamide and related compounds to enhance prothrombinase activity as well as the observation that dithiothreitol reverses the diamide-induced response as well as the activation of prothrombinase by divalent cation ionophores or by collagen + thrombin (Bevers *et al.* 1989). Enhancement of phosphatidylserine exposure (and hence prothrombinase activity) by collagen could, therefore, result from inhibition of aminophospholipid translocase by a mechanism possibly involving reduction in the cellular -SH:-S.S- ratio. This postulate is incorporated in the scheme shown in Fig. 3.5. It may be significant in this regard that an initial lag period characterizes the development of prothrombinase activity induced by exposure of platelets to collagen + thrombin. In this respect the response induced by collagen + thrombin resembles that induced by -SH oxidizing agents such as diamide more closely than that resulting from addition of the divalent cation ionophores (Bevers *et al.* 1989). The scheme shown in Fig. 3.5 readily explains the synergistic relationship between the activation of prothrombinase by collagen and

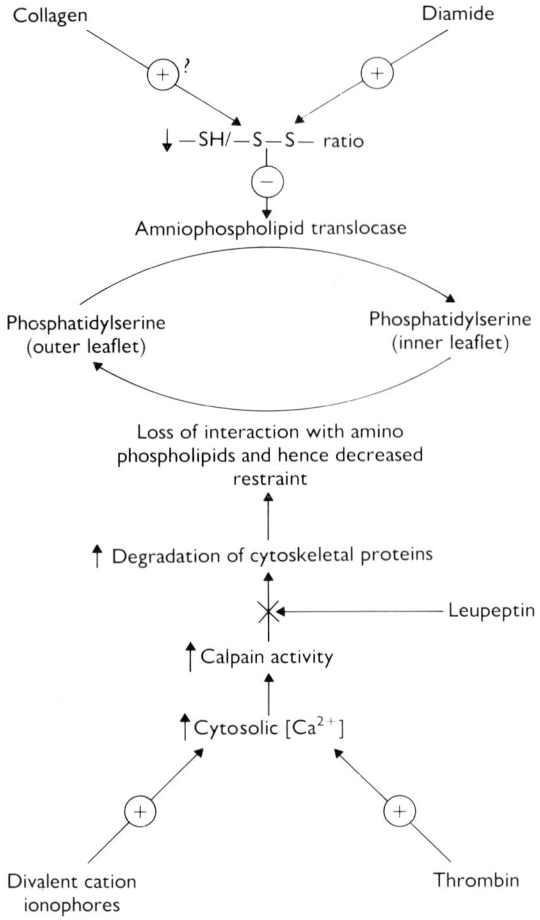

Figure 3.5 Postulated scheme which may explain agonist-induced phosphatidylserine exposure. The scheme is based in part on the data of Verhallen *et al.* (1987, 1988) and Bevers *et al.* (1989). (See note added in press, p. 99.)

thrombin since these two agonists are proposed to act on opposite sides of the translocation cycle.

It is of interest that some features of the mechanisms which are proposed as being involved in the exposure of phosphatidylserine on the platelet surface, e.g. cytoskeletal degradation, calpain activation, are similar to events implicated in the response of hepatocytes to oxidative stress induced by addition of agents such as menadione or cystamine. In this latter system a decrease in the reduced: oxidized glutathione ratio is postulated to cause a sustained increase in cytosolic [Ca^{2+}] by blocking Ca^{2+} efflux from the cell and hence to lead to calpain activation and cytoskeletal degradation. Morphological changes on the cell surface, e.g. bleb formation, are observed as a consequence of exposure of hepatocytes to oxidative stress but phospholipid distribution between the two leaflets of the plasma membrane does not seem to have been examined (Cotgreave *et al.* 1988).

Platelet activation by adrenaline

Platelet activation induced by most conventional excitatory agonists can be adequately explained by the ability of those agonists to increase either average cytosolic [Ca^{2+}] and/or plasma membrane [1,2-diacylglycerol] (Table 3.1). Adrenaline is, however, an exception since it is generally recognized that this agonist itself induces neither of these responses although increases in average cytosolic [Ca^{2+}] and in [1,2-diacylglycerol] *induced by other agonists* are enhanced by addition of adrenaline (Thompson *et al.* 1986; Bushfield *et al.* 1987). These latter effects adequately explain the well-documented response in which adrenaline enhances aggregation and/or secretion induced by other excitatory agonists.

The capacity of adrenaline to induce aggregation *in the absence of such agonists* is more controversial and has recently been questioned (Kinlough-Rathbone & Mustard, 1986). However, comprehensive recent studies have confirmed that fibrinogen receptor expression, fibrinogen binding and aggregation do result from the addition of adrenaline under conditions where possible contributions from other excitatory agonists have been eliminated (Petty & Scrutton, 1989; Shattil *et al.* 1989). The signal transduction mechanism responsible for mediating this latter response is not well defined. According to conventional dogma (Fain & Garcia-Sainz, 1980) a decrease in intracellular cAMP might be expected to mediate the response since aggregation induced by adrenaline involves occupancy of an α_2-adrenoceptor (Grant & Scrutton, 1979). Although adrenaline decreases platelet cAMP levels when added in the presence of an inhibitory agonist (Haslam, 1975) there is no evidence that this effect is responsible for inducing aggregation (Haslam *et al.* 1978). Adrenaline has also been reported to increase localized intracellular [Ca^{2+}] as measured using aequorin as a probe (Ware *et al.* 1986) (Table 1) and this effect could in principle explain the observed response (see Ca^{2+}-driven responses). The situation is further complicated by evidence which indicates that more than one type of α_2-adrenoceptor may be present on the platelet. For example, in platelets obtained from certain patients with myeloproliferative diseases apparent absence of the ability to aggregate in response to adrenaline is associated with selective loss of an α_2-adrenoceptor population which is detected using dihydroergocryptine, but not yohimbine, as a radioligand. In such platelets adrenaline still enhances aggregation induced by other agonists (the pro-aggregatory response), due presumably to its ability to enhance increases in average cytosolic [Ca^{2+}] and in [1,2-diacylglycerol], and also inhibits adenylate cyclase (Swart *et al.* 1984). Hence the data suggest that a unique α_2-adrenoceptor (α_{2x}) working via an as yet undefined signal transduction system mediates aggregation induced by adrenaline itself. The pro-aggregatory response and the inhibition of adenylate cyclase induced by this agonist would appear from these data to be mediated by a more conventional α_2-adrenoceptor (α_{2y}) albeit one which can enhance indirectly the extent of activation of phosphoinositide phosphodiesterase in addition to its more direct effect on the activity of adenylate cyclase. This interpretation is not, however, in accord with studies using a range of α_2-adrenoceptor agonists and antagonists which indicate that the α_2-adrenoceptor responsible for inhibition of adenylate cyclase is distinct from that which mediates the aggregatory and pro-aggregatory responses induced by adrenaline (Clare *et al.* 1984). Much further work is needed to resolve these discrepancies and to define how signal transduction from the platelet α_2-adrenoceptor(s) relates to that characteristic of platelet receptors for other excitatory agonists.

Conclusions

In this chapter we have attempted to indicate the current status of understanding of the signal transduction mechanisms used by well-described platelet excitatory and inhibitory agonists and to relate some of the mechanisms in a semi-quantitative way, to the responses induced by these agonists. Although susbstantial progress has been made in recent years large areas of uncertainty still remain even in this well-studied area. Little attention has been paid to the role of platelets in responses other than those of haemostasis and of the repair of vascular damage although it has been recognized for many years that this cell has such other roles, e.g. in inflammation. It is, therefore, not surprising that the signal transduction mechanisms responsible for mediating these latter responses have not been examined. Investigations in this area may provide a satisfying rationale for production of 12-lipoxygenase metabolites by platelets and for the ability of this cell to perform processes such as phagocytosis (Mustard & Packham, 1968) and cytocidal responses (Cesbron *et al.* 1987).

References

Adunyah, S.E. & Dean, W.L. (1987) Regulation of human platelet membrane Ca^{2+} transport by cAMP- and calmodulin-dependent phosphorylation. *Biochim Biophys Acta* **930**, 401–409.

Agranoff, B.W., Murthy, P. & Segiun, E.B. (1983) Thrombin-induced phosphodiesteractic cleavage of phosphatidylinositol-bis-phosphate in human platelets. *J Biol Chem* **258**, 2076–2078.

Athayde, C.M. & Scrutton, M.C. (1990) Guanine nucleotides and Ca^{2+}-dependent lysosomal secretion in electropermeabilised human platelets. *Eur J Biochem* **189**, 647–655.

Authi, K.S. & Crawford, N.V. (1985) Inositol-1,4,5-trisphosphate-induced release of sequestered Ca^{2+} from highly purified human platelet intracellular membranes. *Biochem J* **230**, 247–253.

Baldassare, J.J. & Fisher, G.J. (1986) Regulation of membrane-associated and cytosolic phospholipase C activities in human platelets by guanosine triphosphate. *J Biol Chem* **261**, 11942–11944.

Banga, H.S., Simons, E.R., Brass, L.F. & Rittenhouse, S.E. (1986) Activation of phospholipases A_2 and C in human platelets exposed to epinephrine: role of glycoproteins IIb and IIIa and dual role of epinephrine. *Proc Natl Acad Sci USA* **83**, 9197–9201.

Banga, H.S., Walker, R.K., Winberry, L.K. & Rittenhouse, S.E. (1988) Platelet adenylate cyclase and phospholipase C are affected differentially by ADP-ribosylation. Effects on thrombin-mediated responses. *Biochem J* **252**, 297–300.

Barrowman, M.M., Cockcroft, S. & Gomperts, B.D. (1986) Two roles for guanine nucleotides in the stimulus secretion sequence of neutrophils. *Nature* **319**, 504–507.

Berridge, M.J. (1987) Inositol trisphosphate and diacylglycerol: two interacting second messengers. *Ann Rev*

Biochem **56**, 159–193.

Bevers, E.M., Comfurius, P. & Zwaal, R.F.A. (1983) Changes in membrane phospholipid distribution during platelet activation. *Biochim Biophys Acta* **736**, 57–66.

Bevers, E.M., Tilly, R.H.J., Senden, J.M.G., Comfurius, P. & Zwaal, R.F.A. (1989) Exposure of endogenous phosphatidylserine at the outer surface of stimulated platelets is reversed by restoration of aminophospholipid translocase activity. *Biochemistry* **28**, 2382–2387.

Biden, T.J. & Wolheim, C.B. (1986) Ca^{2+} regulates the inositol tris/tetrakisphosphate pathway in intact and broken preparations of insulin-secreting RINm5F cells. *J Biol Chem* **261**, 11 931–11 934.

Bishop, W.R. & Bell, R.M. (1986) Attenuation of sn-1, 2-diacylglycerol second messengers. *J Biol Chem* **261**, 12 513–12 519.

Brass, L.F. (1984) The effect of Na^+ on Ca^{2+} homeostasis in unstimulated platelets. *J Biol Chem* **259**, 12 571–12 575.

Brass, L.F. (1988) G Proteins and the generation of second messengers in platelets. *ISI Atlas of Science: Biochemistry*, pp. 343–354. ISI, Philadelphia.

Brass, L.F. & Laposata, M. (1987) Diacylglycerol causes Ca^{2+} release from the platelet dense tubular system: comparisons with Ca^{2+} release caused by inositol-1,4,5-tris phosphate. *Biochem Biophys Res Commun* **142**, 7–14.

Brass, L.F., Laposata, M., Banga, H.S. & Rittenhouse, S.E. (1986) Regulation of the phosphoinositide hydrolysis pathway in thrombin-stimulated platelets by a pertussis toxin-sensitive guanine-nucleotide binding protein. Evaluation of its contribution to platelet activation and comparisons with the adenylate cyclase inhibitory protein, G_i. *J Biol Chem* **261**, 16 838–16 847.

Brass, L.F., Shaller, C.C. & Delmonte, E.J. (1987) Inositol-1,4,5-trisphosphate-induced granule secretion in platelets. Evidence that activation of Phospholipase C mediated by thromboxane receptors involves a guanine nucleotide binding protein-dependent mechanism distinct from that of thrombin. *J Clin Invest* **79**, 1269–1275.

Brass, L.F., Woolkakis, M.J. & Manning, D.R. (1988) Interactions in platelets between G proteins and the agonists that stimulate phospholipase C and inhibit adenylyl cyclase. *J Biol Chem* **263**, 5348–5355.

Bushfield, M., McNicol, A. & MacIntyre, D.E. (1985) Inhibition of platelet-activating-factor-induced human platelet activation by prostaglandin D_2. Differential sensitivity of platelet transduction processes and functional responses to inhibition by cyclic AMP. *Biochem J* **232**, 267–271.

Bushfield, M., McNicol, A. & MacIntyre, D.E. (1987) Possible mechanisms of the potentation of blood platelet activation by adrenaline. *Biochem J* **241**, 671–676.

Carrol, R.C., Butler, R.G., Morris, P.A. & Gerrard, J.M. (1982) Separable assembly of platelet pseudopodal and contractile cytoskeletons. *Cell* **30**, 385–393.

Cesbron, J.Y., Capron, A., Vargaftig, B.B., Lagarde, M., Pincemail, J., Braquet, P., Taelman, H. & Joseph, M. (1987) Platelets mediate the action of diethylcarbamazine on microfilariae. *Nature* **325**, 533–536.

Clare, K.A., Scrutton, M.C. & Thompson, N.T. (1984) Effect of α_2-adrenoceptor agonists and antagonists and of related compounds on aggregation of, and on adenylate cyclase activity in, human platelets. *Br J Pharmacol* **82**, 467–476.

Cobbold, P.M. & Rink, T.J. (1987) Fluoresence and bioluminesence measurement of cytoplasmic free calcium. *Biochem J* **248**, 313–328.

Connolly, T.M. & Limbird, L.E. (1983) Removal of extraplatelet Na^+ eliminates indomethacin-sensitive secretion from human platelets stimulated by epinephrine, ADP and thrombin. *Proc Natl Acad Sci USA* **80**, 5320–5324.

Connolly, T.M., Lawing, W.J. & Majerus, P.W. (1986) Protein kinase C phosphorylates human platelet inositol trisphosphate 5′-phosphomonoesterase, increasing the phosphatase activity. *Cell* **46**, 951–958.

Connor, J. & Schroit, A.J. (1988) Transbilayer movement of phosphatidylserine in erythrocytes: inhibition of transport and preferential labelling of a 31 000 dalton protein by sulfhydryl reactive reagents. *Biochemistry* **27**, 848–851.

Cotgreave, I.A., Moldeus, P. & Orrenius, S. (1988) Host biochemical defense mechanisms against prooxidants. *Ann Rev Pharmacol Toxicol* **28**, 189–212.

Crawford, N.V. & Scrutton, M.C. (1987) Biochemistry of the blood platelet. In Bloom, A.L. & Thomas, D.P. (eds) *Haemostasis and Thrombosis*, 2nd edn, pp. 47–77. Churchill Livingstone, Edinburgh.

Culty, M., Davidson, M.M.L. & Haslam, R.J. (1988) Guanosine-5′-[-thio]-triphosphate and thrombin stimulate the hydrolysis of polyphosphoinositides by phospholipase C in electropermeabilised human platelets. *Eur J Biochem* **171**, 523–533.

Daniel, J.F., Danglemaier, C.A., Selak, M. & Smith, J.B. (1986) ADP stimulates IP_3 formation in human platelets. *FEBS Lett* **206**, 299–303.

Deckmyn, H., Tu, S.-M. & Majerus, P.W. (1986) Guanine nucleotides stimulate soluble phosphoinositide-specific phospholipase C in the absence of membranes. *J Biol Chem* **261**, 16 553–16 558.

Dejesus, M., Fikrig, S. & Detwiler, T. (1972) Phagocytosis-stimulated nitrobluetetrazolium reduction by platelets. *J Lab Clin Med* **80**, 117–124.

Dodds, W.J. (1978) Platelet function in animals: species specificities. In De Gaetano, G. & Garrattini, S. (eds) *Platelets; a multidisciplinary approach*, pp. 45–59. Raven Press, New York.

Edgecombe, M. & Scrutton, M.C. (1987) Relationship between elevation of cyclic-3′,5′-GMP(cGMP) and aggregate formation in human platelets. *Thromb Haemost* **58**, 469.

Edgecombe, M. & Scrutton, M.C. (1988) Agonist-induced increases in platelet cyclic-3′,5′-GMP(cGMP) levels: a role in feedback modulation of the aggregation response? *Br J Haematol* **69**, 127.

El-Mofty, S., Scrutton, M.C., Serroni, A., Nicolini, C. & Farber, J.L. (1975) Early and reversible plasma injury in galactosamine-induced liver cell death. *Am J Pathol* **79**, 579–595.

Fain, J.N. & Garcia-Sainz, J.A. (1980) Role of phosphatidylinositol turnover in α_1-adrenoceptor, and adenylate cyclase inhibition in α_2-adrenoceptor, effects of catecholamines. *Life Sci* **26**, 1183–1194.

Feinberg, H., Sandler, W.C., Scorer, M., LeBreton, G.C., Grossman, B. & Born, G.V.R. (1977) Movement of Na^+ into human platelets induced by ADP. *Biochim Biophys Acta* **470**, 317–324.

Feinstein, M.G., Fiekes, J. & Fraser, C. (1976) An analysis of the mechanism of local anaesthetic inhibition of platelet aggregation and secretion. *J Pharmacol Exp Therap* **197**, 215–228.

Fisher, G.J., Bakshian, S. & Baldassare, J.J. (1985) Activation of human platelets by ADP causes a rapid rise in cytosolic free calcium without hydrolysis of phosphatidylinositol-4,5-bisphosphate. *Biochem Biophys Res Commun* **129**, 958–964.

Fujimura, K. & Phillips, D.R. (1983) Calcium cation regulation of glycoprotein IIb–IIIa complex formation in platelet plasma membranes. *J Biol Chem* **258**, 10 247–10 252.

Funder, J., Hershco, L., Rothstein, A. & Livne, A. (1988) Na^+/H^+ exchange and aggregation of human platelets activated by ADP: the exchange is not required for aggregation. *Biochim Biophys Acta* **938**, 425–433.

Fuse, I. & Tai, H.H. (1987) Stimulations of arachidonate release and inositol-1,4,5-trisphosphate formation are mediated by distinct G-roteins in human platelets. *Biochem Biophys Res Commun* **146**, 659–665.

Gilman, A.G. (1987) G Proteins: transducers of receptor-generated signals. *Ann Rev Biochem* **56**, 615–650.

Grant, J.A. & Scrutton, M.C. (1979) Novel α_2-adrenoceptors primarily responsible for inducing platelet aggregation. *Nature* **277**, 659–661.

Hack, N., Croset, M. & Crawford, N.V. (1986) Studies on the bivalent cation activated ATPase activities of highly purified human platelet surface and intracellular membranes. *Biochem J* **233**, 661–668.

Halenda, S.P. & Rehm, A.G. (1987) Thrombin and C-kinase activators potentiate calcium-stimulated arachidonic acid release in human platelets. *Biochem J* **248**, 471–475.

Hallam, T.J. & Rink, T.J. (1985a) Responses to adenosine diphosphate in human platelets loaded with the fluorescent indicator quin2. *J Physiol* **368**, 131–146.

Hallam, T.J. & Rink, T.J. (1985b) Agonists stimulate divalent cation channels in the plasma membrane of human platelets. *FEBS Lett* **186**, 175–179.

Hallam, T.J. & Rink, T.J. (1989) Receptor-mediated Ca^{2+} entry: diversity of function and mechanism. *Trends Pharmacol Sci* **10**, 8–10.

Hallam, T.J., Sanchez, A. & Rink, T.J. (1984a) Stimulus–response coupling in human platelets. Changes evoked by platelet-activating factor in cytoplasmic free calcium monitored with the fluorescent calcium indicator quin2. *Biochem J* **218**, 819–827.

Hallam, T.J., Thompson, N.T., Scrutton, M.C. & Rink, T.J. (1984b) The role of cytoplasmic free calcium in the responses of quin2-loaded platelets to vasopressin. *Biochem J* **221**, 897–901.

Hallam, T.J., Daniel, J.L., Kendrick-Jones, J. & Rink, T.J. (1985) Relationship between cytoplasmic free calcium and myosin light chain phosphorylation in intact platelets. *Biochem J* **232**, 373–377.

Hallam, T.J., Poenie, M. & Tsien, R.Y. (1986) Homogeneity of ADP- and Thrombin-stimulated rises in $[Ca^{2+}]_i$ in Fura-loaded human platelet populations revealed by fluoresence image processing. *J Physiol* **377**, 123P.

Hallam, T.J., Jacob, R. & Merritt, J.E. (1988) Evidence that agonists stimulate bivalent cation influx into human endothelial cells. *Biochem J* **255**, 179–184.

Hallam, T.J., Jacob, R. & Merritt, J.E. (1989) Influx of bivalent cations can be independent of receptor stimulation in human endothelial cells. *Biochem J* **259**, 125–129.

Haslam, R.J. (1975) Roles of cyclic nucleotides in platelet function. *Ciba Foundation Symp. No. 35* (new series), pp. 121–143.

Haslam, R.J. (1987) Signal transduction in platelet activation. In Verstraete, M., Vermylen, J., Lijnen, R. & Arnout, J. (eds) *Haemostasis and Thrombosis 1987*, pp. 147–174. Leuven University Press, Belgium.

Haslam, R.J. & Davidson, M.M.L. (1984a) Receptor-induced diacylglycerol formation in permeabilised platelets: possible role for a GTP-binding protein. *J Receptor Res* **4**, 605–629.

Haslam, R.J. & Davidson, M.M.L. (1984b) Potentiation by thrombin of the secretion of serotonin from permeabilised platelets equilibrated with Ca^{2+} buffers. Relationship to protein phosphorylation and diacylglycerol formation. *Biochem J* **222**, 351–361.

Haslam, R.J. & Lynham, J.A. (1977) Relationship between phosphorylation of blood platelet proteins and secretion of platelet granule constituents. I. Effects of different aggregating agents. *Biochem Biophys Res Commun* **77**, 714–721.

Haslam, R.J., Davidson, M.M.L. & Desjardins, J.V. (1978) Inhibition of adenylate cyclase by adenosine analogues in broken and intact human platelets: evidence for unidirectional control of platelet function by cyclic-3′,5′,-adenosine monophosphate. *Biochem J* **176**, 83–95.

Haslam, R.J., Salama, S.E., Fox, J.E.B., Lynham, J.A. & Davidson, M.M.L. (1980) Roles of cyclic nucleotides and of protein phosphorylation in the regulation of platelet function. In Rotman, A., Meyer, F.A., Gitler, C. & Silberberg, A. (eds) *Platelets: Cellular Response Mechanisms and their Biological Significance*, pp. 213–231. Wiley, Chichester.

Haslam, R.J., Davidson, M.M.L., Knight, D.E. &

Scrutton, M.C. (1985a) GTP not Cyclic GMP enhances secretion from permeabilised platelets. *Nature* **313**, 821–822.

Haslam, R.J., Williams, K.A. & Davidson, M.M.L. (1985b) Receptor–effector coupling in platelets: roles of guanine nucleotides. In Westwick, J., Scully, M.F., MacIntyre, D.E. & Kakkar, V.V. (eds) *Mechanisms of Stimulus–Response Coupling in Platelets*, pp. 265–280. Plenum Press, New York.

Henderson, A.H., Morgan, R.O. & Newby, A.C. (1987) The inhibition by sodium nitroprusside of ADP-induced calcium influx and calcium mobilisation in human platelets. *J Physiol* **387**, 89P.

Higgs, E.A., Moncada, S., Vane, J.R., Caen, J.P., Michel, H. & Tobelem, G. (1978) Effect of prostacyclin (PGI_2) on platelet adhesion to rabbit arterial subendothelium. *Prostaglandins* **23**, 437–457.

Hill, T.D., Dean, N.M. & Boynton, A.L. (1988) Inositol-1,3,4,5-tetrakisphosphate induces Ca^{2+} sequestration in rat liver cells. *Science* **242**, 1176–1178.

Hirota, K., Hirota, J., Aginlera, G. & Catt, K.J. (1985) Hormone-induced redistribution of calcium-activated phospholipid-dependent protein kinase in pituitary gonadotrophs. *J Biol Chem* **260**, 3243–3246.

Horne, W.C. & Simons, E.R. (1978) Effects of amiloride on the response of human platelets to bovine alpha thrombin. *Thromb Res* **13**, 599–607.

Horne, W.C., Norman, N.E., Schwartz, D.B. & Simons, E.R. (1981) Changes in cytoplasmic pH and in membrane potential in thrombin-stimulated platelets. *Eur J Biochem* **120**, 295–302.

Howell, T.W. & Gomperts, B.D. (1987) Rat mast cells permeabilised with streptolysin-O secrete histamine in response to Ca^{2+} at concentrations buffered in the micromolar range. *Biochim Biophys Acta* **927**, 177–183.

Hrbolich, J.K., Culty, M. & Haslam, R.J. (1987) Activation of phospholipase C associated with rabbit platelet membranes by guanosine-5′-[γ-thio]-triphosphate and by thrombin in the presence of GTP. *Biochem J* **243**, 457–465.

Ignarro, L.J., Adams, J.B., Horowitz, P.M. & Wood, K.S. (1986) Activation of soluble guanylate cyclase by NO-heme exchange. Comparison of heme-containing and heme-deficient forms. *J Biol Chem* **261**, 4997–5002.

Irvine, R.F. & Moor, R.M. (1986) Microinjection of inositol-1,3,4,5-tetrakisphosphate activates sea urchin eggs by a mechanism dependent on external Ca^{2+}. *Biochem J* **240**, 914–920.

Jakobs, K.H., Saur, W. & Schultz, G. (1976) Reduction of adenylate cyclase activity in lysates of human platelets by the alpha-adrenergic component of epinephrine. *J Cyclic Nucleotide Res* **2**, 381–392.

Jakobs, K.H., Bauer, S. & Watanabe, Y. (1985) Modulation of adenylate cyclase of human platelets by phorbol ester. Impairement of the hormone-sensitive inhibitory pathway. *Eur J Biochem* **151**, 425–430.

Johnson, P.C., Ware, J.A., Smith, M., Cliveden, P.B., Dvorak, A.M. & Salzman, E.W. (1985) Measurement of ionised calcium in blood platelets with the photoprotein aequorin: comparison with quin2. *J Biol Chem* **260**, 2069–2076.

Jones, G.D. & Gear, A.R.L. (1988) Subsecond calcium dynamics in ADP- and thrombin-stimulated platelets: a continuous flow approach using Indo l. *Blood* **71**, 1539–1543.

Kaibuchi, K., Takai, Y. & Nishizuka, Y. (1981) Cooperative roles of various membrane phospholipids in the activation of calcium-activated phospholipid-dependent protein kinase. *J Biol Chem* **256**, 7146–7149.

Kaser-Glanzmann, R., Jakabova, M., George, J.N. & Luscher, E.F. (1977) Stimulation of calcium uptake in platelet membrane vesicles by adenosine-3′,5′-cyclic monophosphate and protein kinase. *Biochim Biophys Acta* **466**, 429–440.

Kinlough-Rathbone, R.L. & Mustard, J.F. (1986) Synergism of agonists. In Holmsen, H. (ed.) *Platelet Responses and Metabolism*, Vol. 1, pp. 193–208. CRC Press Inc., Boca Raton, Florida.

King, W.G. & Rittenhouse, S.E. (1989) Inhibition of protein kinase C by staurosporine promotes elevated accumulations of inositol trisphosphates and tetrakisphosphates in human platelets exposed to thrombin. *J Biol Chem* **264**, 6070–6074.

Kishimoto, A., Takai, Y., Mori, T., Kikkawa, U. & Nishizuka, Y. (1980) Activation of calcium and phospholipid-dependent protein kinase by diacylglycerol; its possible relation to phosphatidylinositol turnover. *J Biol Chem* **255**, 2273–2276.

Knight, D.E. & Scrutton, M.C. (1985) Effects of various excitatory agonists on the secretion of 5-hydroxytryptamine from permeabilised human platelets induced by Ca^{2+} in the presence or absence of GTP. *FEBS Lett* **183**, 417–422.

Knight, D.E. & Scrutton, M.C. (1986a) Effects of guanine nucleotides on the properties of 5-hydroxytryptamine secretion from human platelets. *Eur J Biochem* **160**, 183–190.

Knight, D.E. & Scrutton, M.C. (1986b) Gaining access to the cytosol: the technique and some applications of electropermeabilisation. *Biochem J* **234**, 497–506.

Knight, D.E. & Scrutton, M.C. (1987) Secretion of 5-hydroxytryptamine from electropermeabilised human platelets: effects of GTP and cyclic-3′,5′-AMP. *FEBS Lett* **233**, 47–52.

Knight, D.E., Hallam, T.J. & Scrutton, M.C. (1982) Second messenger concentration and agonist selectivity in Ca^{2+}-mediated secretion. *Nature* **296**, 256–257.

Knight, D.E., Niggli, V. & Scrutton, M.C. (1984) Thrombin and activators of protein kinase C modulate secretory responses of permeabilised human platelets induced by Ca^{2+}. *Eur J Biochem* **143**, 437–446.

Krishnamurthi, S., Patel, Y. & Kakkar, V.V. (1988) Inhibition of platelet aggregation, Ca^{2+} mobilisation and granule secretion by guanosine-5′-[β-thio-] diphosphate and GDP in intact platelets. Evidence for an inhibitory mechanism unrelated to inhibition of G-protein-GTP interaction. *Biochem J* **250**, 209–214.

Kucera, G.L. & Rittenhouse, S.E. (1988) Inhibition by GDPβS of agonist-activated phospholipase C in human platelets requires cell permeabilisation. *Biochem Biophys Res Commun* **153**, 417–421.

Lagarde, M. (1987) Role of cyclooxygenase and lipoxygenase metabolites in platelets. In MacIntyre, D.E. & Gordon, J.L. (eds) *Platelets in Biology and Pathology 3*, pp. 269–288. Elsevier/North Holland Biomedical Press, Amsterdam.

Lagarde, M., Menashi, S. & Crawford, N.V. (1981) Localisation of phospholipase A_2 and diglyceride lipase activities in human platelet intracellular membranes. *FEBS Lett* **124**, 23–26.

Lansman, J.B., Hallam, T.J. & Rink, T.J. (1987) Single stretch-activated ion channels in vascular endothelial cells as mechanotransducers. *Nature* **325**, 811–813.

Lanza, F., Beretz, A., Kubina, M. & Cazenave, J.P. (1987) Increased aggregation and secretion responses of human platelets when loaded with the calcium fluorescent probes, quin2 and Fura2. *Thromb Haemost* **58**, 737–743.

Lapetina, E.G., Silio, J. & Ruggiero, M. (1985) Thrombin induces serotinin secretion and aggregation independently of inositol phospholipid hydrolysis and protein phosphorylation in human platelets permeabilised with saponin. *J Biol Chem* **260**, 7078–7083.

LePeuch, C.J., LePeuch, D.A., Katz, S., DeMaille, J.G., Hincke, M.T., Bredoux, R., Enouf, J., Levy-Toledano, S. & Caen, J. (1983) Regulation of calcium accumulation and efflux from platelet vesicles. Possible role for cyclic AMP. *Biochim Biophys Acta* **731**, 456–464.

Lyons, R.M., Stanford, N. & Majerus, P.W. (1975) Thrombin-induced protein phosphorylation in human platelets. *J Clin Invest* **56**, 924–936.

MacIntyre, D.E. & Rink, T.J. (1982) The role of platelet membrane potential in the initiation of platelet aggregation. *Thromb Haemost* **47**, 22–26.

MacIntyre, D.E., McNicol, A. & Drummond, A.H. (1985a) Tumour-promoting phorbol esters inhibit agonist-induced phosphatidate formation and Ca^{2+} flux in human platelets. *FEBS Lett* **180**, 160–164.

MacIntyre, D.E., Bushfield, M. & Shaw, A.M. (1985b) Regulation of platelet cytosolic free calcium by cyclic nucleotides and protein kinase C. *FEBS Lett* **188**, 383–388.

MacIntyre, D.E., Pollock, W.K., Shaw, A.M., Bushfield, M., MacMillan, L.J. & McNicol, A. (1985c) Agonist-induced inositol phospholipid metabolism and Ca^{2+} flux in human platelet activation. *Adv Exp Med Biol* **192**, 127–144.

McGowan, E.B. & Detwiler, T.C. (1986) Modified platelet responses to thrombin. Evidence for two types of receptors or coupling mechanisms. *J Biol Chem* **261**, 739–746.

Marcus, A.J. (1979) Pathways of oxygen utilisation by stimulated platelets and leukocytes. *Sem Haematol* **16**, 188–195.

Mauco, G., Dangelmaier, C.A. & Smith, J.B. (1984) Inositol lipids, phosphatidate and diacylglycerol share stearoylarachidonylglycerol as a common backbone in thrombin-stimulated platelets. *Biochem J* **224**, 933–940.

Mauco, G., Dajeans, P., Chap, H. & Douste-Blazy, L. (1987) Subcellular localisation of inositol lipids in blood platelets as deduced from the use of labelled precursors. *Biochem J* **244**, 757–761.

Mayhaut-Smith, M.P., Sage, S.O. & Rink, T.J. (1990) Receptor-activated single channels in intact human platelets. *J. Biol. Chem.* **265**, 10479–10483.

Milligan, G. (1988) Techniques used in the identification and analysis of function of pertussis toxin-sensitive guanine nucleotide binding proteins. *Biochem J* **255**, 1–13.

Mills, D.C.B. (1982) The role of cyclic nucleotides in platelets. In Kebabian, J.W. & Nathanson, J.A. (eds) *Cyclic Nucleotides*, Part II, *Handbook of Physiology and Pharmacology*, Vol. **58**, pp. 723–761. Springer-Verlag, Heidelberg.

Moncada, S., Palmer, R.M.J. & Higgs, E.A. (1987) Prostacyclin and endothelium-derived relaxing factor: biological interactions and significance. In Verstraete, M., Vermylen, J., Lijnen, R. & Arnout, J. (eds) *Haemostasis and Thrombosis 1987*, pp. 597–618. Leuven, University, Press, Belgium.

Moos, M. & Goldberg, N.D. (1988) Cyclic AMP opposes IP_3-induced calcium release from permeabilised human platelets. *Second Messengers and Phosphoproteins* **12**, 163–170.

Morris, A.P., Gallacher, D.V., Irvine, R.F. & Peterson, O.H. (1987) Synergism of inositol trisphosphate and inositol tetrakisphosphate in activating Ca^{2+}-dependent K^+ channels. *Nature* **330**, 653–655.

Mustard, J.F. & Packham, M.A. (1968) Platelet phagocytosis. *Sem Haematol* **1**, 168–181.

Nachman, R.L., Silverstein, R.L. & Asch, A.S. (1987) Thrombospondin: cell biology of an adhesive protein. In Verstraete, M., Vermylen, J., Lijnen, R. & Arnout, J. (eds) *Haemostasis and Thrombosis 1987*. pp. 81–91. Leuven University Press, Belgium.

Nakano, T., Hanasaki, K. & Arita, H. (1987) Involvement of the Na^+/H^+ antiporter in activation of rat platelets by collagen. *J Biochem* **102**, 677–680.

Nakashima, S., Hattori, H., Shirato, L., Takenaka, A. & Nozawa, Y. (1987) Differential sensitivity of arachidonic acid release and 1,2-diacylglycerol formation to pertussis toxin, GDPβS and NaF in saponin-permeabilised human platelets; possible evidence for distinct GTP binding proteins involving phospholipase C and A_2 activation. *Biochem Biophys Res Comm* **148**, 971–978.

Nishizuka, Y. (1984) The role of protein kinase C in cell surface signal transduction and tumour promotion. *Nature* **308**, 693–698.

O'Rourke, F., Zavoico, G.B. & Feinstein, M.B. (1989) Release of Ca^{2+} by inositol-1,4,5-trisphosphate in platelet membrane vesicles is not dependent on cyclic AMP-dependent protein kinase. *Biochem J* **257**, 715–721.

Palmer, R.M.J., Ferrige, A.G. & Moncada, S. (1987) Nitric oxide release accounts for the biological activity of endothelium-derived relaxing factor. *Nature* **327**, 524-526.

Peerschke, E.B. (1985) The platelet fibrinogen receptor. *Sem Haematol* **22**, 241–259.

Petty, A. & Scrutton, M.C. (1989) Platelet aggregation in whole blood: Is the response to adrenaline, 5-hydroxytryptamine and PAF a direct consequence of stimulation by these agonists? *Thromb Res* **54**, 151–159.

Phillips, D.R. & Baughan, A.K. (1983) Fibrinogen binding to human platelet plasma membranes. *J Biol Chem* **258**, 10 240–10 246.

Pollock, W.K. & Rink, T.J. (1986) Thrombin and ionomycin can raise platelet cytosolic Ca^{2+} to micromolar levels by discharge of internal Ca^{2+} stores: studies using Fura2. *Biochem Biophys Res Commun* **139**, 308–314.

Pollock, W.K., Rink, T.J. & Irvine, R.F. (1986) Liberation of [^{3}H]-arachidonate and changes in cytosolic free calcium in Fura2-loaded human platelets stimulated by ionomycin and collagen. *Biochem J* **235**, 869–877.

Pouyssegur, J. (1985) The growth factor-activatable Na^+/H^+ exchange system: a genetic approach. *Trends Biochem Sci* **10**, 453–455.

Putney, J.W. (1986) A model for receptor-regulated calcium entry. *Cell Calcium* **7**, 1–12.

Quinn, P.J. & Chapman, D. (1980) The dynamics of membrane structure. *CRC Crit Rev Biochem* **8**, 1–117.

Radomski, M.W., Palmer, R.M.J. & Moncada, S. (1987) The role of nitric oxide and cGMP in platelet adhesion to vascular endothelium. *Biochem Biophys Res Commun* **148**, 1482–1489.

Radomski, M.W., Palmer, R.M.J. & Moncada, S. (1990) An L-arginine/nitric oxide pathway present in human platelets regulates aggregation. *Proc Natl Acad Sci, USA* **87**, 5193–5197.

Rasmussen, H. (1981) *Calcium and Cyclic AMP as Synarchic Messengers*, pp. 256–286. Wiley, Chichester.

Rink, T.J. & Sanchez, A. (1984) Effects of prostaglandin I_2 and forskolin on secretion from platelets evoked at basal concentrations of cytoplasmic free calcium by thrombin, collagen, phorbol ester and exogenous diacylglycerol. *Biochem J* **222**, 833–836.

Rink, T.J., Smith, S.W. & Tsien, R.Y. (1982) Cytoplasmic free Ca^{2+} in human platelets: Ca^{2+} thresholds and Ca-independent activation for shape change and secretion. *FEBS Lett* **148**, 21–26.

Rittenhouse-Simmons, S.E. (1979) Production of diglyceride from phosphatidylinositol in activated platelets. *J Clin Invest* **63**, 580–587.

Rittenhouse-Simmons, S.E. (1984) Activation of human platelet phospholipase C by ionophore A23187 is totally dependent on cyclooxygenase products and ADP. *Biochem J* **222**, 103–110.

Rock, C.O. & Jackowski, S. (1987) Thrombin- and nucleotide-activated phosphatidylinositol-4,5-bisphosphate phospholipase C in human platelet membranes. *J Biol Chem* **262**, 5492–5498.

Ruda, E.M. & Scrutton, M.C. (1987) Effect of leupeptin on platelet aggregation, fibrin formation and amidolysis induced by thrombin. *Thromb Res* **47**, 611–619.

Sage, S.O. (1987) Kinetics of ADP-evoked and thrombin-evoked rises in cytoplasmic calcium in human platelets: studies with manganese and nickel. *J Physiol* **396**, 43P.

Sage, S.O. & Rink, T.J. (1986) Effect of ionic substitution on $[Ca^{2+}]_i$ rises evoked by thrombin and PAF in human platelets. *Eur J Pharmacol* **128**, 99–107.

Sage, S.O. & Rink, T.J. (1987) The kinetics of changes in intracellular calcium concentration in Fura2-loaded human platelets. *J Biol Chem* **262**, 16 364–16 369.

Sage, S.O., Merritt, J.E., Hallam, T.J. & Rink, T.J. (1989) Receptor-mediated calcium entry in Fura2-loaded human platelets stimulated with ADP and thrombin. Dual wavelength studies with Mn^{2+}. *Biochem J* **258**, 923–926.

Sanchez, A., Alonso, M.T. & Collazos, J.M. (1988) Thrombin-induced changes of intracellular Ca^{2+} and pH in human platelets. Cytoplasmic alkalinisation is not a prerequisite for calcium mobilisation. *Biochim Biophys Acta* **938**, 497–500.

Scrutton, M.C. & Knight, D.E. (1987) Permeabilised preparations: their use in studies of signal transduction mechanisms. In MacIntyre, D.E. & Gordon, J.L. (eds) *Platelets in Biology and Pathology 3*, pp. 467–492. Elsevier/North Holland Biomedical Press, Amsterdam.

Scrutton, M.C. & Wallis, R.B. (1981) Platelet adrenoceptors. In Gordon, J.L. (ed.) *Platelets in Biology and Pathology 2*, pp. 179–210. Elsevier/North Holland Biomedical Press, Amsterdam.

Seagar, M.J., Takahashi, M. & Catterall, W.A. (1988) Molecular properties of dihydropyridine-sensitive calcium channels. *Ann NY Acad Sci* **522**, 162–175.

Shattil, S.J. & Brass, L.F. (1987) Induction of the fibrinogen receptor on human platelets by intracellular mediators. *J Biol Chem* **262**, 992–1000.

Shattil, S.J., Hoxie, J.A., Cunningham, M. & Brass, L.F. (1985) Changes in the platelet membrane glycoprotein IIb/IIIa complex during platelet activation. *J Biol Chem* **260**, 11 107–11 114.

Shattil, S.J., Budzynski, A. & Scrutton, M.C. (1989) Epinephrine induces platelet fibrinogen receptor expression, fibrinogen binding and aggregation in whole blood in the absence of other excitatory agonists. *Blood* **73**, 150–158.

Shukla, S.D. (1985) Platelet activating factor-stimulated formation of inositol triphosphate in platelets and its regulation by various agents including Ca^{2+}, indomethacin, CV-3988 and forskolin. *Arch Biochem Biophys* **240**, 674–681.

Siess, W. (1989) Molecular mechanisms of platelet activation. *Pharmacol Rev* **69**, 58–128.

Siess, W. & Binder, H. (1985) Thrombin induces the rapid formation of inositol bis-phosphate and inositol tris-phosphate in human platelets. *FEBS Lett* **180**, 107–112.

Siffert, W. & Akkerman, J.W.N. (1987) Activation of sodium-proton exchange is a prerequisite for Ca^{2+} mobilisation in human platelets. *Nature* **325**, 456–458.

Siffert, W. & Akkerman, J.W.N. (1988) Na^+/H^+ exchange as a modulator of platelet activation. *Trends Biochem Sci* **13**, 148–151.

Siffert, W., Siffert, G., Scheid, P., Riemens, T., Gorter, G. & Akkerman, J.W.N. (1987) Inhibition of Na^+/H^+ exchange reduces Ca^{2+} mobilisation without affecting the initial cleavage of phosphatidylinositol-4,5-bisphosphate in thrombin-stimulated platelets. *FEBS Lett* **212**, 123–126.

Siffert, W., Siffert, G., Scheid, P. & Akkerman, J.W.N. (1989) Activation of Na^+/H^+ exchange and Ca^{2+} mobilisation start simultaneously in thrombin-stimulated platelets. Evidence that platelet shape change disturbs early rises of BCECF fluoresence which causes an underestimate of actual cytosolic alkalinisation. *Biochem J* **258**, 521–527.

Simpson, A.W.M. & Rink, T.J. (1987) Elevation of pH_i is not an essential step in calcium mobilisation in Fura2-loaded platelets. *FEBS Lett* **222**, 144–148.

Simpson, A.W.M., Hallam, T.J. & Rink, T.J. (1986) Low concentrations of the stable prostaglandin endoperoxide U44069 stimulate shape change in quin2-loaded platelets without a measurable increase in $[Ca^{2+}]_i$. *FEBS Lett* **201**, 301–305.

Sims, P.J., Wiedmer, T., Esmon, C.T., Weiss, H.J. & Shattil, S.J. (1989) Assembly of the platelet prothrombinax complex is linked to vesiculation of the platelet plasma membrane. Studies in Scott syndrome: an isolated defect in platelet procoagulant activity. *J Biol Chem* **264**, 17049–17057.

Sune, A., Bette-Bobillo, P., Bienvenue, A., Fellman, P. & Devaux, P.F. (1987) Selective outside-inside translocation of aminophospholipids in human platelets. *Biochemistry* **26**, 2972–2978.

Swart, S., Pearson, D., Wood, J.K. & Barnett, D.B. (1984) Functional significance of the platelet α_2-adrenoceptor in patients with myeloproliferative disorders. *Thromb Res* **33**, 531–541.

Sweatt, J.D., Connolly, T.M., Cragoe, E.J. & Limbird, L.E. (1986) Evidence that Na^+/H^+ exchange regulates receptor-mediated phospholipase A_2 activation in human platelets. *J Biol Chem* **261**, 8667–8673.

Takai, Y., Kaibuchi, K., Matsubara, T. & Nishizuka, Y. (1981) Inhibitory action of guanosine-3′,5′-monophosphate on thrombin-induced phosphatidylinositol turnover and protein phosphorylation in human platelets. *Biochem Biophys Res Commun* **101**, 61–67.

Thompson, N.T. & Scrutton, M.C. (1985) Intracellular Ca^{2+} fluxes in human platelets. *Eur J Biochem* **147**, 421–427.

Thompson, N.T., Scrutton, M.C. & Wallis, R.B. (1986) Synergistic responses in human platelets: comparison between aggregation, secretion and cytosolic Ca^{2+} concentration. *Eur J Biochem* **161**, 399–408.

Touqui, L., Rothbut, B., Shaw, A.M., Fradin, A., Vargaftig, B.B. & Russo-Marie, F. (1986) Platelet activation — a role for a 40K anti-phospholipase protein indistinguishable from lipocortin. *Nature* **321**, 177–180.

Tsien, R.Y. (1981) A non-disruptive technique for loading calcium buffers and indicators into cells. *Nature* **290**, 527–528.

Tsien, R.Y., Pozzan, T. & Rink, T.J. (1982) Calcium homeostasis in intact lymphocytes: cytoplasmic free calcium monitored with a new intracellularly trapped fluorescent indicator. *J Cell Biol* **94**, 325–334.

Tyers, M., Rachubinski, R.A., Stewart, M.I., Varrichio, A.M., Shorr, R.G.I., Haslam, R.J. & Harley, C.B. (1988) Molecular cloning and expression of the major protein kinase C substrate of platelets. *Nature* **333**, 470–473.

Verhallen, P.J.F., Bevers, E.M., Comfurius, P. & Zwaal, R.J.A. (1987) Correlation between calpain-mediated cytoskeletal degradation and platelet procoagulant activity. *Biochim Biophys Acta* **903**, 206–217.

Verhallen, P.J.F., Bevers, E.M., Comfurius, P. & Zwaal, R.F.A. (1988) Fluoride-dependent Ca^{2+}-induced platelet procoagulant activity shows that calpain is involved in increased phospholipid transbilayer movement. *Biochim Biophys Acta* **942**, 150–158.

Vickers, J.D., Kinlough-Rathbone, R.L. & Mustard, J.F. (1984) Accumulation of the inositol phosphates in thrombin-stimulated washed rabbit platelets in the presence of lithium. *Biochem J* **224**, 399–405.

Waldman, S.A. & Murad, F. (1987) Cyclic GMP synthesis and function. *Pharmacol Rev* **39**, 163–196.

Ware, J.A., Johnson, P.C., Smith, M. & Salzman, E.W. (1985) Aequorin detects increased cytoplasmic calcium in platelets stimulated with phorbol ester or diacylglycerol. *Biochem Biophys Res Commun* **133**, 98–104.

Ware, J.A., Johnson, P.C., Smith, M. & Salzman, E.W. (1986) Effect of common agonists on cytoplasmic ionised calcium concentrations in platelets. *J Clin Invest* **77**, 878–886.

Ware, J.A., Smith, M., Fossel, E.T. & Salzman, E.W. (1988) Cytoplasmic Mg^{2+} concentration in platelets: implications for determination of Ca^{2+} with aequorin. *Am J Physiol* **255**, H855–859.

Watson, S.P. & Hambleton, S. (1989) Phosphorylation-dependent and -independent pathways of platelet aggregation. *Biochem J* **258**, 479–485.

Watson, S.P., Reep, B., McConnell, R.T. & Lapetina, E.G. (1985) Collagen stimulates $[^3H]$-inositol trisphosphate formation in indomethacin-treated human platelets. *Biochem J* **226**, 869–877.

Watson, S.P., McNally, J., Shipman, L.J. & Godfrey, P.P. (1988) The action of the protein kinase C inhibitor, staurosporine, on human platelets. Evidence against a regulatory role for protein kinase C in the formation of inositol trisphosphate by thrombin. *Biochem J* **249**, 345–350.

Wiedmer, T., Shattil, S.J., Cunningham, M. & Sims, P.J. (1990) Role of calcium and calpain in complement-induced vesiculation of the platelet plasma membrane and in the exposure of the platelet factor V_a receptor. *Biochem* **29**, 623–632.

Williams, K.A., Murphy, W. & Haslam, R.J. (1987) Effects of activation of protein kinase C on the agonist-induced stimulation and inhibition of cyclic AMP formation in intact human platelets. *Biochem J* **243**, 667–678.

Yamaguchi, A., Suzuki, H., Tanoue, K. & Yamazaki, H. (1986) Simple method of aequorin loading into platelets using dimethylsulfoxide. *Thromb Res* **44**, 165–174.

Zavoico, G.B. & Cragoe, E.J. (1988) Ca^{2+} mobilisation can occur independent of acceleration of Na^+/H^+ exchange in thrombin-stimulated platelets. *J Biol Chem* **263**, 9635–9639.

Zavoico, G.B., Halenda, S.P., Sha'afi, R.I. & Feinstein, M.B. (1985) Phorbol myristate acetate inhibits thrombin-stimulated Ca^{2+} mobilisation and phosphatidylinositol-4,5-bisphopsphate hydrolysis in human platelets. *Proc Natl Acad Sci USA* **82**, 3859–3862.

Zschauer, A., van Breeman, C., Buhler, F.R. & Nelson, M.T. (1988) Calcium channels in thrombin-activated human platelet membrane. *Nature* **334**, 703–706.

Note added in press

Recent studies (Sim *et al.* 1989; Wiedmer *et al.* 1990) suggest that some parts of Fig. 3.5 may not be correct. They indicate that there is no causal link between Ca^{2+}-induced cytoskeletal protein degradation and the exposure of phosphatidyl serine in the outer leaflet of the plasma membrane as proposed in Fig. 3.5.

4: Experimental Techniques for the Assessment of Platelet Function

Gillian R. May, Caroline M. Herd and Clive P. Page

Introduction

It has been known for almost a century that blood platelets are essential elements in haemostasis and that abnormal platelet function may contribute to a variety of pathophysiological conditions including thrombosis (Born, 1985), atherosclerosis (Woolf, 1981), myocardial infarction (Moore *et al.* 1976), stroke (Del Zoppo *et al.* 1986) and pulmonary embolism (Malik, 1983; see Chapter 10). More recently, it has been recognized that platelets also have non-haemostatic functions physiologically (Page, 1988) and that inappropriate activation of platelets may be involved in inflammatory conditions (e.g. rheumatoid arthritis) (Nachman & Weksler, 1980) and allergic diseases (e.g. bronchial asthma) (Gresele *et al.*, 1988; see Chapter 6).

Due to the undoubted importance of platelets in health and disease, many methods for studying platelet function, both *in vitro* and *in vivo* have been established both for the investigation of platelet function *per se* but also for the detection of novel drugs that can influence platelet behaviour.

Methods of monitoring platelet function

In vitro

Platelets can readily be isolated from whole blood for study *in vitro*. In 1962, Born introduced the technique whereby platelet aggregation within a cuvette is measured as an increase in light transmission through a stirred platelet suspension. This method has allowed detailed analysis of platelet aggregation *in vitro* and has facilitated delineation of some of the underlying biochemical pathways. At least three independent pathways of platelet aggregation have been identified; adenosine diphosphate (ADP) dependent, thromboxane A_2 dependent and platelet activating factor (PAF) dependent (Vargaftig *et al.* 1981). Additionally, a plethora of pharmacological agents have been identified as having an inhibitory activity on platelet aggregation *in vitro*, raising the possibility that such substances may have potential as antithrombotic agents (Didisheim & Fuster, 1978; Butler, see Chapter 12). However, the majority of substances that inhibit platelet aggregation *in vitro* fail to retard, or prevent, thrombosis in intact animals (Didisheim & Fuster, 1978; Butler, see Chapter 12) suggesting the participation of other blood elements in the induction and development of thrombosis.

The Born Aggregometer functions only with translucent cell suspensions, thus only permitting the study of platelet–platelet interactions. A whole blood aggregometer has since been developed (Cardinal & Flower, 1980) and studies of platelets in this experimental system may provide an assessment of platelet behaviour *in vitro* that is more predictive of the behaviour of platelets in their natural environment. However, this method which measures changes in electronic impedence between two electrodes also requires the presence of the anticoagulant citrate, which by the nature of its mode of action reduces calcium availability. Since calcium ions are necessary for platelet activation (Ardlie, 1982), the reduced calcium concentration required *in vitro* is non-physiological. Moreover, small changes in citrate concentration have dramatic effects upon the resulting platelet aggregation (Tsao *et al.* 1976). Adenosine diphosphate normally induces irreversible aggregation *in vitro*, but if the calcium concentration is increased to physiological levels, ADP can only induce a reversible primary wave of aggregation.

In vivo, ADP induces a reversible thrombocytopenia (Born & Cross, 1963), suggesting that many of the studies investigating the effects of ADP on platelet aggregation in the Born Aggregometer do not necessarily mimic the behaviour of platelets in the circulation. Therefore, there is an obvious need for predictive *in vivo* techniques for the evaluation of platelet function.

In vivo

There are numerous techniques for looking at platelet function *in vivo*. Some involve studying platelet interactions with either artificial surfaces (Gryglewski *et al.* 1978) or with areas of vessel wall damage induced either mechanically (Grouse *et al.* 1982; Buchanan & Hirsch, 1984; Menys & Davies, 1984; Shand *et al.* 1987) or electrically (Bourgain & Six, 1974; Shishido & Katori, 1981; Hladovec, 1986; Massad *et al.* 1987). These techniques provide useful information about platelet function in certain pathological thrombotic conditions and can be used to look at the effects of various antithrombotic agents. However, it is often difficult to assess the thrombotic response and, therefore, the antithrombotic potential of drugs with such techniques. Other techniques enable one to study platelet aggregation itself *in vivo* using platelet activating agents and therefore to look at similar aspects of platelet function that are possible with *in vitro* techniques such as the Born Aggregometer.

Born and Cross (1963) observed that the administration of a platelet agonist such as ADP produced a transient thrombocytopaenia in experimental animals. This transient thrombocytopaenia reflects aggregates being formed, becoming trapped in the microvasculature and then platelets recirculating as they disaggregate. Using this very simple technique for looking at platelet function it is already apparent that there is a difference between the response to ADP *in vivo*, which is transient, and the response to ADP in the Born Aggregometer, which is irreversible except at very low concentrations. However, a drawback of this technique is that it requires blood sampling and this, therefore, limits the number of observations one can make in each animal. There are also constraints on how close together samples can be taken which then reflects how readily the kinetics of a response to a platelet activating agent can be followed.

Another technique that has been used to study platelet activation *in vivo* is the aortic 'filter-loop' technique described by Hornstra in 1970. This involves placing a microfilter (pore size 20 μm) in continuity with the arterial circulation of anaesthetized rats and continuously recording blood pressure, both before and behind the filter. Platelet activating agents such as ADP are infused into the circulation before the filter and any aggregates formed will become trapped in this filter. This will have the effect of increasing pressure before, and decreasing pressure behind, the filter, thereby allowing aggregation to be assessed quantitatively by a calculated 'aggregation index'. Disaggregation can also be followed in this way. This has been used by several workers to investigate various antiplatelet agents (Hornstra, 1971; Roba *et al.* 1976; Hall *et al.* 1979; Bee *et al.* 1980). However, this technique is very cumbersome and highly invasive. The animals must be heparinized in order to allow the blood to pass through the filter and in many cases only the first two administrations of a platelet activating agent such as ADP produce comparable aggregation indices; thereafter there is a significant reduction in the size of the response. Again this limits the number of observations that can be made in each animal with the result that extensive studies on platelet function with this technique and the technique of Born and Cross become time-consuming and expensive due to the large numbers of animals required before statistical analysis is possible.

In 1974, Wu and Hoak described a technique for estimating circulating aggregates as a way of diagnosing thrombotic disease in man and this was adapted for use in experimental animals (Pinon, 1984). Blood samples are taken and fixed with a formalin buffer so that a ratio of free platelets and platelet aggregates can be determined. This can be used to assess intravascular platelet aggregation in response to platelet activating agents or to look at the presence or absence of circulating platelet aggregates in animal models of pathological conditions such as atherosclerosis. It is very important that the blood samples are taken carefully with this technique so that the aggregates present, that enable the aggregation index to be calculated, are indeed circulating aggregates and are not formed during the sampling procedure, and also that the withdrawal of blood itself does not break up any aggregates that had been formed in the circulation.

Again, a drawback of this technique, as for measuring thrombocytopaenia is that it is necessary to withdraw blood so that a limiting factor is how many samples can be taken from an individual animal and how close together it is practically possible to take them. The latter problem has been circumvented by another technique to investigate platelet function *in vivo*. Smith and Freuler

(1973) describe a technique whereby the numbers of circulating platelets can be continuously monitored, thereby allowing the kinetics of a platelet response to be fully examined. This technique uses the Technicon Autocounter which is an automated system for counting platelets and white blood cells. Arterial blood is continuously withdrawn from the experimental animal at a slow rate (0.1 ml/minute) using a special double-tipped cannula so that anticoagulant (citrate) can be mixed with the blood after it has been withdrawn from the animal and, thereby, not interfere with the response of platelets to the agent being studied. The red cells are lysed and the platelets are counted optically. This technique has several advantages over the aortic filter-loop technique of Hornstra. For instance, the filter loop cannot be used with certain platelet agonists such as collagen as the collagen fibrils themselves will obstruct the microfilter. In addition, as mentioned before, the animals must be heparinized so that the blood will pass through the filter. Continuous platelet counting does not require systemic anticoagulant and it can be used to investigate a wide variety of platelet agonists in a wider variety of experimental animals. However, it is nevertheless an invasive technique requiring the removal of blood from the animal, thereby limiting the duration of investigations in individual animals in order to retain reproducibility.

A non-invasive technique for the continuous monitoring of platelet function in the circulation has been described by Page *et al.* (1982). This technique involves radiolabelling platelets and then externally monitoring them using scintillation detectors. It has been adapted from the clinical procedure whereby radiolabelled blood elements can be externally imaged with gamma camera devices. Intravenous (i.v.) administration of a platelet agonist will cause aggregates to be formed and these will become trapped in the microvasculature of the pulmonary circulation. They will then be detected as an increase in radioactive counts by a scintillation detector placed over the thoracic region. This technique is extremely reproducible, many observations can be made in individual animals and the kinetics of each response can be followed very closely (every second if necessary). It also has the advantage that several different anatomical regions can be monitored simultaneously and so platelet function in different vascular beds can be assessed. In addition, the response of other blood elements can be investigated just as easily (for example erythrocytes, neutrophils, fibrinogen, albumin) making it possible to build-up a comprehensive picture of the involvement of a variety of different blood elements in a particular response.

Radiolabelling of blood platelets

Use of the gamma-emitting isotope ^{51}chromium as a label for blood platelets was described by Aas and Gardner in 1958. Platelets that are ^{51}Cr-labelled have been shown to be evenly distributed within the platelet population (Busch & Olson, 1973), to function normally *in vitro* (Butler *et al.* 1979) and to have the same survival time as unlabelled platelets *in vivo*. The retention of ^{51}Cr-labelled platelets within the pulmonary vasculature, assessed histologically, has provided a quantitative index of platelet activation *in vivo* (Pinckard *et al.* 1977; Butler *et al.* 1979). In addition to histological evaluation, platelet counts in blood samples were assessed using a gamma scintillation counter. Whilst this test system has been used productively for the evaluation of aggregatory stimuli and of inhibitors of platelet aggregation *in vivo* (Butler *et al.* 1979), this method has the disadvantage of being both time-consuming and expensive. It requires the sacrifice of a relatively large number of animals to define a time course for a response, or to provide dose–response relationships. Furthermore, using a simple gamma detector connected to a chart recorder, a number of investigators had previously reported the accumulation of radioactivity in the thoracic area (thought to be associated with the retention of platelet aggregates within the pulmonary vasculature) following i.v. administration of thrombin as a model of pulmonary embolism (Busch & Saldeen, 1973). Armed with the knowledge that platelet agonists induce entrapment of platelet aggregates within the pulmonary vasculature, we established a technique for automating the detection of the fate of radiolabelled platelets in the circulation.

The use of ^{51}Cr as a platelet label has been largely superseded by ^{111}indium complexes such as oxine (8-hydroxyquinoline) or tropolone (2-hydroxy,2,4,6-cyclo-heptatienone). ^{111}Indium-oxine has been utilized extensively to assess platelet function in both experimental animals and clinical studies (Thakur *et al.* 1976; Goodwin *et al.* 1978; Heaton *et al.* 1979). Platelets may be labelled using ^{111}In-oxine without a change in physiological function, and have a half-life similar to their unlabelled counterparts within the circulation of man and experimental animals (Thakur *et al.* 1976; Goodwin *et al.* 1978; Heaton *et al.* 1979). Greater than 90% of the ^{111}In-oxine accumulates in the cytosol of most mammalian platelets and is not released when the platelets are activated *in vitro* (Thakur *et al.* 1976; Baker *et al.* 1982). The lifespan of ^{111}In-labelled platelets is comparable to ^{51}Cr-labelled platelets. However, ^{111}In has advantages over ^{51}Cr as it has a higher labelling efficiency, a shorter half-life and higher energy gamma emissions making it easier to monitor the platelet content of different anatomical regions of the body externally, using either complex imaging devices (Thakur *et al.* 1976; Goodwin *et al.* 1978; Heaton *et al.* 1979) or simple detector systems (Page *et al.* 1982; Morley *et al.* 1983; Barrett *et al.* 1984; Oyekan & Botting, 1986; Smith *et al.* 1989).

Method of labelling platelets

For *in vivo* aggregometery, platelets are isolated from blood anticoagulated with acid citrate (3.8%) from either a donor animal or the animal to be studied. Platelet-rich plasma (PRP) is obtained by centrifugation at 200 g for 10 minutes. As ^{111}In binds avidly to proteins and other cells, radiolabelling of platelets with this isotope is carried out in a plasma-free environment. The PRP is centrifuged at

600 g for 10 minutes in an excess of calcium-free Tyrode's buffer containing prostaglandin (PGE_1) to prevent spontaneous aggregation (Shio & Ramwell, 1972). Plasma proteins are readily decanted and the remaining platelet pellet is resuspended in modified Tyrode's buffer and incubated with 25–50 μCi of ^{111}In-oxine (Amersham international PLC) for 1.5 minutes at 37°C. Further centrifugation at 600 g for 10 minutes allows unbound radioactivity in the supernatant to be removed. The isotopically labelled platelets are resuspended in 1 ml of modified Tyrode's buffer for intravenous administration.

Monitoring of radiolabelled platelets

Continuous recording of isotopically labelled platelets *in vivo* is achieved using collimated sodium iodide crystal detectors with appropriate spectrometers to monitor radioactivity, a special purpose microcomputer co-processor to log and process experimental data, a commercial microcomputer (IBMXT) to define the experimental protocol and a printer to provide permanent records (Page *et al.* 1982; Morley *et al.* 1983; Barrett *et al.* 1984). A diagramatic representation of this system is depicted in Fig. 4.1. Radioactive counts are monitored continuously in various anatomical regions by separate detectors. For example, one detector may be located over the thoracic region whilst a second detector may be located over another region of interest (e.g. the abdomen, leg or head) for purpose of comparison. Signals from these two detectors are amplified within the spectrometer and signals are logged by the recording system which is specifically designed for the collection and processing of such experimental data (AIMS 8000 system, MUMED, UK).

Administration of labelled platelets

A platelet suspension is infused slowly into the superficial foot vein of the guinea pig (Page *et al.* 1982; Morley *et al.* 1983; Barrett *et al.* 1984), tail vein of the rat (Oyekan & Botting, 1986), radial vein in dogs (Page *et al.* 1982) or primates (Arnoux *et al.* 1988) or the ear vein of the rabbit (May *et al.* 1990; Thiemermann *et al.* 1990; Herd, 1991). Following administration of radiolabelled platelets, a considerable increase in the count rates is recorded by both detectors, and within 30 minutes the counts stabilize, as the labelled platelets equilibrate with the endogenous population. The basal count rates in the various anatomical regions represent the relative distribution of blood and remain relatively constant for prolonged periods of time (hours).

Data collection and analysis

The monitor screen displays the counts per second for each probe. Prior to initiation of an experiment, the experimental details such as the animal weight

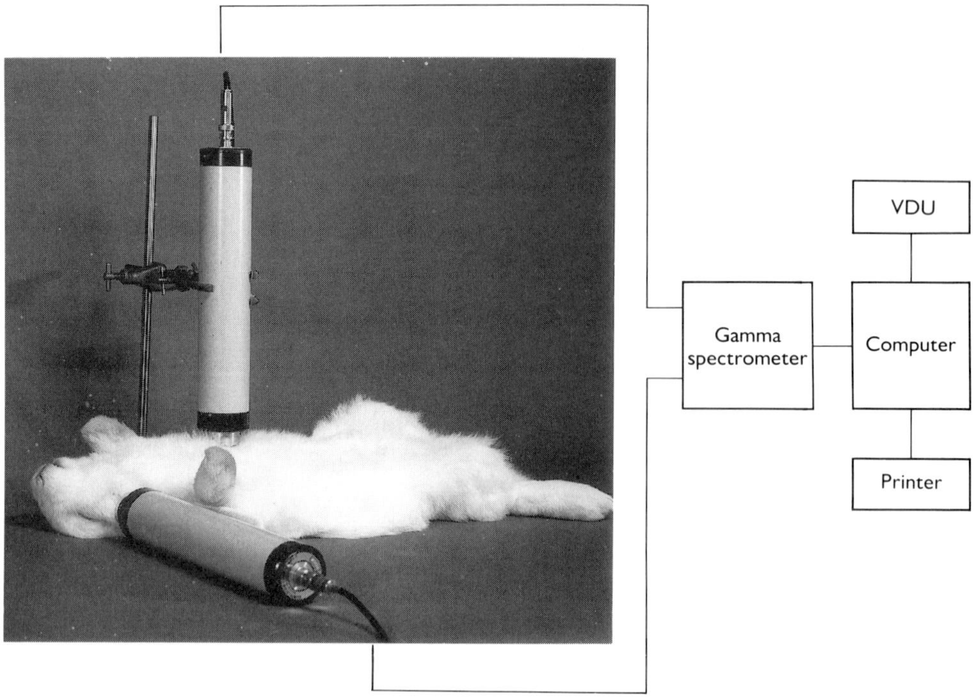

Figure 4.1 This shows the location of the scintillation detectors over the thoracic and cranial regions of an anaesthetized rabbit. The radioactive counts detected by these probes are estimated with a dual-channel gamma spectrometer (Nuclear Enterprises NE 461) and logged with the aid of a special application interface with a microcomputer.

and drugs used can be specified via the IBM computer keyboard. Additionally, the frequency and overall duration of the periods of observation are computed. The counts can be collected from the various anatomical regions over a number of consecutive time-steps (up to 250) of variable duration (1–2000 seconds) depending on the agonist used and the kinetics of the response. For example, to record the effects of a bolus injection of the platelet agonist ADP in the guinea pig, rat or rabbit, we use 240 sequential steps of 1 second duration (4 minutes in total) with one probe over the thoracic region and another probe over the abdomen. The platelet response to ADP is rapid and transient, the maximum accumulation in the lung being achieved within the first minute and prestimulated counts re-established soon after.

Intravenous administration of a diverse range of aggregatory stimuli (e.g. ADP, collagen, arachidonic acid, PAF, thrombin, 5-hydroxytryptamine (5-HT), antigen) evoke increases in the counts recorded by the thoracic probe. Such an increase can be attributed to retention of platelets within the pulmonary vasculature as confirmed by histological evidence of platelet aggregates within all levels of the pulmonary vasculature of lungs from animals sacrificed when thoracic counts are elevated (Butler *et al.* 1979; Dewar *et al.* 1984). In addition to this, there is a fall in the count rate in the abdominal probe which for ADP, parallels the time course of thrombocytopenia (Barrett *et al.* 1984). The time course of thrombocytopenia is similar to that observed with the method of Smith and Freuler (1973).

Such responses are not a reflection of changes in blood flow or blood pooling within the thoracic region as the administration of platelet agonists do not produce any significant increase in the counts recorded over the thoracic region when

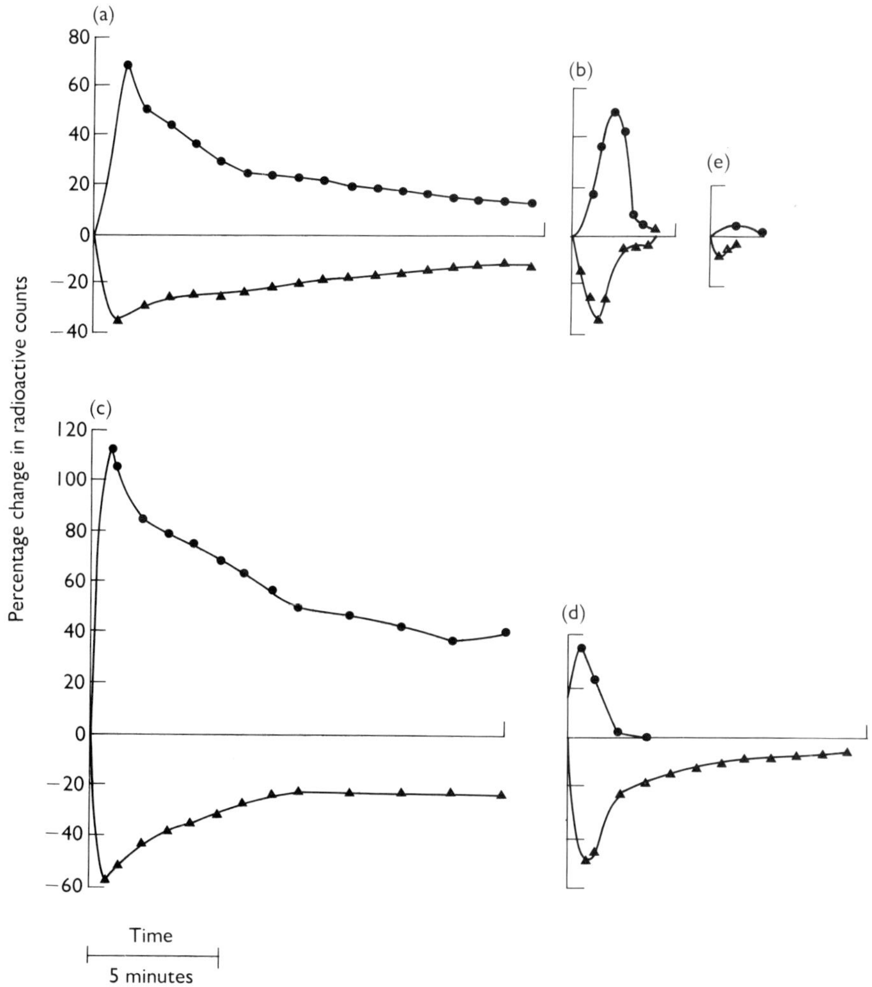

Figure 4.2 Changes in thoracic (●) and cranial (▲) platelet-associated radioactivity over time following i.v. administration of bolus doses of (a) collagen (100 μg/kg), (b) ADP (10 μg/kg), (c) thrombin (32 iu/kg), (d) PAF (0.1 μg/kg), and (e) saline in individual rabbits. Changes are expressed as percentage change in radioactive counts as compared with pre-injection levels.

radiolabelled red blood cells are used (see Fig. 4.2). Each stimulus of platelet aggregation produces a unique profile as illustrated in Fig. 4.2.

In total contrast to the *in vitro* situation, most doses of platelet aggregatory stimuli produce reversible aggregation, except when the coagulation cascade is simultaneuosly activated to elicit clot formation (as assessed by [^{125}I]fibrinogen accumulation), as can be observed following i.v. administration of high doses of thrombin (Barrett *et al.* 1984). The occurrence of platelet disaggregation allows repeated administrations to be made in the same experimental animal and permits studies of dose–response relationships using a single animal as its own control (Fig. 4.3). The complete time course of platelet aggregation and disaggregation can be accurately monitored and therefore alterations in the kinetics of the responses in the presence of drugs can be studied. Reproducibility of responses to certain aggregatory stimuli is high both between, and within, experimental animals (Page *et al.* 1982; Oyekan & Botting, 1986; Bhardwaj *et al.* 1988; Smith *et al.* 1989). Such reproducibility readily permits the detection of phenomena such as tachyphylaxis, as observed following repeated administration of PAF at 30-minute intervals (Page *et al.* 1983a), although this phenomenon is not evident when intervals of 60 minutes are used (unpublished results). The spontaneous disaggregation of platelet aggregates within the pulmonary vasculature suggests that there is an endogenous mechanism for limiting platelet aggregation *in vivo* although it is unlikely to be secondary to the generation of PGI_2 as the disaggregation produced is not altered in animals treated with nonsteroidal anti-inflammatory drugs (NSAIDs) (Bhardwaj *et al.* 1988). However, endothelium derived relaxation factor (EDRF) has been postulated as limiting the extent of platelet aggregation induced by ADP (Bhardwaj *et al.* 1988; Humphries *et al.* 1990) and collagen (Humphries *et al.* 1990) and is a substance known to be released by endothelial cells in response to thrombotic stimuli (see Vanhoutte & Shimokawa, 1989). It remains plausible that the release of nitric oxide (NO) by pulmonary endothelial cells may therefore contribute to this disaggregation phenomenon a suggestion recently confirmed by the use of inhibitors of endogenous NO generation (May

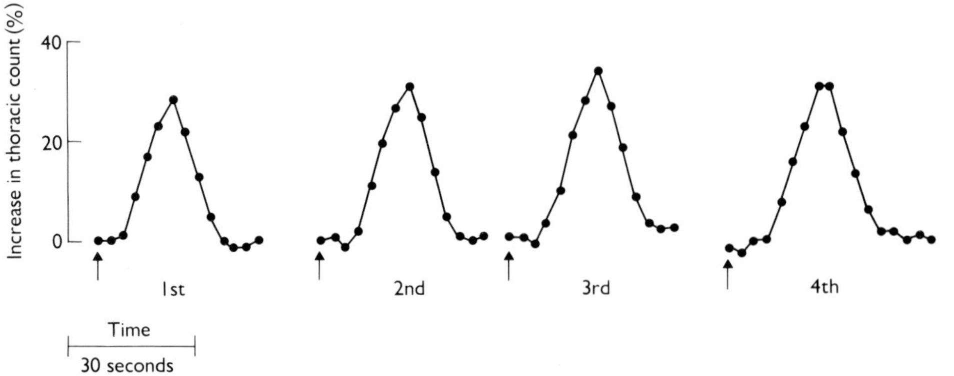

Figure 4.3 Responses to repeated challenge of ^{111}indium-oxine-labelled platelets in the rabbit *in vivo* with ADP (56 μg/kg i.v.) at 15-minute intervals.

et al. 1991). Furthermore, other investigators have reported that local fibrinolytic activity may result in disaggregation (Oyekan & Botting, 1988).

Platelet aggregometry *in vivo* can be studied in a variety of experimental animals and has been employed to study platelet function in guinea pigs (Page *et al.* 1982; Morley *et al.* 1983; Page *et al.* 1983a; Dewar *et al.* 1984; Beijer *et al.* 1987), rats (Curtis *et al.* 1985; Oyekan & Botting, 1986; Bhardwaj *et al.* 1988), dogs (Page *et al.* 1982), primates (Arnoux *et al.* 1988) and rabbits (May *et al.* 1990; Thiemermann *et al.* 1990; Herd, 1991). It is well known that there is considerable species variation in the responsiveness of platelets to aggregatory stimuli *in vitro* (Burke *et al.* 1983; Mallarkey & Smith, 1985). This can be extended to platelet aggregometry *in vivo*; for example, PAF is an exceedingly potent activator of guinea pig platelets *in vitro* (Vargaftig *et al.* 1981) and dose-related increases in platelet activation in response to intravenous injections of PAF can be monitored *in vivo* (Page *et al.* 1982; Page *et al.* 1983a). Conversely, rat platelets are totally insensitive to PAF *in vitro* (Namm *et al.* 1982) and similarly using *in vivo* aggregometry, no effect of PAF can be observed (unpublished observations). These observations support the observation that rat platelets lack PAF receptor sites (Inarrea *et al.* 1984). In contrast ADP and collagen, which activate platelets from the dog, rat and guinea pig *in vitro*, also produce responses *in vivo* in these species (Page *et al.* 1982). However, platelet aggregometry has also thrown up anomalous results. For example, 5-HT has no aggregatory effect on rat platelets *in vitro*, yet induces dose-related accumulation of platelets in the pulmonary vasculature of rats *in vivo* following i.v. administration (Oyekan & Botting, 1986).

Since the technique of *in vivo* aggregometry is non-invasive and given that ^{111}indium-labelled platelets have a normal half-life in the circulation, the reactivity of platelets to a given stimulus can be studied repeatedly over days, weeks or even months, thereby allowing the determination of altered platelet reactivity following various treatments, such as modifications of dietary lipids (to induce atherosclerosis), induction of diabetes or treatment with pharmacological agents suspected of having either pro- or antithrombotic properties. For example, rats with alloxan-induced diabetes have an altered platelet reactivity compared to control animals (Curtis *et al.* 1985). Similarly, the influence of endogenous factors such as hormones on platelet behaviour *in vivo* have been demonstrated by utilizing cross-over experiments where, for example, the platelets from female animals have been re-injected into male animals and vice versa in order to determine the influence of the sex hormones on platelet function (Oyekan & Botting, 1986).

Although the majority of studies using this technique have adopted administration of platelet agonists by intravenous injection, administration by other routes may also be employed. For example, inhalation of endotoxin by guinea pigs results in a progressive accumulation of platelets over a period of several hours (Beijer *et al.* 1987), whilst in the baboon, intratracheal administration of PAF elicits a more rapid, but reversible accumulation of platelets within the pulmonary vasculature (Arnoux *et al.* 1988). Both observations indicate that platelet behaviour can be modified by the introduction of agents directly into the airways, an observation of considerable interest in the context of understanding bronchial asthma where it is known that inhalation of antigen by allergic asthmatics results in the activation of platelets (Knauer *et al.* 1981; Gresele *et al.* 1988; see Chapter 6) sometimes resulting in trapping of the micro-aggregates within the microvasculature of the lung (Beasley *et al.* 1989). Furthermore, we have recently demonstrated that intracarotid administration of platelet agonists will induce platelet activation within various vascular beds that can be detected using external scintillation detectors (May *et al.* 1990). In particular, intracarotid administration of thrombin has been shown to elicit a dose-related and largely irreversible accumulation of platelets within the cranial vasculature that may be a novel method to investigate the contribution of platelets to thrombo-embolic disorders in the cerebral vascular system.

Anti-aggregatory agents

Intravenous administration of PGI_2 (50–500 ng/kg) as a bolus injection elicits a dose-related inhibition of ADP- and collagen-induced platelet accumulation into the thoracic region of the guinea pig (Page *et al.* 1982; Morley *et al.* 1983; Humphries *et al.* 1989), an observation which is consistent with the proposal that this substance has potent anti-aggregatory activity (Moncada & Vane, 1981). The sensitivity of platelets to PGI_2 using *in vivo* aggregometry is comparable to the sensitivity of platelets to this anti-aggregatory prostanoid observed in the clinical situation (Szczeklik & Gryglewski, 1985). Platelet behaviour assessed by *in vivo* aggregometry may, therefore, reflect platelet behaviour in normal circulating blood and thus provide a useful test system to evaluate the physiological control of platelet function in the circulation.

PGI_2 has a short biological half-life within the circulation (Moncada & Vane, 1981), hence the anti-aggregatory effect of this prostanoid *in vivo* is transient (Morley *et al.* 1983). However, synthetic PGI_2 analogues exist which are not so rapidly metabolized (Morley *et al.* 1983) and *in vivo* aggregometry is a convenient method to determine the duration of action of these antiplatelet drugs. Thus FCE 21292 and FCE 21258 could be shown to inhibit ADP-induced platelet accumulation for up to 1.5 hours (Morley *et al.* 1983).

The use of *in vivo* aggregometry has also highlighted that there are differences between platelet behaviour *in vitro* and *in vivo*. Notable examples are the pro-aggregatory or potentiating effects of adrenaline on platelet aggregation *in vitro*. In contrast, infusion of adrenaline *in vivo* has no pro-aggregatory effects but rather inhibits ADP-induced platelet aggregation in the rat (Botting & Oyekan, 1986; Oyekan & Botting, 1986). This inhibitory effect of adrenaline can be prevented by prior treatment with α- but not β-adrenoceptor antagonists (Botting & Oyekan, 1986). It is not yet known how this effect of adrenaline is brought about but it may well be related to the ability of adrenaline to increase fibrinolytic activity (Oyekan & Botting, 1988).

In vivo platelet aggregometry has been used to evaluate other classes of potential and established antithrombotic drugs (Table 4.1). It has been demonstrated that thromboxane synthetase inhibitors or thromboxane antagonists such as L-640,035 inhibit platelet accumulation induced by arachidonic acid (Barrett *et al.* 1986) or the prostaglandin endoperoxide analogue U44069, (Chan *et al.* 1984) respectively. The inability of L-640,035 to reduce platelet accumulation induced by i.v. ADP, supports the concept that thromboxane does not play a major role in ADP-induced platelet activation *in vivo* (Chan *et al.* 1984). This suggests that inhibitors of platelet activation may have very selective profiles which can be determined by *in vivo* aggregometry.

Detection of anticoagulant drugs

Heparin and related anticoagulants are widely prescribed pharmaceuticals for the treatment of thrombotic disorders yet there are conflicting reports on the effect of this class of drug on platelet function (Mustard & Packham, 1975). In the majority of *in vivo* techniques for studying platelet function, systemic anticoagulants are mandatory, thereby precluding an analysis of the effects of these agents on platelet behaviour within the circulation. As our described method of *in vivo* aggregometry is surgically non-invasive, systemic anticoagulants are not required, thus allowing the determination of the effects of anticoagulants on platelet function *in vivo* (Barrett *et al.* 1984). In this experimental system, low doses of heparin (30–100 iu/kg) have been shown to inhibit platelet accumulation induced by thrombin, an observation consistent with the anticoagulant activity of this molecule (Barrett *et al.* 1984). The anticoagulant property of heparin in these experiments can be confirmed directly by continuous monitoring of ^{125}iodine-labelled fibrinogen which will accumulate in response to thrombin over the same dose range as that required to induce platelet accumulation (Barrett *et al.* 1984). Such fibrinogen accumulation is inhibited by the same dose range of heparin that is required to inhibit platelet accumulation induced by thrombin (Barrett *et al.* 1984).

However, doses of heparin that inhibit thrombin-induced platelet accumulation and activation of the coagulation cascade have no significant effect on platelet accumulation induced by other platelet agonists such as ADP, collagen or PAF (Barrett *et al.* 1984). Furthermore, these other stimuli of platelet activation do not initiate the coagulation cascade (as assessed by ^{125}iodine-labelled fibrinogen accumulation *in vivo*) suggesting that substantial platelet activation may occur in the circulation independently of the coagulation cascade (Barrett *et al.* 1984). If this interpretation is correct, it follows that conventional anticoagulant therapy may not be optimal for minimizing thrombotic episodes. However, larger doses of heparin (100–500 iu/kg) will elicit a dose-related inhibitory effect on platelet activation *in vivo*, whether induced by ADP, collagen or PAF (Barrett *et al.* 1984). These observations indicate that commercial heparin preparations may possess both anticoagulant and antiplatelet activity. Whether these distinct properties are attributable to defined entities within the heparin molecule has yet to be

Table 4.1 The modulation of agonist-induced platelet accumulation in a variety of species by various pharmacological agents *in vivo*

Platelet agonist	Drug	Effect on platelet accumulation	Species	Reference
ADP	PGI_2	Inhibition	Guinea-pig	Page *et al.* (1982)
	PGI_2	Inhibition	Guinea-pig	Humphries *et al.* (1989)
	PGI_2 analogues			
	FCE 21292	Inhibition	Guinea-pig	Morley *et al.* (1983)
	FCE 21258	Inhibition		
	Heparin			
	High dose	Inhibition	Guinea-pig	Barrett *et al.* (1984)
	Low dose	No effect		
	TX antagonist			
	L-640,035	No effect	Guinea-pig	Chan *et al.* (1984)
	Adrenaline	Inhibition	Rat	Oyekan and Botting (1986)
	EDRF (carbachol-induced release)	Inhibition	Rat	Bhardwaj *et al.* (1988)
	EDRF (substance P-induced release)	Inhibition	Guinea-pig	Humphries *et al.* (1990)
	Endothelin-1	Inhibition	Rabbit	Thiemermann *et al.* (1990)
	PAF antagonists			
	SRI 63-441	No effect	Guinea-pig	Smith *et al.* (1989)
	SRI 63-441	No effect	Rabbit	Herd (1991)
	Brotizolam	No effect		
	Inhibitor of NO synthesis			
	L-NAME	Potentiation	Rabbit	May *et al.* (1991)
Collagen	Heparin			
	High dose	Inhibition	Guinea-pig	Barrett *et al.* (1984)
	Low dose	No effect		
	Indomethacin	No effect	Guinea-pig	Butler *et al.* (1986)
	Aspirin	No effect		
	Aspirin	Inhibition	Guinea-pig	Smith *et al.* (1989)
	Aspirin	Inhibition	Rabbit	Herd (1991)
	Diclofenac	Inhibition	Guinea-pig	Butler *et al.* (1986)
	TX synthetase inhibitors			
	CGS 13080	Inhibition		
	N(1-carboxyheptyl) imidazole	Inhibition		
	Dazoxiben	Inhibition		
	EDRF (substance P-induced release)	Inhibition	Guinea-pig	Humphries *et al.* (1990)
	Endothelin-1	Inhibition	Rabbit	Thiemermann *et al.* (1990)
	PAF antagonist			
	SRI 63-441	No effect	Guinea-pig	Smith *et al.* (1989)
	SRI 63-441	No effect	Rabbit	Herd (1991)
PAF	Heparin			
	Low dose	No effect	Guinea-pig	Barrett *et al.* (1984)
	High dose	Inhibition		
	Heparin (high dose)	Inhibition	Rabbit	Herd (1991)
	Aspirin	No effect	Guinea-pig	Smith *et al.* (1989)
	Aspirin	Potentiation	Rabbit	Herd (1991)
	Indomethacin	Potentiation		
	Endothelin-1	Inhibition	Rabbit	Thiemermann *et al.* (1990)

Table 4.1 Continued

Platelet agonist	Drug	Effect on platelet accumulation	Species	Reference
	PAF antagonist			
	SRI 63-441	Inhibition	Guinea-pig	Smith *et al.* (1989)
	SRI 63-441	Inhibition	Rabbit	Herd (1991)
	Brotizolam	Inhibition		
	PGI_2 analogue			
	Iloprost	Inhibition		
	Ketotifen	No effect	Baboon	Arnoux *et al.* (1988)
	Pyribenzamine	No effect		
	Inhibitor of NO synthesis			
	L-NAME	Potentiation	Rabbit	May *et al.* (1991)
Thrombin	Heparin (low dose)	Inhibition	Guinea-pig	Barrett *et al.* (1984)
	Endothelin-1	No effect	Rabbit	Thiemermann *et al.* (1990)
	Inhibitor of NO synthesis			
	L-NAME	Potentiation	Rabbit	May *et al.* (1991)
Arachidonic acid	Indomethacin	Inhibition	Guinea-pig	Barrett *et al.* (1986)
	Aspirin	Inhibition		
	Diclofenac	Inhibition		
	TX synthetase inhibitors			
	CGS 12970			
	Low dose	Inhibition		
	High dose	Potentiation and blood pooling		
	CGS 13080			
	Low dose	No effect		
	High dose	Potentiation and blood pooling		
	N(1-carboxyheptyl) imidazole	Inhibition		
U44069	TX antagonist			
	L-640,035	Inhibition	Guinea-pig	Chan *et al.* (1984)
Antigen challenge	PGI_2	Inhibition	Guinea-pig	Pretolani *et al.* (1986)
	Leukotriene C and D antagonist			
	FPL 55712	No effect		
	Aspirin + mepyramine + methysergide	No effect		
Endotoxin	PAF antagonists			
	CV 3988	Inhibition	Guinea-pig	Beijer *et al.* (1987)
	Brotizolam	Inhibition		
	BN 52021	Inhibition		
	Indomethacin	No effect		
	Heparin	Inhibition		
	PGI_2 analogue			
	ZX 36374	Inhibition		

determined. Study of synthetic heparin fragments by *in vivo* aggregometry could resolve this issue and may indicate more selective use of heparin and related molecules. It has been noted during these experiments that no concentration of heparin induced platelet aggregation *per se* nor did heparin potentiate platelet aggregation in response to any other activation stimulus; this is in marked contrast to the reports of heparin-induced potentiation of platelet aggregation *in vitro* (Eika, 1972; Mohammad *et al.* 1981), further illustrating that platelet behaviour *in vitro* does not necessarily reflect the behaviour of this blood element within the circulation.

The use of radiolabelled platelets has been extended to investigate possible non-haemostatic functions of platelets. The activation of platelets by a variety of substances (e.g. collagen, Forssman antiserum, PAF, ADP or antigen) is associated with bronchoconstriction which is dependent upon platelet activation, since bronchoconstrictor responses are suppressed in animals pretreated with antiplatelet antiserum or with drugs known to inhibit the platelet release reaction (Pinckard *et al.* 1977; Butler *et al.* 1979; Vargaftig *et al.* 1980; Chignard *et al.* 1982; Vargaftig *et al.* 1982). In man, aggregation of platelets within the pulmonary vasculature has been reported to be associated with acute respiratory failure and sudden death (Pirkle & Carstens, 1974; Schneider *et al.* 1980). Hence, it has been suggested that bronchoconstriction associated with platelet activation is a consequence of physical obstruction of the pulmonary vessels by platelet emboli (Malik, 1983). Although reflex bronchoconstriction as a consequence of the deposition of emboli is well established in animal models (Mills *et al.* 1969; Widdicombe & Sterling, 1970; Malik, 1983), there is considerable evidence to suggest that this may not be the sole determinant of platelet-dependent bronchospasm. For instance, platelet-dependent bronchoconstriction *in vivo* can be inhibited by drugs which inhibit the platelet release reaction but have no effect upon the extent of platelet aggregation (Vargaftig *et al.* 1980; Chignard *et al.* 1982; Vargaftig *et al.* 1982; Page *et al.* 1984; Page *et al.* 1985; Arnoux *et al.* 1988). Experiments with indium-labelled platelets have confirmed that platelet-dependent bronchoconstriction is associated with platelet accumulation in the pulmonary vasculature, but additionally have demonstrated a clear dissociation between these two response parameters (Page *et al.* 1984; Arnoux *et al.* 1988). Platelet-dependent bronchoconstriction does not follow platelet accumulation within the pulmonary vasculature but rather precedes detectable accumulation (Page *et al.* 1984). This implies that platelet sequestration *per se* is not the stimulus for bronchospasm, but rather some other aspect of platelet activation. Furthermore, there are several classes of drugs including the anti-asthma drugs, ketotifen and theophylline which inhibit this release reaction of platelets *in vitro* and platelet-dependent bronchospasm *in vivo*, but do not affect platelet accumulation within the pulmonary vasculature (Page *et al.* 1985). These observations indicate that platelet-derived mediators contribute to the bronchospasm as well as, or instead of, physical obstruction of pulmonary vessels by platelet aggregates. By dissociating platelet release and aggregation *in vivo*, this test system has led to a novel hypothesis which postulates that platelet activation plays a central role in the pathogenesis of asthma (Morley *et al.* 1984) and casts some doubt upon *in vitro* work which has linked aggregation with the release reaction of platelets. These conclusions do not depend solely upon *in vivo* aggregometry since dissociation of aggregation from the release reaction in platelets has been proposed on the basis of changes of biochemical indices during platelet activation (Rink *et al.* 1983). Such conclusions also demonstrate the importance of measuring products released from platelets in addition to the platelet aggregation itself. This is a major disadvantage of *in vivo* aggregometry as no indices of the platelet release reactions are measured.

Since there is increasing evidence that the platelet has properties appropriate to an inflammatory cell like the neutrophil (Nachman & Weksler, 1980; Page, 1988; Page, 1989; De Gaetano *et al.* 1989), aggregometry *in vivo* has been utilized to investigate accumulation of platelets into inflammatory lesions. Platelet activating factor, in addition to being the most potent agonist for platelet activation, is a very potent inflammatory agent (Morley *et al.* 1983; Archer *et al.* 1984; Pirotzky *et al.* 1984; Archer *et al.* 1985), and has been implicated as a mediator of inflammation and asthma (Page, 1988). An intravenous infusion of PAF to guinea-pigs induces pulmonary platelet accumulation in addition to an increase in the airways' responsiveness to a wide range of spasmogens, an important characteristic of bronchial asthma. This bronchial hyper-responsiveness induced by PAF is dependent upon the presence of circulating platelets (Mazzoni *et al.* 1985; Coyle *et al.* 1990). However, other platelet agonists such as ADP, collagen and the thromboxane mimetic U46619 do not induce bronchial hyper-responsiveness despite producing a similar pulmonary platelet accumulation (Robertson & Page, 1987). This indicates that pulmonary retention of platelets *per se* is not responsible for induction of bronchial hyper-responsiveness.

Local administration of PAF into the subplanter region of the guinea-pig causes a sustained increase in vascular permeability, which is associated with platelet accumulation (Page *et al.* 1983b). This can readily be demonstrated by placing scintillation detectors over the paws of experimental animals and treating one paw with the inflammatory agent and the other with vehicle. The platelet accumulation observed in response to PAF is selective since histamine, which can induce a marked increase in vascular permeability in the paw, is without any effect upon platelet accumulation (Page *et al.* 1983b). In contrast, when PAF is administered locally into the paw of the rat, increased vascular permeability is observed, without evidence of platelet accumulation, which is consistent with the observation that rat platelets are insensitive to PAF *in vitro* (Namm *et al.* 1982).

In conclusion, whilst a range of techniques exist for both the *in vitro* and *in vivo* investigation of platelet function, we feel that measurement of aggregation and disaggregation of platelets *in vivo*, using a computer-based automated isotope monitoring system for the external detection of radiolabelled platelets, provides a novel technique to supercede existing techniques. The methodology allows the investigation of diverse stimuli which produce characteristic response patterns. Established and novel inhibitors of platelet aggregation can be detected. Interactions between platelets and the coagulation cascade can be demonstrated and drug effects analysed in this context. Observations show a closer parallel with clinical evidence than *in vitro* tests of platelet function and this technique can be extended to the investigation of non-haemostatic aspects of platelet function, since this methodology has been employed in the analysis and detection of prophylactic anti-asthma drugs (Page *et al.* 1985). The methodology is flexible and has already been applied to other aspects of the inflammatory reaction, including cell accumulation (Sweatman *et al.* 1987) and plasma protein extravasation (Pirotzky *et al.* 1985).

References

Aas, K.A. & Gardner, F.H. (1958) Survival of blood platelets labelled with chromium. *J Clin Invest* **37**, 1257–1268.

Archer, C.B., Page, C.P., Paul, W., Morley, J. & MacDonald, D.M. (1984) Inflammatory characteristics of platelet activating factor (Paf-acether) in human skin. *Br J Dermatol* **110**, 45–50.

Archer, C.B., Page, C.P., Morley, J.M. & MacDonald, D.M. (1985) Accumulation of inflammatory cells in response to intracutaneous platelet activating factor (Paf-acether) in man. *Br J Dermatol* **112**, 285–290.

Ardlie, N.G. (1982) Calcium ions, drug action and platelet function. *Pharmacol Ther* **18**, 249–270.

Arnoux, B., Denjean, A., Page, C.P., Nolibe, D., Morley, J. & Benveniste, J. (1988) Accumulation of platelets and eosinophils in baboon lung after Paf-acether challenge. *Am Rev Respir Dis* **137**, 855–860.

Baker, J.R.J., Butler, K.D., Eakins, M.N., Pay, G.F. & White, A.M. (1982) Subcellular localization of 111-In in human and rabbit platelets. *Blood* **59**, 351–359.

Barrett, P.A., Butler, K.D., Morley, J., Page, C.P., Paul, W. & White, A.M. (1984) Inhibition by heparin of platelet accumulation *in vivo*. *Thromb Haemost* **51**, 366–370.

Barrett, P.A., Butler, K.D., Shand, R.A. & Wallis, R.B. (1986) Intrathoracic platelet accumulation in the guinea-pig induced by intravenous administration of arachidonic acid — effect of cyclooxygenase and thromboxane synthetase inhibitors. *Thromb Haemost* **56**, 311–317.

Beasley, R., Roche, W.R., Roberts, J.A. & Holgate, S.T. (1989) Cellular events in the bronchi in mild asthma and after bronchial provocation. *Am Rev Respir Dis* **139**, 806–817.

Bee, D., Leach, E., Martin, J.F. & Suggett, A.J. (1980) The effects of vincristine on the platelet aggregation studied by a filter loop technique in the rat. *Br J Pharmac* **69**, 227–231.

Beijer, L., Botting, J., Crook, P., Oyekan, A.O., Page, C.P. & Rylander, R. (1987) The involvement of platelet activating factor in endotoxin-induced pulmonary platelet recruitment in the guinea-pig. *Br J Pharmac* **92**, 803–808.

Bhardwaj, R., Page, C.P., May, G.R. & Moore, P.K. (1988) Endothelium derived relaxing factor inhibits platelet aggregation in human whole blood and in the rat in vivo. *Eur J Pharmacol* **157**, 83–92.

Born, G.V.R. (1962) Quantitative investigations into the aggregation of blood platelets. *Proc Physiol Soc* 67P–68P.

Born, G.V.R. (1985) Physiological and pathological involvements of platelets. In Neri Serneri, G.G., McGiff, J., Paoletti, R. & Born, G.V.R. (eds) *Advances in Prostaglandin Thromboxane and Leukotriene Research*, Vol. 13, pp. 1–11, Raven Press, New York.

Born, G.V.R. & Cross, M.J. (1963) Effect of adenosine diphosphate on the concentration of platelets in circulating blood. *Nature* **197**, 974–976.

Botting, J.H. & Oyekan, A.O. (1986) Inhibition of intravascular platelet aggregation in rats by adrenaline. *Br J Pharmacol* **89**, 752P.

Bourgain, R.H. & Six, F. (1974) A continuous registration method in experimental arterial thrombosis in the rat. *Thromb Res* **4**, 599–607.

Buchanan, M.R. & Hirsch, J. (1984) Effect of aspirin and salicylate on platelet–vessel wall interaction in rabbits. *Arteriosclerosis* **4**, 403–406.

Burke, S.E., Lefer, A.M., Nicolaou, K.C., Smith, G.M. & Smith, J.B. (1983) Responsiveness of platelets and coronary arteries from different species to synthetic thromboxane and prostaglandin endoperoxide analogues. *Br J Pharmac* **78**, 287–292.

Busch, C. & Olson, P.S. (1973) Density of 51-Cr-labelled platelets within the circulating dog platelet population. *Thromb Res* **3**, 1–11.

Busch, C. & Saldeen, T. (1973) Amount of fibrin in different organs after intravenous, intraportal and intraaortal injection of thrombin in the rat. *Thromb Diath Haemorr* **29**, 87–93.

Butler, K.D., Pay, G.M., Roberts, J.M. & White, A.M.

(1979) The effect of sulphinpyrazone and other drugs on the platelet response during the active arthus reaction in guinea pigs. *Thromb Res* **15**, 319–340.

Butler, K.D., Shand, R.A. & Wallis, R.B. (1986) The effects of modulation of prostanoid metabolism on the thoracic platelet accumulation induced by intravenous administration of collagen in the guinea-pig. *Thromb Haemost* **56**, 263–267.

Cardinal, D.C. & Flower, R.J. (1980) The electronic aggregometer: a novel device for assessing platelet behaviour in blood. *J Pharmacol Meth* **3**, 135–158.

Chan, C.C., Nathaniel, D.G., Yusko, P.J., Hall, R.A. & Ford-Hutchinson, A.W. (1984) Inhibition of prostanoid-mediated platelet aggregation *in vivo* and *in vitro* by 3-hydroxymethyl-dibenzo(b,f)thiepin 5,5-dioxide (L-640,035). *J Pharmacol Exp Ther* **229**, 276–282.

Chignard, M., Wal, F., Lefort, J. & Vargaftig, B.B. (1982) Inhibition by sulphinpyrazone of the platelet-dependent bronchoconstriction due to platelet activating factor (Paf-acether) in the guinea pig. *Eur J Pharmacol* **78**, 71–79.

Coyle, A.J., Spina, D. & Page, C.P. (1990) PAF-induced bronchial hyperresponsiveness in the rabbit: contribution of platelets and airway smooth muscle. *Br J Pharmacol* **97**, 550P.

Curtis, L.D., Oyekan, A.O., Botting, J.H. & Betteridge, D.J. (1985) Enhanced *in vivo* platelet aggregation in experimental diabetes. *Diabetes* **34** (Suppl. 1), 215A.

De Gaetano, G., Cerletti, C., Nanni-Costa, M.P. & Poggi, A. (1989) The blood platelet as an inflammatory cell. *Eur Respir J* **2** (Suppl. 6), 441s–445s.

Del Zoppo, G.J., Copeland, B.R., Harker, L.A., Waltz, T.A., Zyroff, J., Hanson, S.R. & Battenberg, E. (1986) Experimental acute thrombotic stroke in baboons. *Stroke* **17**, 1254–1265.

Dewar, A., Archer, C.B., Paul, W., Page, C.P., MacDonald, D.M. & Morley, J. (1984) Cutaneous and pulmonary histopathological responses to platelet activating factor (Paf-acether) in the guinea-pig. *J Pathol* **144**, 25–35.

Didisheim, P. & Fuster, V. (1978) Actions and clinical status of platelet-suppressive agents. *Sem Haematol* **15**, 55–72.

Eika, C. (1972) Platelet refractory state induced by heparin. *Scand J Haematol* **9**, 665–672.

Goodwin, D.A, Bushberg, J.T., Doherty, P.W., Lipton, M.J., Conley, F.K., Diamanti, C.I. & Meares, C.F. (1978) Indium 111 labelled autologous platelets for location of vascular thrombi in humans. *J Nucl Med* **19**, 626–634.

Gresele, P., Ribaldi, E., Grasselli, S., Todiso, T. & Nenci, G.G. (1988) Evidence for platelet activation in allergic asthma. *Agents and Actions Suppl* **21**, 119–128.

Grouse, H.M., Kinlough-Rathbone, R.L., Richardson, M., Jorgensen, L., Moore, S. & Mustard, J.F. (1982). Thrombin generation and fibrin formation following injury to rabbit neointima. Studies of vessel wall reactivity and platelet survival. *Lab Invest* **46**, 605–612.

Gryglewski, R.J., Korbut, R., Ocetkiewicz, A., Splawinski, J., Wojtaszek, B. & Swies, J. (1978) Lungs as a generator of prostacyclin — Hypothesis on physiological significance. *Nauyn Schmeiderberg Arch Pharmacol* **304**, 45–50.

Hall, D.W.R., Funcke, A.B.H. & Jaitly, K.D. (1979) some biological activities of a series of 9a-homo-9,11-epoxy prostanoic acid analogues. *Prostaglandins* **18**, 317.

Heaton, W.A., Davis, H.H., Welch, M.J., Mathias, C.J., Joist, J.H., Sherman, L.A. & Siegal, B.A. (1979) Indium-111: a new radionuclide label for studying human platelet kinetics. *Br J Haematol* **42**, 613–622.

Herd, C.M. (1991) Pharmacological modulation of PAF-induced platelet accumulation in the pulmonary circulation of the rabbit. *Br J Pharmacol* (in press).

Hladovec, J. (1986) A new model of arterial thrombosis. *Thromb Res* **41**, 659–664.

Hornstra, G. (1970) Method to determine the degree of ADP-induced platelet aggregation in circulating rat blood ('Filter-loop technique'). *Br J Haematol* **19**, 321–329.

Hornstra, G. (1971) Degree and duration of prostaglandin E_1-induced inhibition of platelet aggregation in the rat. *Eur J Pharmacol* **15**, 343–349.

Humphries, R.G., O'Connor, S.E. & Tomlinson, W. (1989) Differential inhibition of collagen and ADP-induced platelet aggregation by prostacyclin *in vivo*. *Br J Pharmacol* **96**, 167P.

Humphries, R.G., Tomlinson, W., O'Connor, S.E. & Leff, P. (1990) Inhibition of collagen- and ADP-induced platelet aggregation by substance P *in vivo*: Involvement of endothelium-derived relaxing factor. *J Cardiovasc Pharmacol* **16**, 292–297.

Inarrea, P., Gomez-Cambronero, J., Nieto, M. & Sanchez-Crespo, M. (1984) Characteristics of the binding of platelet-activating factor to platelets of different animal species. *Eur J Pharmacol* **105**, 309–315.

Knauer, K.A., Lichtenstein, L.M., Franklin Adkinson Jr, N. & Fish, J.E. (1981) Platelet activation during antigen-induced airway reactions in asthmatic subjects. *New Engl J Med* **304**, 1404.

Malik, A.B. (1983) Pulmonary microembolism. *Physiol Rev* **63**, 1115–1207.

Mallarkey, G. & Smith, G.M. (1985). A comparative study of the involvement of the prostaglandin H2/thromboxane A2 pathway in intravascular platelet aggregation. *Br J Pharmacol* **84**, 424–430.

Massad, L., Plotkine, M., Capdeville, C. & Boulu, R.G. (1987) Electrically induced arterial thrombosis model in the conscious rat. *Thromb Res* **48**, 1–10.

May, G.R., Herd, C.M., Butler, K.D. & Page, C.P. (1990) Radioisotopic model for investigating thromboembolism in the rabbit. *J Pharmacol Meth* **24**, 19–35.

May, G.R., Crook, P., Moore, P.K. & Page, C.P. (1991) Endothelium-derived nitric oxide is an endogenous regulator of platelet and neutrophil activation within

the pulmonary circulation. *Br J Pharmacol (in press)*.
Mazzoni, L., Morley, J., Page, C.P. & Sanjar, S. (1985) Induction of airway hyper-reactivity by platelet activating factor in the guinea pig. *J Physiol* **365**, 107P.
Menys, V.C. & Davies, J.A. (1984) A thromboxane antagonist, EP092, reduces the incorporation of platelets into fibrin-rich thrombi in rabbits. *Clin Sci* **66**, 22P.
Mills, J.E., Sellick, H. & Widdicombe, J.G. (1969) Lung irritant receptors in pulmonary microembolism, anaphylaxis and drug induced bronchoconstriction. *J Physiol* **203**, 337–357.
Mohammad, S.F., Anderson, W.H., Smith, J.B., Chuang, Y.K. & Mason, R.G. (1981) Effects of heparin on platelet aggregation and release and thromboxane A_2 production. *Am J Pathol* **104**, 132–141.
Moncada, S. & Vane, J. R. (1981) Prostacyclin: its biosynthesis, action and clinical potential. *Phil Trans R Soc London Ser B* **294**, 305–328.
Moore, S., Belbeck, L.W. & Evans, G. (1976) Myocardial lesions associated with partial, compared to complete, thrombotic occlusion of a coronary artery. *Circulation* **54**, 202–212.
Morley, J. Page, C.P., Paul, W., Monjelli, N., Ceserani, R. & Gandolfi, C. (1983) A comparative study of prostacyclin and two analogues (FCE 21258 and FCE 21292) in various *in vitro* and *in vivo* systems. *Prostaglandins Leuk Med* **11**, 391–399.
Morley, J., Sanjar, S. & Page, C.P. (1984) The platelet in asthma. *Lancet* **ii**, 1142–1144.
Mustard, J.F. & Packham, M.A. (1975) Platelets, thrombosis and drugs. *Drugs* **9**, 19–76.
Nachman, R.L. & Weksler, B.B. (1980) The platelet as an inflammatory cell. In Weissmann, G. (ed.) *The Cell Biology of Inflammation*, pp. 145–162. Elsevier/North Holland, Amsterdam.
Namm, D.H., Tadepalli, A.S. & High, J.A. (1982) Species specificity of the platelet responses to 1-O-alkyl-2-acetyl-*sn*-glycero-3-phosphocholine. *Thromb Res* **25**, 341–350.
Oyekan, A.O. & Botting, J.H. (1986) A minimally invasive technique for the study of intravascular platelet aggregation in anaesthetized rats. *J Pharmacol Meth* **15**, 271–277.
Oyekan, A.O. & Botting, J.H. (1988) The influence of adrenaline and gender difference on adenosine diphosphate-induced aggregation of platelets in the rat. *Thromb Haemost* **56**, 263–267.
Page, C.P. (1988) The involvement of platelets in non-thrombotic processes. *Br Pharmacol Sci* **9**, 66–71.
Page, C.P. (1989) The platelet as an inflammatory cell. *Immunopharmacology* **17**, 51–59.
Page, C.P., Paul, W. & Morley, J. (1982) An *in vivo* model for studying platelet aggregation and disaggregation. *Thromb Haemost* **47**, 210–213.
Page, C.P., Paul, W. & Morley, J. (1983a) *In vivo* aggregation of guinea-pig platelets in response to synthetic platelet activating factor (Paf-acether). Agents and Actions **13**, 506–507.
Page, C.P., Paul, W. & Morley, J. (1983b) Continuous monitoring of plasma protein extravasation and cell accumulation *in vivo*. *Br J Dermatol* **109**, 103–105.
Page, C.P., Paul, W. & Morley, J. (1984) Platelets and bronchospasm. *Int Arch Allergy Appl Immunol* **74**, 347–351.
Page, C.P., Tomiak, R.H.H., Sanjar, S. & Morley, J. (1985) Suppression of Paf-acether responses: an anti-inflammatory effect of anti-asthma drugs. *Agents and Actions* **16**, 33–35.
Pinckard, R.N., Halonen, M., Palmer, J.D., Butler, C., Shaw, J.O. & Henson, P.M. (1977) Intravascular aggregation and pulmonary sequestration of platelets during IgE induced systemic anaphylaxis in the rabbit: Abrogation of lethal anaphylactic shock by platelet depletion. *J Immunol* **119**, 2185–2193.
Pinon, J.F. (1984) *In vivo* study of platelet aggregation in rats. *J Pharmacol Meth* **12**, 79–84.
Pirkle, H. & Carstens, P. (1974) Pulmonary platelet aggregates associated with sudden death in man. *Science* **185**, 1062–1064.
Pirotzky, E., Page, C.P., Roubin, R., Pfister, A., Paul, W., Bonnet, J. & Benveniste, J. (1984) Paf-acether induced plasma exudation is independent of platelets and neutrophils in rat skin. *Microcirc Endothelium and Lymphatics* **1**, 107–122.
Pirotzky, E., Page, C.P., Morley, J. & Benveniste, J. (1985) Vascular permeability induced by Paf-acether (platelet activating factor) in the isolated perfused rat kidney. *Agents and Actions* **6**, 17–18.
Pretolani M., Page, C.P., Lefort, J., Lagente, V. & Vargaftig, B.B. (1986) Pharmacological modulation of the respiratory and haematological changes accompanying anaphylaxis in the guinea-pig. *Eur J Pharmacol* **125**, 403–409.
Rink, T.J., Simpson, A.W.M. & Hallam, T.J. (1985) Stimulus-secretion coupling: studies with human platelets. In Dumonte, J.E., Hanprecht, B. & Nunez J. (eds) *Hormones and Cell Regulation*, Vol. 9. pp. 305–324. Inserm, European Symposium. Elsevier Bismedical Science Publishers, Amsterdam.
Roba, J., Claeys, M. & Lambelin, G. (1976) Antiplatelet and antithrombogenic effects of suloctidil. *Eur J Pharmacol* **37**, 265–274.
Robertson, D.N. & Page, C.P. (1987) Effect of platelet agonists on airway reactivity and intrathoracic platelet accumulation. *Br J Pharmacol* **92**, 105–111.
Schneider, R.C., Zapol, W.M. & Carvalho, A.C. (1980) Platelet consumption and sequestration in severe acute respiratory failure. *Am Rev Respir Dis* **122**, 445–451.
Shand, R.A., Butler, K.D., Davies, J.A., Menys, V.C. & Wallis, R.B. (1987) The kinetics of platelet and fibrin deposition on to damaged rabbit carotid arteries *in vivo*: involvement of platelets in the initial deposition of fibrin. *Thromb Res* **45**, 505–515.
Shio, H. & Ramwell, P.W. (1972) Prostaglandin E_1 in platelet harvesting: An *in vitro* study. *Science* **175**, 506.
Shishido, M. & Katori, M. (1981) A quantitative method

using continuous recording of platelet thrombus size in hamster cheek pouch. *Microvasc Res* **22**, 199–209.

Smith, D., Sanjar, S., Herd, C. & Morley, J. (1989) *In vivo* method for the assessment of platelet accumulation. *J Pharmacol Meth* **21**, 45–59.

Smith, G.M. & Freuler, F. (1973) The measurement of intravascular aggregation by continuous platelet counting. *Bibl Anat* **12**, 229–234.

Sweatman, W.J.F., Brandon, D.R., Cranstone, S., Gooderham, R. & Walker, J.R. (1987) Indium-111-radiolabelled guinea pig peripheral leukocytes, *in vivo* distribution and response to leukotriene B_4. *J Pharmacol Meth* **18**, 227–237.

Szczeklik, A. & Gryglewski, R.J. (1985) Prostaglandins in therapy of cardiovascular disease. *Adv Prostaglandins Thromboxane Leukotriene Res* **13**, 345–354.

Thakur, M.L., Welch, M.J., Joist, J.H. & Coleman, R.E. (1976) Indium-111 labeled platelets: studies on preparation and evaluation of *in vitro* and *in vivo* functions. *Thromb Res* **9**, 345–357.

Thiemermann, C., May, G.R., Page, C.P. & Vane, J.R. (1990) Endothelin-1 inhibits platelet aggregation *in vivo*: a study with 111-indium-labelled platelets. *Br J Pharmacol* **99**, 303–308.

Tsao, C.H., Lo, R. & Raymono, J. (1976) Critical importance of citrate-blood ratio in platelet aggregation studies. *Am J Clin Pathol* **65**, 518–522.

Vanhoutte, P.M. & Shimokawa, H. (1989) Endothelium-derived relaxing factor and coronary vasospasm. *Circulation* **80**, 1–9.

Vargaftig, B.B., Lefort, J., Chignard, M. & Benveniste, J. (1980) Platelet activating factor induced a platelet dependent bronchoconstriction unrelated to the formation of prostaglandin derivatives. *Eur J Pharmacol* **65**, 185–192.

Vargaftig, B.B., Chignard, M. & Benveniste, J. (1981) Present concepts on the mechanisms of platelet aggregation. *Biochem Pharmacol* **30**, 263–271.

Vargaftig, B.B., Lefort, J., Wal, F., Chignard, M. & Medeiros, M.C. (1982) Interference of non-steroidal anti-inflammatory drugs associated to anti-histamine and anti-serotonin agents with the bronchial and platelet effects of platelet activating factor (Paf-acether). *Eur J Pharmacol* **82**, 121–130.

Widdicombe, J.G. & Sterling, G.M. (1970) The autonomic nervous system and breathing. *Arch Intern Med* **126**, 337–357.

Woolf, N. (1981) Thrombosis and atherosclerosis. In Bloom, A.L. & Thomas, D.P. (eds) *Haemostasis and thrombosis*, pp. 527–554, Churchill Livingstone,

Wu, K.K. & Hoak, J.C. (1974) A new method for the quantitative detection of platelet aggregates in patients with arterial insufficiency *Lancet* **ii**, 924–926.

5: The Involvement of Platelets in the Allergic Response

Michel Joseph

Introduction

After decades of dogma considering allergy as a two-partner tragedy between IgE and mast cells, our knowledge of the physiopathological mechanisms of immediate hypersensitivity reactions has considerably improved in the past few years. Several cell populations have now been identified as being involved in the immediate and delayed phases of allergic reactions. Besides mast cells and basophils, other cells, such as eosinophils, mononuclear phagocytes, or neutrophils, have been described as active participants in the allergic response as well as a plethora of chemical mediators. The platelet has recently been added to the list of cells potentially involved in the immunological mechanisms of allergy (Capron, A. *et al.* 1987; Gresele *et al.* 1987; Page, 1988), partly as a consequence of the demonstration of surface receptors for IgE on this cell type (Cines *et al.* 1986; Joseph *et al.* 1986).

A receptor for IgE on blood platelets

The identification of a specific receptor for IgE on blood platelets came from the analysis of effector mechanisms in antiparasite immunity (Capron, A. *et al.* 1986), and more particularly from the demonstration of cytotoxic functions by platelets from patients infected with the helminth *Schistosoma mansoni* (Joseph *et al.* 1983). These studies indicated that human platelets can bind IgE *in vitro* and that the cross-linking of surface-bound IgE with anti-IgE or the specific antigens induced platelet activation and secretion. Further experiments led to the demonstration of a specific receptor for the Fc fragment of IgE (FcεRII) on the platelet membrane, different from the high-affinity receptor described for IgE (FcεRI) on mast cells and basophils (Joseph *et al.* 1986). Furthermore, the platelet IgE receptor clearly appeared as distinct from the previously described IgG-binding sites. Scatchard analysis of the FcεRII identified between 600 and 1000 binding sites for IgE per platelet with an affinity constant of $3 \times 10^7 M^{-1}$. In normal subjects 20% of platelets were IgE positive, this percentage increased to a mean of 35% in allergic patients and up to 50% for patients with schistosomiasis or filariasis. Several lines of evidence pointed to similarities between the platelet IgE receptor and the FcεRII on monocytes, macrophages, and eosinophils. In particular a monoclonal antibody (BB10), raised against the eosinophil IgE receptor, inhibited the binding of IgE to platelets and their subsequent IgE-dependent activation (Capron, M. *et al.* 1986). The cross-linking of surface-bound IgE could also be achieved with an IgE-binding factor known as histamine releasing factor (HRF), released by macrophages and platelets themselves. Purification and subsequent gel analysis of the platelet IgE receptor has provided evidence of two subunits of 43 and 30 kDa, the latter differing from the smaller subunit in eosinophils and monocytes generally identified as a 23–25 kDa molecule.

The existence of such a receptor on platelets, together with the increased percentage of this receptor in allergic patients, suggested the possibility of a direct participation of platelets in allergy. In fact, the precise involvement of platelets in immediate hypersensitivity reactions (during either early or late phase) has not been clearly determined. However, several converging observations have shown that these blood elements are able to participate in allergic diseases, and more particularly in asthma (Gresele *et al.* 1987; Chapter 6). Indirect arguments have been collected which concern *in vitro* and *in vivo* manifestations of platelet activation, modifications of platelet physiology, the platelet dependence of several clinical or physiopathological manifestations, and finally the platelet dependence of certain cellular aspects of the allergic response.

Signs of platelet activation *in vitro* in allergic disease

Platelets isolated from patients with allergic asthma (to house dust, mites or grass pollens), or platelets from patients with *Hymenoptera* venom hypersensitivity react *in vitro* to specific allergens or to IgE-specific ligands (such as anti-IgE antibody) by producing cytotoxic mediators — measured as death of the parasite larvae (Joseph *et al.* 1983) — or oxygen-derived free radicals — measured by luminol-luciferin chemiluminescence (Joseph *et al.* 1986). Anti-IgG, as well as non-specific allergens, were unable to induce such effects. Due to the presence of IgE receptors on at least 20% of the thrombocyte population, platelets isolated from healthy donors could be passively sensitized with IgE antibody by pre-incubation in the serum of allergic patients. The addition of specific allergens or anti-IgE induced effector functions demonstrated by the death of *Schistosoma mansoni* and by free-radical-dependent chemiluminescence. Here again, anti-IgG was inactive on such platelets, whereas the role of bound IgE in the platelet reactivity was confirmed by isotype-specific adsorption of antibody from the serum of allergic donors: adsorption of IgE, but not that of IgG, could abrogate the ability of serum, from allergic patients, to induce normal platelets to have cytotoxic activity. The participation of IgE in this activation process was further corroborated by the inhibitory role of polyclonal (Spiegelberg, 1984) and monoclonal antibodies (Capron, M. *et al.* 1986) against the FcεRII on the passive sensitization and activation of normal platelets by serum from allergic patients.

If platelets have a general role in allergy, their IgE-dependent selective functions might also be triggered through IgE-independent mechanisms in other clinically similar disorders, such as asthmatic syndromes of non-immunological origin. In this context, aspirin-induced asthma appeared as a good model for investigating such an hypothesis. Whereas, until recently, no *in vitro* abnormality and no involvement of any cell population or humoral factor could be identified in this severe subset of asthmatics, platelets isolated from patients with aspirin-induced asthma exhibited *in vitro* an abnormal response to aspirin, generating oxygen metabolites and cytotoxic mediators in the presence of acetylsalicylic acid or various non-steroidal anti-inflammatory drugs (NSAIDs), such as indomethacin or flurbiprofen (Ameisen *et al.* 1985). Neither blood leukocytes, nor purified leukocyte populations from the same patients, could be triggered to have cytotoxic activity in the presence of aspirin or other NSAIDs. The involvement of IgE in this abnormal response was ruled out by several lines of evidence, among them the inability of serum from patients to passively sensitize platelets from healthy donors to NSAIDs, and the absence of an inhibitory effect of polyclonal or monoclonal antibodies against the FcεRII. Investigations into the mechanism of this platelet response showed it to be related to the inhibitory effect of aspirin and NSAIDs on cyclooxygenase. Briefly, the abnormal response of platelets from aspirin-sensitive patients might be due to the reduced binding of endogenous prostaglandin H_2(PGH_2) endoperoxides to their platelet receptor, an indirect consequence of the NSAID-induced inhibition of cyclooxygenase that lowered PGH_2 synthesis. Although the precise nature of the specific platelet abnormality remains to be defined in platelets from such patients, endoperoxides might play a crucial regulatory role which NSAIDs can disturb. One possibility is that PGH_2 might be involved in the control of the synthesis and/or of the biological effect of platelet lipoxygenase products (Ameisen, 1986).

In the framework of allergic and inflammatory disorders other biological mediators that trigger platelet activation have also been demonstrated. C reactive protein has been demonstrated to be a potent inducer of platelet activation. Platelets collected during the acute phase of experimental infection of rodents by schistosomes were highly cytotoxic for schistosome larvae, and normal platelets from rat and man could be triggered into effector cells by highly purified C reactive protein (Bout *et al.* 1986).

More recently, the neuropeptide substance P was shown to trigger platelet activation directly (Damonneville *et al.* 1990), opening new perspectives of neuroimmunological interactions. Interestingly, the amino acid sequence of substance P actively involved in platelet activation appeared confined to the N-terminal region of the molecule, as for the stimulation of T lymphocyte proliferation, whereas amino acids of the C-terminal portion induced histamine release from mast cells. The synthesis of various peptides derived from the sequence of substance P has led to the identification of the 5–11 amino acid sequence as the most active site of the molecule. In competition experiments, it was also demonstrated that platelet activation by substance P could be inhibited by IgE, and that this competitive inhibition might be related to the existence of limited but significant conformational homology between the primary structure of substance P and the domain of the ε chain.

To go further in the context of inflammatory cell interactions possibly implicated in immediate hypersensitivity reactions, lymphokines were also described as active in stimulating platelets: cytotoxic functions were elicited into normal human platelets by the addition of supernatants from mitogen- or antigen-stimulated $CD4^+$ T cells. The physicochemical properties of the activating factor(s) strongly suggested that IFN_γ was probably one of the lymphokines inducing platelet cytotoxicity. The neutralization of the killer effect induction by monoclonal and polyclonal anti-IFN_γ antibodies, the presence of IFN_γ in the $CD4^+$ lymphocyte supernatants, and, finally, the direct induction of the cytotoxic effect by recombinant IFN_γ clearly demonstrated that this lymphokine was one of the factors responsible for the induction of platelet cytotoxic functions (Pancré *et al.* 1987). The *in vivo* relevance of this effect was demonstrated in the rat model: the passive transfer of normal rat platelets treated with rat recombinant IFN_γ to normal syngeneic recipients on the day of a challenge infection led to a high degree of protection. Moreover, IFN_γ could also act on the IgE-dependent platelet cytotoxicity by enhancing the IgE receptor expression on the platelet membrane (Pancré *et al.* 1988). The possibility of an activation process with this lymphokine was strengthened by the demonstration that human IFN_γ was able to bind to an estimate of 150–200 high-affinity specific receptors on human platelets with a K_D of 2×10^{-10} M (Molinas *et al.* 1987). A second inducing factor of platelet cytotoxicity, exhibiting a neutral pI, was also evidenced in $CD4^+$ stimulated T lymphocyte supernatants. This factor was identified as tumour necrosis factor (TNF). Indeed, recombinant TNF_β, and to a lesser extent TNF_α induced normal platelets into cytotoxic effectors against *S. mansoni* larvae (Damonneville *et al.* 1988). An additive effect of TNF and IFN_γ was observed in this model.

Besides these *in vitro* parameters of activation, during immediate hypersensitivity reactions, platelets exhibit *in vivo* manifestations of reactivity which will now be briefly summarized.

Signs of platelet activation *in vivo* in allergic responses

In allergic disorders, platelet activation has often been considered as occurring indirectly through the effects of platelet activating factor (PAF). Platelet activating factor is released by a variety of IgE sensitized cells that express either $Fc_\varepsilon RI$ (mast cells, basophils) or $Fc_\varepsilon RII$ (macrophages, eosinophils). This phospholipid is also released by stimulated endothelial cells and by activated platelets themselves (reviewed by Barnes *et al.* 1988). In rabbit, PAF induces the release of platelet factor 4 (PF4) both *in vitro* and *in vivo* (McManus *et al.* 1979). Similarly, the IgE-induced anaphylaxis in the rabbit led to the release of PF4 into the plasma.

Platelet Factor 4 and β-thromboglobulin (β-TG) were observed in the plasma of asthmatic patients after allergen challenge, whereas these mediators were not found when bronchospasm was produced by an IgE-independent stimulus such as methacholine (Knauer *et al.* 1981). The same platelet-specific factors were identified by several authors in the plasma and broncho-alveolar lavage fluids of asthmatics after bronchoprovocation tests (Gresele *et al.* 1982, 1985; Metzger *et al.* 1983). However, other investigators have not confirmed these observations (Cella & Girolami, 1981; Greer *et al.* 1984; Durham *et al.* 1985).

Thrombocytopenia has been reported after asthmatic attacks, reflecting platelet activation during allergic reactions (Storck *et al.* 1955), and circulating platelet aggregates were observed in the rabbit during anaphylactic shock (Pinckard *et al.* 1977), and in man after bronchoprovocation tests (Gresele *et al.* 1982; Traietti *et al.* 1984). The significance of these observations is debatable: however, they can be put together with the pulmonary sequestration of platelet aggregates in allergic animals (Pinckard *et al.* 1977; Page *et al.* 1984). Extravascular migration of platelets has been demonstrated in the lungs of guinea pigs after intravenous injection of PAF (Lellouch-Tubiana *et al.* 1985), and in the lungs of baboons after intratracheal injection of the phospholipid (Arnoux *et al.* 1988). In man, platelets have been observed in broncho-alveolar lavage fluids in early and late phases, but in larger amounts immediately after allergen challenge (Metzger *et al.* 1985, 1986, 1987). Post mortem studies carried out on patients dying in *status asthmaticus*, revealed the presence of a greater number of megakaryocytes, than could be found in control lungs (Slater *et al.* 1985). The injection of anti-IgE antibody in the skin and of antigen intravenously generated platelet accumulation at the site of Arthus reaction in the rabbit (Kravis & Henson, 1977). The same occurred after intradermal injection of PAF in the guinea-pig (Morley *et al.* 1983).

Changes in platelet physiology

Qualitative differences have been reported for platelets from allergic patients compared with healthy donors. First, platelets from atopic patients and allergic animals exhibited hypoaggregability to various aggregating agents *in vitro* (Fishel & Zwemer, 1970; Solinger *et al.* 1973; Henson & Pinckard, 1977; Maccia *et al.* 1977; Gallagher *et al.* 1978; Rao & Walsh, 1983; Thompson *et al.* 1984). However, this decrease of platelet aggregability was reversible, platelet aggregation returning to normal curves after specific desensitization. Then, in association with hypoaggregability, an increased bleeding time was noticed in allergic patients, reported in the case of symptomatic pollinic rhinitis (Gallagher *et al.* 1978), in the case of anaphylactic shock to *Hymenoptera* venom (Smith *et al.* 1980), and in the case of allergic asthma together with a reduced aggregability and sensitivity to PAF *in vitro* (Szczeklik *et al.* 1986). Some authors, however, have not observed these modifications of platelet reactivity (Harwell *et al.* 1973; McDonald *et al.* 1974; Greer *et al.* 1984). Finally, a decrease of the platelet regeneration time together with an increase of the platelet consumption (Gresele *et al.* 1987), also estimated as a fall in the half-life of circulating platelets in asthmatics (4.7 ± 1.3 days) compared with normal individuals (8.9 ± 1.0 days) (Taytard *et al.* 1986) has been reported although such changes have not been observed by others (Ind *et al.* 1985). Platelet half-life returned to normal values after ketotifen treatment of asthmatics (Taytard *et al.* 1987).

In *Hymenoptera* venom hypersensitivity, platelets from patients undergoing specific immunotherapy by rush desensitization lost their specific reactivity to allergens *in vitro*, becoming unable to generate free radicals and cytotoxic mediators, in contrast with the properties they exhibited before desensitization. The *in vitro* sensitivity of platelets exactly correlated the sensitivity of patients to venom (Tsicopoulos *et al.* 1988a, 1990). Recent experiments favour the possible involvement of lymphokines in the observed modification of platelet reactivity. Indeed, lymphocyte supernatants obtained from patients after rush desensitization were able to down-regulate platelet reactivity. Similarly, sera obtained from desensitized patients were able to suppress the IgE-dependent platelet activation (Tsicopoulos *et al.* 1989). Physicochemical characterization of the suppressive factor present in lymphocyte supernatants and in serum showed properties very similar to those previously described for a lymphokine able to suppress platelet activity (Pancré *et al.* 1986). It was shown that ConA- and antigen-stimulated $CD8^+$ T lymphocytes released a factor able to inhibit the IgE-dependent platelet generation of cytotoxic mediators and of oxygen metabolites. This platelet activity suppressive lymphokine (PASL) was identified as an acid- and heat-stable polypeptide of 15–20 kDa with a pI of 4.6. The factor was specifically absorbed by platelet membrane suggesting its action through the binding to a receptor. Besides its apparent similarity with the factor present in the serum of allergic patients undergoing rush desensitization, the *in vivo* relevance of PASL could be established by a complete abolition of the protection normally conferred toward a challenge infection with schistosome worms by the intravenous passive transfer of platelets from immune to normal rats, after PASL-treatment of transferred platelets (Pancré *et al.* 1989). The molecular cloning of PASL is presently underway.

In aspirin-sensitive asthma, platelets lose their abnormal reactivity to aspirin and their associated cytotoxic functions during the refractory period induced in patients by the daily ingestion of high doses of aspirin. In other words, at the very period when patients became clinically insensitive to aspirin, their platelets were deactivated. Inversely, platelets recovered their full reactivity as soon as the oral treatment with aspirin was stopped and patients were aspirin-sensitive again (Ameisen *et al.* 1985).

Platelet-dependence of anaphylactic shock or bronchoconstriction

Besides the observations reported above, platelets seem also to be involved in physiological effects of allergen challenge, either in the anaphylactic reaction, or in the bronchospasm induced in sensitized animals or allergic patients by the specific allergens. The lethal shock induced by the intravenous injection of bovine serum albumin in rabbits sensitized to this protein was abrogated by platelet depletion (Pinckard *et al.* 1977). Similarly the bronchoconstriction produced by the intravenous injection of ovalbumin in sensitized guinea-pigs (Page *et al.* 1984) was inhibited by the antiplatelet treatment of the animals (Lellouch-Tubiana *et al.* 1988). Furthermore, bronchial hyper-reactivity could be associated with platelet activation since allergic rabbits challenged by inhalation of allergen presented a dramatically reduced bronchial hyper-reactivity and a suppression of the late phase reaction after platelet depletion (Coyle *et al.* 1990).

The role of PAF in such effects is far from being clearly understood. However, its participation is strongly suggested by several observations. Platelet activating factor induced acute responses of the respiratory tract following intravenous injection or intratracheal instillation in man (Gateau *et al.* 1984) and in animals (Halonen *et al.* 1980; Vargaftig *et al.* 1980; Denjean *et al.* 1983), associated with thrombocytopenia. Here again specific platelet depletion or the inhibition of platelet activation by prostacyclin suppressed the effects of both PAF and antigen challenge in the lungs of rabbits and guinea-pigs (Halonen *et al.* 1981; Vargaftig & Benveniste, 1983; Coyle *et al.* 1990; Lellouch-Tubiana *et al.* 1988). Compounds able to inhibit platelet degranulation also blocked the airway smooth muscle contraction induced by PAF *in vitro* (Schellenberg *et al.* 1983). *In vitro*, PAF contracted surgical human bronchi only in the presence of platelets, whereas neither PAF nor platelets alone could produce the bronchospasm (Schellenberg *et al.* 1983). In the rat, whose platelets have no receptor for PAF, the intravenous injection of the phospholipid is unable to induce a bronchoconstriction (Vargaftig & Benveniste, 1983; Barnes *et al.* 1988).

Platelet-dependence of cell influx or activation

The cell interactions underlying the physiopathological processes of allergy and associated inflammatory reactions may involve the participation of platelets in the recruitment of various other leukocytes involved in the immunological conflict arising from the contact between allergens and sensitized tissues. One of the most clearly established examples of this cell–cell interaction is the platelet-dependence of the eosinophil recruitment in the lung of experimental animals following the administration of PAF or specific allergens: inhibition of platelet activation by prostacyclin or depletion with antiplatelet serum significantly lowered the eosinophil infiltration into the pulmonary tissue of guinea-pigs (Lellouch-Tubiana *et al.* 1988). In the allergic rabbit, specific platelet depletion led to a 63% decrease of the allergen-induced eosinophil influx into the lung, together with the disappearance of the late phase reaction already discussed above (Coyle *et al.* 1990). In the guinea-pig, PAF generated a platelet-independent increase of the airway and arterial pressure, but this effect was potentiated by the addition of thrombocytes: the participation of endothelial cells in this mechanism has been postulated

(Hamasaki *et al.* 1984). Platelet factor 4 has been shown to stimulate histamine release from human basophils (Brindley *et al.* 1983), and another platelet factor demonstrated similar effects on human circulating basophils and pulmonary mast cells (Knauer *et al.* 1984; Orchard *et al.* 1986). This factor was produced spontaneously or following stimulation by specific allergens or anti-IgE from allergic patient platelets; it was distinct from platelet derived growth factor (PDGF) and from PF4, and was heat- and acid-stable (Knauer *et al.* 1984). A positive immediate reaction to intradermal injection of this platelet derived histamine releasing factor (PDHRF), was presented by 75% of allergic asthmatics, of which 25% exhibited a late reaction. These subjects had also non-specific bronchial hyper-responsiveness as measured by their sensitivity to metacholine (Fisher *et al.* 1988). Patients with intrinsic asthma or allergic rhinitis had negative intradermal reaction to PDHRF (IDR) (Weiss *et al.* 1988). The analysis of the platelet-dependence of cell recruitment and activation is presently at its very beginning. It will certainly provide new insights into the concept of the potential implication of thrombocytes in the immunological and inflammatory mechanisms of allergic disorders.

Platelets and anti-allergy drugs

If platelets are involved in certain aspects of the immediate hypersensitivity reaction, drugs with anti-allergic properties should exhibit some effects on platelet reactivity. Likewise, compounds demonstrating the ability of inhibiting platelets in IgE-dependent conditions should be considered as possibly active in the regulation of allergic disorders, and thus as potential drugs in the treatment of allergy.

In fact, disodium cromoglycate (Lomudal®) and nedocromil sodium (Tilade®) inhibited very significantly *in vitro* and *ex vivo* the IgE-dependent activation of platelets from allergic patients (Thorel *et al.* 1988; Tsicopoulos *et al.* 1988b). Similarly, cetirizine (Zyrtec®, a new anti-allergic compound) also very significantly blocked the IgE-induced generation of cytotoxic mediators by platelets from patients with mite asthma or with *Hymenoptera* venom hypersensitivity (De Vos *et al.* 1989). These observations focus on the need of widening to all IgE-positive cell populations (including platelets) the analysis of anti-allergy and anti-inflammatory drug effects. Results obtained in this field will allow new applications to the therapeutic management of such pathologies. An example of such a development was shown by the high capacity of nedocromil sodium to inhibit the abnormal response to NSAIDs of platelets from aspirin-sensitive asthmatics (ASA) both *in vitro* and *ex vivo* after nedocromil sodium inhalation (Joseph *et al.* 1987; Marquette *et al.* 1990). *In vitro* the generation of cytotoxic mediators by ASA-platelets incubated with aspirin was inhibited by nedocromil sodium at concentrations at least 500 times lower than disodium cromoglycate, i.e. at therapeutic concentrations of the drug. When platelets were recovered from ASA-patients 15 minutes after inhalation of Tilade® they were shown to be insensitive to aspirin. Inversely, Lomudal® inhalation by these patients had no effect on the *in vitro* reactivity of ASA platelets possibly because the drug is not absorbed.

These compounds had already shown inhibiting activities on other cells potentially involved in IgE-dependent activation processes, such as eosinophils (Leprevost *et al.* 1988), macrophages and monocytes (Thorel *et al.* 1988; Tsicopoulos *et al.* 1988b). It is, therefore, likely that part of their therapeutic efficacy is actually supported by their activity on non-mast cell leukocytes. The investigations undertaken in this area will simultaneously increase our fundamental knowledge on immunopathological processes of immediate hypersensitivity and improve our approach in developing new therapeutic agents for the management of allergic diseases. We would like to conclude this brief review of possible platelet implications in allergy with the concept that, if platelets are finally to be demonstrated as active partners in allergic disorders, they should not to be considered as the only participants and will have to be integrated therefore in the general cell network which is progressively defined for allergy and associated inflammatory reactions.

Acknowledgements

I wish to thank all those who have contributed to the development of investigations on platelets in our laboratory, the first of which is Professor André Capron, and, immediately behind, my skillfull technician and friend Han Vorng. Then, in alphabetical order, I would like to thank Jean-Claude Ameisen, Claude Auriault, Daniel Bout, Monique Capron, Jean-Yves Cesbron, Martine Damonneville, Jean-Pierre Kusnierz, Philippe Lassalle, Didier Monté, Véronique Pancré, André-Bernard Tonnel, Gérard Torpier and Anne Tsicopoulos.

References

Ameisen, J.C. (1986) Aspirin sensitive asthma: a model for a role of platelets in hypersensitivity reactions. *Ann Inst Pasteur Immunol* **137D**, 141–147.

Ameisen, J.C., Capron, A., Joseph, M., Maclouf, J., Vorng, H., Pancré, V., Fournier, E., Wallaert, B. & Tonnel, A.B. (1985) Aspirin-sensitive asthma: abnormal platelet response to drugs inducing asthmatic attacks. Diagnostic and physiopathological implications. *Int Arch Allergy Appl Immunol* **78**, 438–448.

Arnoux, B., Denjean, A., Page, C.P., Nolibe, B., Morley, J. & Benveniste, J. (1988) Accumulation of platelets and eosinophils in baboon lung after PAF-acether challenge. Inhibition by ketotifen. *Am Rev Respir Dis* **137**, 855–860.

Barnes, P.J., Chung, K.F. & Page C.P. (1988) Platelet-activating factor as a mediator of allergic disease. *J Allergy Clin Immunol* **81**, 919–934.

Bout, D., Joseph, M., Pontet, M., Vorng, H., Deslée, D. & Capron, A. (1986) Rat resistance to schistosomiasis: Platelet-mediated cytotoxicity induced by C-reactive protein. *Science* **231**, 153–156.

Brindley, L.L., Sweet, J.M. & Goetzl, E.J. (1983) Stimulation of histamine release from human basophils by human platelet factor 4. *J Clin Invest* **72**, 1218–1233.

Capron, A., Dessaint, J.P., Capron, M., Joseph, M., Ameisen, J.C. & Tonnel, A.B. (1986) From parasites to allergy: a second receptor for IgE. *Immunology Today* **7**, 15–18.

Capron, A., Joseph, M., Ameisen, J.C., Capron, M., Pancré, V. & Auriault, C. (1987) Platelets as effectors in immune and hypersensitivity reactions. *Int Arch Allergy Appl Immunol* **82**, 307–312.

Capron, M., Jouault, T., Prin, L., Joseph, M., Ameisen, J.C., Butterworth, A.E., Papin, J.P., Kusnierz, J.P. & Capron, A. (1986) Functional study of a monoclonal antibody to IgE Fc receptor (FcεRII) of eosinophils, platelets, and macrophages. *J Exp Med* **164**, 72–89.

Cella, G. & Girolami, A. (1981) Platelet activation in antigen-induced bronchoconstriction. *New Engl J Med* **305**, 892–893.

Cines, D.B., van der Keyl, H. & Levinson, A.I. (1986) *In vitro* binding of an IgE protein to human platelets. *J Immunol* **136**, 3433–3440.

Coyle, A.J., Page, C.P., Atkinson, L., Flanagan, R. & Metzger, W.J. (1990) The requirement for platelets in allergen-induced late asthmatic airway obstruction, eosinophil infiltration and heightened airways responsiveness in allergic rabbits. *Am Rev Resp Dis* **142**, 587–593.

Damonneville, M., Wietzerbin, J., Pancré, M., Joseph, M., Capron, A. & Auriault, C. (1988) Recombinant tumor necrosis factors mediate platelet cytotoxicity to *Schistosoma mansoni* larvae. *J Immunol* **140**, 3962–3965.

Damonneville, M., Monté, D., Auriault, C., Gras-Masse, R., Tartar, A., Joseph, M. & Capron, A. (1990) The neuropeptide substance P stimulates the effector functions of platelets. *Clin Exp Immunol* **81**, 346–351.

Denjean, A., Arnoux, B., Masse, R., Lockart, A. & Benveniste, J. (1983) Acute effects of intratracheal administration of platelet-activating factor in baboons. *J Appl. Physiol* **55**, 799–804.

De Vos, C., Joseph, M., Leprevost, C., Vorng, H., Tomassini, M., Capron, M. & Capron, A. (1989) Inhibition of human eosinophil chemotaxis and of the IgE-dependent stimulation of human blood platelets by cetirizine. *Int Arch Allergy Appl Immunol* **88**, 212–215.

Durham, S.R., Dawes, J. & Kay, A.B. (1985) Platelets in asthma. *Lancet* **ii**, 36.

Fishel, C.W. & Zwemer, R.J. (1970) Aggregation of platelets from *B. pertussis*-infected mice and atopically sensitive human individuals. *Fed Proc* **29**, 640.

Fisher, R., Weiss, M., Kagey-Sobotka, A. & Lichtenstein, L.M. (1988) Response to platelet-derived histamine releasing factor (PD-HRF) is associated with allergic but not non-allergic asthma. *New Engl Regional Proc* **9**, 249.

Gallagher, J.S., Bernstein, I.L., Maccia, C.A., Splanski, G.L. & Glück, H.I. (1978) Cyclic platelet dysfunction in IgE-mediated allergy. *J Allergy Clin Immunol* **62**, 229–235.

Gateau, O., Arnoux, B., Deriaz, H., Viars, P. & Benveniste, J. (1984) Acute effects of intratracheal administration of paf-acether (platelet-activating factor) in humans. *Am Rev Respir Dis* **129**, 3A.

Greer, I.A., Winter, J.H., Gaffney, D., Regan, K., Belch, J.J.F., Boyd, G. & Forbes, C.D. (1984) Platelets in asthma. *Lancet* **ii**, 1479.

Gresele, P., Todisco, T., Merante, F. & Nenci, G.G. (1982) Platelet activation and allergic asthma. *New Engl J Med* **306**, 549.

Gresele, P., Grasselli, S., Todisco, T. & Nenci, G.G. (1985) Platelets and asthma. *Lancet* **i**, 347.

Gresele, P., Ribaldi, E., Grasseli, S., Todisco, T. & Nenci, G.G. (1987) Evidence for platelet activation in allergic asthma. *Agents and Actions Suppl* **21**, 119–128.

Halonen, M., Palmer, J.D., Lohman, I.C., McManus, L.M. & Pinckard, R.N. (1980) Respiratory and circulatory alterations induced by acetyl glyceryl ether phosphorylcholine, a mediator of IgE anaphylaxis in the rabbit. *Am Rev Respir Dis* **122**, 915–924.

Halonen, M., Palmer, J.D., Lohman, I.C., McManus, L.M. & Pinckard, R.N. (1981) Differential effects of platelet depletion on the physiologic alterations of IgE anaphylaxis and acetyl glyceryl ether phosphorylcholine infusion in the rabbit. *Am Rev Respir Dis* **124**, 416–421.

Hamasaki, Y., Mojarad, M., Saga, T., Tai, H.H. & Said, S.I. (1984) Platelet-activating factor raises airway and vascular pressures and induces edema in lungs perfused with platelet-free solutions. *Am Rev Respir Dis* **129**, 742–746.

Harwell, W.B., Patterson, J.T., Lieberman, P. & Beachey, E. (1973) Platelet aggregation in normal and atopic subjects. *J Allergy Clin Immunol* **51**, 274–284.

Henson, P.M. & Pinckard, R.N. (1977) Basophil-derived platelet-activating factor (PAF) as an *in vivo* mediator of acute allergic reactions: demonstration of specific desensitization of platelets to PAF during IgE-induced anaphylaxis in the rabbit. *J Immunol* **119**, 2179–2184.

Ind, P.W., Peters, A.M., Malik, F., Lavender, J.P. & Dollery, C.T. (1985) Pulmonary platelet kinetics in asthma. *Thorax* **41**, 290–294.

Joseph, M., Auriault, C., Capron, A., Vorng, H. & Viens, P. (1983) A new function for platelets: IgE-dependent killing of schistosomes. *Nature* **303**, 810–812.

Joseph, M., Capron, A., Ameisen, J.C., Capron, M., Vorng, H., Pancré, V., Kusnierz, J.P. & Auriault, C. (1986) The receptor for IgE on blood platelets. *Eur J Immunol* **16**, 306–312.

Joseph, M., Marquette, C.H., Thorel, T., Vorng, H., Tonnel, A.B. & Capron, A. (1987) Comparative effect of nedocromil sodium and sodium cromoglycate on the abnormal response to aspirin of platelets from aspirin-sensitive asthmatics. In *Proceedings of the 6th Congress of the European Society of Pneumology*, 31 August–5 September, Amsterdam (Abstract).

Knauer, K.A., Lichtenstein, L.M., Adkinson, N.F. & Fish, J.E. (1981) Platelet activation during antigen-induced airway reactions in asthmatic subjects. *New Engl J Med* **304**, 1404–1407.

Knauer, K.A., Kagey-Sobotka, A., Adkinson, N.F. & Lichtenstein, L.M. (1984) Platelet augmentation of IgE-dependent histamine release from human basophils and mast cells. *Int Arch Allergy Appl Immunol* **74**, 29–35.

Kravis, T.C. & Henson, P.M. (1977) Accumulation of platelets at sites of antigen-antibody-mediated injury: a possible role for IgE antibody and mast cells. *J Immunol* **118**, 1569–1573.

Lellouch-Tubiana, A., Lefort, J., Pirotzky, E., Vargaftig, B.B. & Pfister, A. (1985) Ultrastructural evidence for extravascular platelet recruitment in the lung upon intravenous injection of platelet activating factor (Paf-acether) to guinea-pigs. *Br J Exp Pathol* **66**, 345–355.

Lellouch-Tubiana, A., Lefort, J., Simon, M.T., Pfister, A. & Vargaftig, B.B. (1988) Eosinophil recruitment into guinea pig lungs after PAF-acether and allergen administration. Modulation by prostacyclin, platelet depletion, and selective antagonists. *Am Rev Respir Dis* **137**, 948–954.

Leprevost, C., Capron, M., De Vos, C., Tomassini, M. & Capron, A. (1988) Inhibition of eosinophil chemotaxis by a new antiallergic compound (cetirizine). *Int Arch Allergy Appl Immunol* **87**, 9–13.

McDonald, J.R., Tan, E.M., Stevenson, D.D. & Vaughan, J.H. (1974) Platelet aggregation in asthmatics and normal subjects. *J Allergy Clin Immunol* **54**, 200–208.

McManus, L.M., Morley, C.A., Levine, S.P. & Pinckard, R.N. (1979) Platelet Activating Factor (PAF) induced release of Platelet Factor 4 (PF4) *in vitro* and during IgE anaphylaxis in the rabbit. *J Immunol* **123**, 2835–2841.

Maccia, C.A., Gallagher, J.S., Ataman, G., Glück, H.I., Brooks, S.M. & Bernstein, I.L. (1977) Platelet thrombopathy in asthmatic patients with elevated immunoglobulin E. *J Allergy Clin Immunol* **59**, 101–108.

Marquette, C.H., Joseph, M., Tonnel, A.B., Vorng, H., Lassalle, P., Tsicopoulos, A. & Capron, A. (1990) The abnormal *in vitro* response to aspirin of platelets from aspirin-sensitive asthmatics is inhibited after inhalation of nedocromil sodium but not of sodium cromoglycate. *Br J Clin Pharmac* **29**, 525–531.

Metzger, W.J., Henriksen, R.A., Zaleski, A. & Donnelley, A. (1983) Evidence for platelet release and thrombin generation in early and late asthmatic response. *Clin Res* **33**, 164.

Metzger, W.J., Hunninghake, G.W. & Richerson, H.B. (1985) Late asthmatic responses: inquiry into mechanisms and significance. *Clin Rev Allergy* **3**, 145–165.

Metzger, W.J., Richerson, H.B., Worden, K., Monick, M. & Hunninghake, G.W. (1986) Bronchoalveolar lavage of allergic asthmatic patients following allergen bronchoprovocation. *Chest* **89**, 477–483.

Metzger, W.J., Sjoerdsma, B.A., Richerson, H.B., Moseley, P., Zavala, D., Monick, M. & Hunninghake, G.W. (1987) Platelets in bronchoalveolar lavage from asthmatic patients and allergic rabbits with allergen-induced late phase responses. *Agents and Actions Suppl* **21**, 151–159.

Molinas, F.C., Wietzerbin, J. & Falcoff, E. (1987) Human platelets possess receptors for a lymphokine: demonstration of high specific receptors for hu IFN_{γ}. *J Immunol* **138**, 802–806.

Morley, J., Page, C.P. & Paul, W. (1983) Inflammatory actions of Paf-acether in guinea pig skin. *Br J Pharmacol* **80**, 503–509.

Orchard, M.A., Kagey-Sobotka, A., Proud, D. & Lichtenstein, L.M. (1986) Basophil histamine release induced by a substance from stimulated human platelets. *J Immunol* **136**, 2240–2244.

Page, C.P. (1988) The involvement of platelets in non-thrombotic processes. *Trends Pharmacol Sci* **9**, 66–71.

Page, C.P., Paul, W. & Morley, J. (1984) Platelets and bronchospasm. *Int Arch Allergy Appl Immunol* **74**, 347–350.

Pancré, V., Auriault, C., Joseph, M., Cesbron, J.Y., Kuznierz, J.P. & Capron, A. (1986) A suppressive lymphokine of platelet cytotoxic functions. *J Immunol* **137**, 585–591.

Pancré, V., Joseph, M., Mazingue, C., Wietzerbin, J., Capron, A. & Auriault, C. (1987) Induction of platelet cytotoxic functions by lymphokine: role of gamma interferon. *J Immunol* **138**, 4490–4495.

Pancré, V., Joseph, M., Capron, A., Wietzerbin, J., Kusnierz, J.P., Vorng, H. & Auriault, C. (1988) Recombinant human immune interferon induces increased IgE receptor expression on human platelets. *Eur J Immunol* **18**, 829–832.

Pancré, V., Joseph, M., Capron, A., Delannoye, A., Vorng, H. & Auriault, C. (1989) Characterization of a suppressive factor of platelet cytotoxic functions in human and rat schistosomiasis mansoni. *Clin Exp Immunol* **76**, 417–421.

Pinckard, R.N., Halonen, M., Palmer, J.D., Butler, C., Shaw, J.O. & Henson, P.M. (1977) Intravascular aggregation and pulmonary sequestration of platelets during IgE-induced systemic anaphylaxis in the rabbit: abrogation of lethal anaphylactic shock by platelet depletion. *J Immunol* **119**, 2185–2193.

Rao, A.K. & Walsh, P.N. (1983) Acquired qualitative platelet disorders. *Clin Haematol* **12**, 201–238.

Schellenberg, R.R., Walker, B. & Snyder, F. (1983) Platelet-dependent contraction of human bronchus by platelet-activating factor. *J Allergy Clin Immunol* **71**, 145.

Slater, D., Martin, J. & Trowbridge, A. (1985) The platelet in asthma. *Lancet* **i**, 110.

Smith, P.L., Sobotka, A.K., Bleecker, E.R., Traystman, R., Kaplan, A.P., Gralnick, H., Valentine, M.D., Permutt, S. & Lichtenstein, L.M. (1980) Physiologic manifestations of human anaphylaxis. *J Clin Invest* **66**, 1072–1080.

Solinger, A., Bernstein, I.L. & Glück, H.I. (1973) The effect of epinephrine on platelet aggregation in normal and atopic subjects. *J Allergy Clin Immunol* **51**, 29–34.

Spiegelberg, H.L. (1984) Structure and function of Fc receptors for IgE on lymphocytes, monocytes and macrophages. *Adv Immunol* **35**, 61–88.

Storck, H., Hoigné, R. & Killer, F. (1955) Thrombocytes in allergic reactions. *Int Arch Allergy* **6**, 372–384.

Szczeklik, A., Milner, P.C., Birch, J., Watkins, J. & Martin, J.P. (1986) Prolonged bleeding time, reduced platelet aggregation, altered PAF-acether sensitivity, and increased platelet mass are a trait of asthma and hay fever. *Thromb Haemost* **56**, 183–187.

Taytard, A., Guenard, H., Vuillemin, L., Bourot, J.L., Vergeret, J., Ducassou, D., Piquet, Y. & Freour, P. (1986) Platelet kinetics in stable asthmatic subjects.

Am Rev Respir Dis **134**, 983–985.

Taytard, A., Vuillemin, L., Guenard, H., Rio, P., Vergeret, J. & Ducassou, D. (1987) Platelet kinetic in stable asthmatic patients: effect of ketotifen. *Am Rev Respir Dis* **135**, 388A.

Thompson, P.J., Hanson, J.M., Bilani, H., Turner-Warwick, M. & Morley, J. (1984) Platelets, platelet activating factor and asthma. *Am Rev Respir Dis* **129**, 3A.

Thorel, T., Joseph, M., Tsicopoulos, A., Tonnel, A.B. & Capron, A. (1988) Inhibition by nedocromil sodium of IgE-mediated activation of human mononuclear phagocytes and platelets in allergy. *Int Arch Allergy Appl Immun* **85**, 232–237.

Traietti, P., Marmaggi, S., Dardes, N., Moscatelli, B., Bologna, E. & Vulterini, S. (1984) Circulating platelet activation in respiratory diseases: differences between arterial and venous blood in cold and asthmatic patients. *Respiration* **46** (Suppl. 1), 62–63.

Tsicopoulos, A., Tonnel, A.B., Wallaert, B., Joseph, M., Ameisen, J.C., Ramon, P., Dessaint, J.P. & Capron, A. (1988a) Decrease of IgE-dependent platelet activation in Hymenoptera hypersensitivity after specific rush desensitization. *Clin Exp Immunol* **71**, 433–438.

Tsicopoulos, A., Lassalle, P., Joseph, M., Tonnel, A.B., Thorel, T., Dessaint, J.P. & Capron, A. (1988b) Effect of disodium cromoglycate on inflammatory cells bearing the Fc epsilon receptor type II (FcεRII). *Int J Immunopharmacol* **10**, 227–236.

Tsicopoulos, A., Tonnel, A.B., Wallaert, B., Joseph, M. & Capron, A. (1989) A circulating suppressive factor of platelet cytotoxic functions after rush immunotherapy in Hymenoptera venom hypersensitivity. *J Immunol* **142**, 2683–2688.

Tsicopoulos, A., Tonnel, A.B., Wallaert, B., Joseph, M. & Capron, A. (1990) Short term decrease of skin test sensitivity after rush desensitization in Hymenoptera venom hypersensitivity. *Clin Exp Allergy* **20**, 289–294.

Vargaftig, B.B., Lefort, J., Chignard, M. & Benveniste, J. (1980) Platelet-activating factor induces a platelet-dependent bronchoconstriction unrelated to the formation of prostaglandin derivatives. *Eur J Pharmacol* **55**, 185–192.

Vargaftig, B.B. & Benveniste, J. (1983) Platelet-activating factor today. *Trends Pharmacol Sci* **4**, 341–343.

Weiss, H., Fisher, R.H., Kagey-Sobotka, A., Proud, D., Lichtenstein, L.M. & Adkinson Jr, N.F. (1988) *In vivo* response to platelet derived histamine releasing factor. *J Allergy Clin Immunol* **81**, 224 (Abstract).

6: The Platelet in Asthma

Paolo Gresele

Introduction

Platelets owe most of their present popularity to the central role they play in haemostasis, thrombosis and atherosclerosis. Platelets, however, participate in numerous other physiological and pathological processes and this has gained them the label of multifunctional cells (Gordon & Milner, 1976). Asthma is one of the conditions for which evidence pointing towards the participation of platelets is accumulating.

The basic clinical characteristic of asthma is represented by hyper-responsiveness of tracheobronchial smooth muscle to various stimuli, resulting in the widespread narrowing of the airways. It is becoming evident that inflammation of the airways and the ensuing damage to the epithelium are fundamental requisites for the development of bronchial hyper-reactivity (Barnes, 1988). Many inflammatory, cytotoxic and smooth-muscle contracting mediators may be implicated in the pathogenesis of asthma and several cell types can participate in the inflammatory reaction and in the production of these mediators. Certain inflammatory cells, such as eosinophils, are predominantly involved in this process (Frigas & Gleich, 1986; Barnes, 1988) and some inflammatory mediators, such as platelet activating factor (PAF, Paf-acether, acetyl glyceryl ether phosphorylcholine (AGEPC), antihypertensive polar renomedullary lipid (APRL)), seem to play a central role (Page *et al.* 1985; Benveniste, 1987; Page, 1988b).

Platelet activating factor appears to represent the most likely mediator linking platelet activation to allergic bronchoconstriction. Possible sources of this mediator are several inflammatory cells in the lung, such as alveolar macrophages, neutrophils or eosinophils. Alveolar macrophages from asthmatic patients have been found to be able to release PAF upon stimulation with the specific allergen to which the patient is sensitized (Arnoux *et al.* 1983); eosinophils isolated from patients with hypereosinophilia, including asthmatic patients, produce enormous amounts of PAF (Lee *et al.* 1984). Other cells and tissues can produce PAF: isolated lungs of guinea-pigs release PAF when challenged with an antigen through the airways (Fitzgerald *et al.* 1986); endothelial cells are a good source of PAF; in addition, platelets themselves are able to produce PAF (Chignard *et al.* 1987).

Platelets can participate in allergic asthma in several ways: they can act as inflammatory cells, produce powerful spasmogenic substances, and interact with other cells that are potentially involved in asthma.

In this overview the following topics will be examined:

1 the biochemical and metabolic characteristics of platelets which may be relevant to asthma and inflammation;

2 the current knowledge on the interactions between platelets and other cells potentially involved in bronchoconstriction;

3 the evidence for platelet involvement in experimental models of asthma; and

4 the currently available data on platelet participation in clinical asthma.

Platelets in allergy and inflammation

Platelets in inflammation

Platelet participation in inflammation was recognized many years ago when platelet accumulation at sites of tissue damage was first described (Cotran, 1965). Several studies have confirmed the presence of platelets at localized sites of inflammatory lesions or in inflammatory exudates (Zawilska *et al.* 1973; Kravis & Henson, 1977; Yaron & Djaldetti, 1978). In addition, microthrombosis in small vessels of inflamed tissues has also been observed in conditions characterized by chronic inflammatory reactions, such as in rheumatoid arthritis (Kulka *et al.*, 1955; Schumacher, 1975).

On the other hand, platelets can directly elicit an inflammatory reaction. The subcutaneous injection of a platelet pellet *in vivo* in the rat was shown to cause intense edema, neutrophil infiltration and the accumulation of myofibroblasts; in the same setting, the injection of homogenates of brain, heart or kidney induced a much milder reaction (Braunstein *et al.* 1980). A strong inflammatory reaction, with swelling, redness and tenderness, lasting several hours was also described after injection of extracts of platelets into the skin of normal humans; neutrophils and eosinophils did not induce inflammatory responses while basophils only produced an early, histamine-like response (Day *et al.* 1975). Inflammatory reactions have also been detected at the site where platelet aggregates get trapped in the microcirculation (Jorgensen *et al.* 1970).

The meaning of these initial observations was later clarified by a series of discoveries on the mechanisms which lead to platelet activation during immunological and/or allergic reactions and by the identification of a series of inflammatory activities of platelets (Henson & Ginsberg, 1981; Oxholm & Winther, 1986; Capron *et al.* 1987; de Gaetano *et al.* 1987).

Immunological activation of platelets

Several immunologically generated factors can activate platelets and/or induce the release of their granules, such as immunoglobulins, immune complexes, complement components, some lymphokines and PAF.

Immunoglobulins can activate platelets in different ways: either antibodies directed against surface antigens can stimulate platelets (Henson & Ginsberg, 1981) or aggregated immunoglobulins or immune-complexes interact with a specific Fc receptor located on the platelet membrane (Cheng & Hawiger, 1979). Besides the Fc–IgG receptors mentioned, receptors for IgE have recently been characterized on human blood platelets. These receptors appear to be similar to those previously described on macrophages and eosinophils as far as the affinity constant (3×10^7 M) and the number (600–1000 binding sites per cell) are concerned (Capron *et al.* 1987). The presence of these receptors on platelets is related to the cytocidal action exerted by platelets on some parasites. During this process IgE-activated platelets release oxygen free radicals; interestingly, this release is not accompanied by platelet aggregation (Ameisen *et al.* 1985).

Complement fractions, such as C3b or the C5b–C9 complex, directly cause aggregation or potentiate platelet stimulation induced by thrombin (Polley & Nachman, 1979; Henson & Ginsberg, 1981; Polley & Nachman, 1981). In addition, the activation of the complement cascade on the platelet membrane, leading to platelet lysis, can also provoke the release of granule constituents (Henson & Ginsberg, 1981; Sundsmo & Fair, 1983).

A few reports have claimed that some lymphokines, soluble mediators released by lymphocytes upon immunological stimulation, possess platelet activating properties (Lavell *et al.* 1975; Coeugniet, 1979; see Chapter 5); however, contrasting data have appeared (Oxholm & Winther, 1986), thus this subject requires further clarification.

Platelet activating factor, an ether-linked phospholipid, is generated during immunological reactions by human monocytes, macrophages, polymorphonuclear cells, endothelial cells, etc. (Hanahan, 1986). It is a potent mediator of inflammation and one of the most potent inducers of platelet aggregation and release so far identified.

Some of the above-mentioned immunologically generated factors can synergize in stimulating platelets, as is the case for aggregated IgG and PAF (Valone, 1986).

Platelets exert their pro-inflammatory activities upon activation and degranulation by releasing several potent vasoactive and chemotactic mediators.

Platelet-derived mediators

Among the substances released by platelets which may trigger or boost the inflammatory reaction are: serotonin 5-hydroxytryptamine (5-HT), histamine (rabbit platelets), platelet-derived growth factor (PDGF), a cationic protein called 'permeability factor', another cationic protein able to split the fifth complement component (C5) to generate a fragment with potent chemotactic activity, some acid hydrolases, glycosidases, cathepsins, catalase, PAF, prostaglandin E_2 (PGE_2),

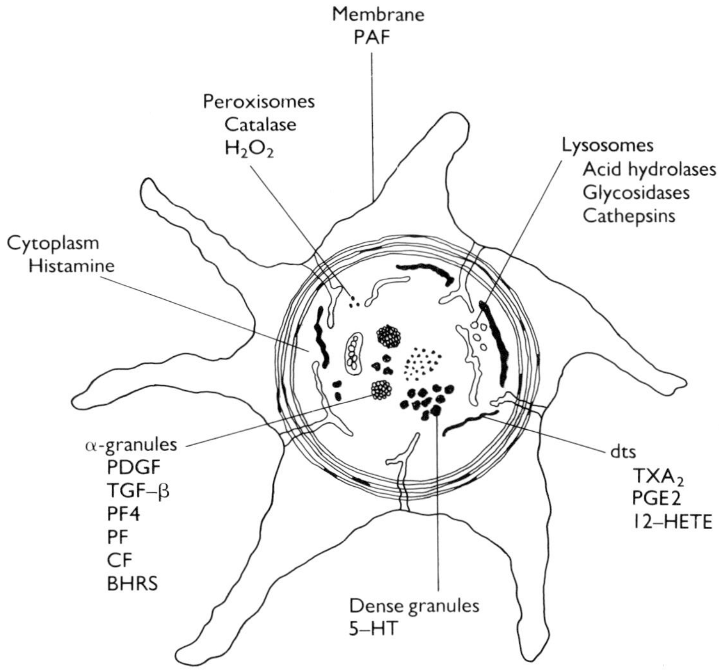

Figure 6.1 Schematic representation of an activated platelet. A series of substances released or synthesized upon stimulation, and which may be involved in allergy inflammation, are indicated. The localization of some of the substances is tentative.

PAF = platelet activating factor; dts = dense tubular system; TXA_2 = thromboxane A_2; PGE_2 = prostaglandin E_2; 12-HETE = 12-hydroxyeicosatetraenoic acid; 5-HT = 5-hydroxytryptamine (serotonin); PDGF = platelet-derived growth factor; TGF-β = transforming growth factor beta; PF4 = platelet factor 4; PF = permeability factor; CF = chemotactic factor; BHRS = basophil histamine-releasing substance; H_2O_2 = hydrogen peroxide.

thromboxane A_2 (TXA_2), 12-hydroxyeicosatetraenoic acid (12-HETE) and hydrogen peroxide (Gordon & Milner, 1976; Oxholm & Winther, 1986; de Gaetano *et al.* 1987) (Fig. 6.1).

Serotonin, which is stored in large amounts in human platelets (Da Prada *et al.* 1981), may participate in inflammation through its vasoconstrictive action (short-lived vasoconstriction is one of the signs of inflammation), and through its capacity to increase vascular permeability (Majno & Palade, 1961); stimulation of fibroblast growth is another action that this amine can explicate in chronic inflammatory reactions (Boucek & Alvarez, 1970).

Platelets also contain histamine. Indeed, the release of histamine from rabbit platelets had already been discovered in the 1950s (Humphrey & Jaques, 1955), well before basophils were identified as the cells most rich in histamine. Human platelets, however, do not appear to release relevant amounts of histamine (Humphrey & Jaques, 1954), which has a cytoplasmic (i.e. extragranular) localization (Da Prada *et al.* 1981). Human platelets present histamine-binding sites (mainly of the H1 type) on their surface (Hallberg *et al.* 1984). The functional role of these putative receptors has not yet been fully elucidated, but it has been suggested that their stimulation may have inhibitory influences on platelets (Mazza *et al.* 1980), possibly through an increase of cyclic adenosine monophosphate (cAMP) synthesis (Klysner *et al.* 1980). Recent studies, however indicate that in human platelets histamine plays an intracellular role as a second messenger mediating platelet aggregation (Saxena *et al.* 1989).

Although human platelets do not release large amounts of histamine themselves, they have recently been demonstrated to be able to stimulate the release of this amine from basophils and mast cells through an IgE-dependent mechanism (Knauer *et al.* 1984). The histamine-releasing substance is liberated upon stimulation with thrombin, collagen and PAF; it is a heat-stable, acid-stable molecule with a molecular weight above 30 000 and it does not appear to be related to platelet factor 4 (PF4) or PDGF (Knauer *et al.* 1984; Orchard *et al.* 1985).

Platelets can also release cationic proteins which enhance vascular permeability, possibly by acting on mast cells (Nachman *et al.* 1972); in addition, a 'permeability factor' that causes mast cells to release histamine has also been described (Holmsen & Weiss, 1979). Platelet α-granules contain an additional cationic protein that cleaves the fifth component of complement to form a factor which is chemotactic for polymorphonuclear leucocytes (Weksler & Coupal, 1973).

Platelet factor 4 (PF4) a protein contained in α-granules and released upon stimulation, has also a number of properties which may be of importance in allergy and inflammation. It stimulates human basophils to release histamine in a concentration-dependent manner (Brindley *et al.* 1983); it is chemotactic for polymorphonuclear leucocytes and for monocytes (Deuel *et al.* 1981); it modulates the activity of some enzymes which may be liberated at localized sites of inflammation, such as collagenase or elastase (Hiti-Harper *et al.* 1978; Lonky & Wohl, 1981); finally, recently PF4 was shown to exert a powerful chemotactic effect for eosinophils and to be able to increase the expression on these cells of Fc-IgG and Fc-IgE receptors (Chihara *et al.* 1988). All these pro-inflammatory actions of PF4 appear even more intriguing if one considers that this protein not only appears in the circulation upon platelet activation, but it can also enter the vessel wall upon close contact between platelets and subendothelium (Goldberg *et al.* 1980) and thus it can act at the very site of the allergic or inflammatory reaction.

Platelet-derived growth factor, a basic protein also contained in α-granules, may exert a role in inflammation by affecting the vascular tone (Berk *et al.* 1986), by displaying a chemotactic activity towards monocytes, neutrophils (Deuel *et al.* 1982) and fibroblasts (Grotendorst *et al.* 1981), by activating monocytes (Tzeng *et al.* 1985) and through its growth factor activity which might contribute to the bronchial smooth muscle hypertrophy which is a feature of the asthmatic lung at autopsy (Page, 1988a).

Platelet α-granules contain other growth factors, among which is transforming growth factor beta (TGF-β): this substance can attract and activate monocytes during inflammation and vascular injury (Wahl *et al.* 1987).

Acid hydrolases and cathepsins, which are contained in small amounts in lysosomes in human platelets, may be secreted in response to strong stimuli (Niewiarowski, 1977); these substances may exert their activity in inflammation by exerting cytotoxic and tissue-degrading effects.

Catalase is contained in platelet peroxisomes (Oxholm & Winther, 1986); this enzyme can play a role in the decomposition of tissues to which activated platelets attach themselves.

In addition to the substances contained in platelets and released upon stimulation, a number of molecules are synthesized and liberated when platelets become activated. Among them are products of the metabolism of arachidonic acid, such as thromboxane A_2 (TXA_2), which is a powerful vasoconstrictor and a bronchial smooth muscle contractor (Samuelsson *et al.* 1978) and which is also able to enhance cholinergic transmission (Chung *et al.* 1985); prostaglandin E_2 (PGE_2), which is a vasodilator and a well-known inflammatory mediator; 12-HETE which is chemotactic for eosinophils (Goetzl *et al.* 1977). In addition, rabbit platelets have been reported to be able to release a slow releasing substance of anaphylaxis (SRS-A)-like substance (Mencia-Huerta *et al.* 1981). Platelets also possess the metabolic machinery which enable them to produce PAF (Chignard *et al.* 1987), which is considered to be one of the most powerful pro-inflammatory agents and a potential mediator of allergic bronchoconstriction (Page, 1988b; Mencia-Huerta *et al.* 1989; Pretolani *et al.* 1989).

Interactions between platelets and other cells relevant to asthma

Platelets do not carry out their activities as isolated elements in the bloodstream but, on the contrary, are in continuous, dynamic interaction with other blood cells and with components of the vessel wall. These interactions can asssume different forms: exchange of metabolic substrates for the synthesis of biologically active products; enzymatic activation; functional modulation.

Exchange of metabolic substrates

The exchange of metabolic intermediates between platelets and other cells was demonstrated several years ago when it was shown that part of the prostaglandin endoperoxides used by endothelial cells for the synthesis of prostacyclin could come from platelets (Marcus *et al.* 1980). Such an exchange of cyclic endoperoxides can also take place between platelets and white blood cells (Defreyn *et al.* 1982; Mehta *et al.* 1985).

The exchange of substrates between platelets and leucocytes, however, is not limited to products of the cyclooxygenase pathway but extensively involves the lipoxygenase metabolic pathway (Marcus *et al.* 1986). A series of lipoxygenase products may be of relevance for inflammation and bronchoconstriction.

One example of metabolic interaction between platelets and leucocytes is represented by the transferal from stimulated platelets of arachidonic acid to neutrophils which utilize it for the synthesis of 5-HETE and leukotriene (LT) B_4 (Marcus *et al.* 1982). Although not directly spasmogenic on bronchial smooth muscle, LTB_4 can play a role in asthma through its potent pro-inflammatory actions. On the other hand, platelets may produce LTC_4 from LTA_4 synthesized by leucocytes. Indeed, platelets, which are devoid of 5-lipoxygenase, contain the enzyme glutathion-S-transferase which can transform LTA_4 into LTC_4 (Maclouf *et al.* 1987), a powerful bronchial smooth muscle spasmogenic substance, claimed to be a possible mediator of allergic asthma (O'Byrne, 1988). The metabolic co-operation between platelets and leucocytes can also involve the synthesis of PAF: indeed, mixtures of leucocytes and platelets stimulated with leucocyte- and platelet-specific stimuli produce much more PAF than the different cell types isolated (Coeffier *et al.* 1984).

Enzymatic activation

Leucocytes can produce increased amounts of leukotrienes in the presence of activated platelets because 12-hydroxyperoxyeicosatetraenoic acid (12-HPETE), produced by platelets, can stimulate the activity of leucocyte 5-lipoxygenase (Maclouf *et al.* 1982). Indeed, that the interaction between leucocytes, platelets and possibly other blood cells affects the amounts and the kinetics of the synthesis of leukotrienes is confirmed by experiments carried out in whole blood where LTB_4 is produced in larger amounts and over a prolonged period as compared with isolated leucocytes (Gresele *et al.* 1986). Another platelet product which can stimulate the synthesis of LTB_4 by leucocytes is PAF (Lin *et al.* 1982).

Functional modulation

Functional interactions between platelets and leucocytes have also been described. Platelet activation is potentiated by neutrophils through the production of hydrogen peroxide and oxygen free radicals (Canoso *et al.* 1974), peptide LTs (Mehta *et al.* 1986) or 'neutrophilin' (Chignard *et al.* 1986) which might indeed be cathepsin G (de Gaetano *et al.* 1987).

Platelet activating factor, released by leucocytes, is also a powerful inducer of platelet aggregation: platelet activation is observed when mixtures of leucocytes and platelets are stimulated with leucocyte-specific stimuli; this aggregation can be blocked by PAF-antagonists (Oda *et al.* 1986). In this regard, it is of interest to note that eosinophils from patients with eosinophilia release enormous amounts of PAF as compared to normal eosinophils (Lee *et al.* 1984).

On the other hand, platelets or platelet-released substances may stimulate a number of leucocyte activities, such as adhesiveness, chemotaxis, cytotoxicity and aggregation (de Gaetano *et al.* 1987). Although most of these interactions have been demonstrated in *in vitro* studies, it is of interest to note that in experimental animals the lung injury provoked by neutrophils following complement activation is partly mediated by platelets: platelet depletion reducing the lesions in certain experimental models (Tvedten *et al.* 1985; Ward *et al.* 1986).

Platelets can also interact functionally with smooth muscle cells of the human bronchi. Indeed, it has been shown that human bronchial smooth muscle spirals stimulated by PAF in the presence of human platelets contract, while PAF alone is without effect (Schellenberg *et al.* 1983). Although platelets normally do not come into contact with smooth muscle cells of the bronchial wall, they can be found extravascularly, in close contact with contracted smooth muscle cells, in particular conditions, such as after the i.v. injection of PAF in guinea-pigs (Lellouch-Tubiana *et al.* 1985). Although it is not yet known how platelets can reach extravascular sites it may be relevant to recall that these blood elements can migrate upon appropriate stimuli (Lowenhaupt *et al.* 1973); this migration can be influenced by products liberated by immunologically competent cells (Coeugniet, 1979). Whether these *in vitro* findings and *in vivo* observations in the animal are relevant to human asthma is not clear; however, it is interesting to observe that degranulated platelets have been recovered in the broncho-alveolar lavage fluid of asthmatic patients after specific allergenic challenge (Metzger *et al.* 1985, 1987). This observation suggests that platelets can migrate through the vessel wall even in allergic humans upon antigenic stimulation; whether this migration is essential for bronchial smooth muscle cells to contract remains to be established.

Finally, complex functional interactions involving platelets, eosinophils and endothelial cells have recently been reported (Chihara *et al.* 1989). The eosinophil chemotactic activity of platelet-released products can be suppressed when endothelial cells are simultaneously present, possibly through a heparin-like activity; however, the modulatory activity of endothelial cells may be diminished by interleukin-1 and this may be of importance in allergic reactions such as bronchial asthma (Chihara *et al.* 1989).

The platelet in asthma: studies in the animal

It has been known for several years that the intravenous injection of some platelet agonists provokes thrombocytopenia associated with bronchospasm in several animal species (Vaage & Hauge, 1977; Lefort & Vargaftig, 1978; Vargaftig & Lefort, 1979). The same phenomenon is observed when sensitized rabbits or guinea-pigs are challenged with a specific antigen; platelet involvement does not appear to be incidental because platelet depletion can abolish the lethal consequences of the allergen challenge (Pinckard *et al.* 1977; Halonen *et al.* 1981). The interdependence of platelet activation and bronchoconstriction in these models appears to be confirmed by the histological finding of platelet aggregates within the pulmonary vasculature (Pinckard *et al.* 1977; Butler & Smith, 1981).

Platelet localization in the lungs, in association with bronchospasm, has also been demonstrated by the use of radiolabelled platelets after allergen challenge (Page *et al.* 1984).

The same phenomena described above after allergen challenge have been reproduced by injecting PAF intravenously into guinea-pigs (Vargaftig *et al.* 1980; Page *et al.* 1984). Platelets play a central role in the bronchoconstrictor action of PAF: rats, whose platelets do not respond to PAF, do not undergo bronchoconstriction upon intravenous injection of PAF (Vargaftig & Benveniste, 1983).

Participation of platelets in allergen- or PAF-induced bronchospasm does not appear to be the consequence of a mechanical embolization within the pulmonary circulation because the inhibition of the platelet release reaction in the presence of continued aggregate embolization in the pulmonary vasculature suppresses bronchospasm (Chignard *et al.* 1982; Vargaftig *et al.* 1982). In addition, in experiments comparing the time course of aggregate localization to the lung and the increase in airway resistance it was noted that maximal bronchoconstriction always preceded maximal platelet accumulation (Page *et al.* 1983, 1984). It therefore seems that platelets, activated during allergen-triggered reactions, release (a) product(s) which contributes to bronchospasm.

Platelet-released products, such as PF4, have been found in the bloodstream after allergen challenge in sensitized animals and the same phenomenon is observed when PAF is used instead of the allergen (McManus *et al.* 1979).

The findings described above demonstrate a remarkable similarity of the effects of allergen and PAF in inducing bronchoconstriction and platelet activation in animals. The inter-relationship between platelets and PAF in allergic bronchoconstriction is also indicated by the observation that platelets collected from sensitized rabbits in the period following exposure to the allergen are hyporesponsive *in vitro* to PAF (Henson & Pinckard, 1977), the development of specific tachyphylaxis after previous exposure to PAF being a well-recognized phenomenon (Vargaftig & Benveniste, 1983).

Another piece of experimental evidence for the participation of PAF in respiratory anaphylaxis is provided by the reduction of acute bronchoconstriction and the associated thrombocytopenia obtained with a PAF-receptor antagonist (BN 52021) in sensitized guinea-pigs challenged with ovalbumin (Braquet *et al.* 1985).

Most of the studies described above have attempted to establish a relationship between platelets and acute bronchospasm, assuming that the latter is a key characteristic of asthma. However, as already mentioned, it has become clear lately that the central features of asthma are bronchial hyper-responsiveness and late asthmatic reactions, both of which are dependent on inflammation of the airways (Page, 1987; Barnes, 1988; Mencia-Huerta, *et al.* 1989). The most recent studies in experimental animal models of asthma have therefore centred their attention on the relationships between platelets, PAF and inflammatory changes of the airways.

It has been proved that PAF administration to normal animals or antigen challenge in sensitized animals causes an increased bronchial responsiveness to various spasmogens such as methacholine (Chung *et al.* 1986; Daffonchio *et al.* 1987; Coyle *et al.* 1988); these effects in guinea-pigs are abolished by platelet depletion (Page, 1988a). Platelet activating factor antagonism with BN 52021 also reduces both allergen-induced late asthmatic reactions and bronchial hyper-reactivity in sensitized animals (Coyle *et al.* 1988; Page *et al.* 1988a). It is also suggested that prophylactic anti-asthma drugs, including disodium cromoglycate (DSCG), Ketotifen, steroids and theophylline, inhibit the platelet-dependent bronchial hyper-responsiveness provoked by PAF administration to experimental animals (Page 1988a,b).

Platelet-activating-factor- or allergen-challenge provoke eosinophil infiltration into the lungs of normal and allergic animals, respectively (Coyle *et al.* 1988; Lellouch-Tubiana *et al.* 1988). Eosinophil accumulation in lungs after allergen inhalation appears to be a feature of patients with allergic asthma (De Monchy *et al.* 1985; Metzger *et al.* 1985). Interestingly, the eosinophil influx into the lungs provoked by aerosolized or i.v. antigen in guinea-pigs is inhibited by PAF-antagonists (Coyle *et al.* 1988; Lellouch-Tubiana *et al.* 1988). Selective platelet depletion with an antiplatelet antiserum reduces PAF and antigen-induced eosinophil infiltration into the lungs of experimental animals, as does prostacyclin, at concentrations totally inhibiting platelet activation (Lellouch-Tubiana *et al.* 1988) suggesting that platelets are central to allergen- and PAF-induced eosinophil infiltration. Besides eosinophil infiltration, extravascular platelet recruitment appears also to be an important histological feature of the experimental inflammatory reactions of the allergic lung (Lellouch-Tubiana *et al.* 1987).

Radiolabelled platelets localize in the lung after intravenous allergen- or PAF-challenge (Page *et al.* 1982, 1984) and they probably undergo diapedesis because they tend to be retained in the lung much longer than after the intravenous injection of adenosine diphosphate (ADP) or U46619 (Robertson & Page, 1987). Confirmation of platelet diapedesis is provided by the following observations: degranulated platelets are found in the close vicinity of bronchial smooth muscle cells after PAF or allergen-administration (Lellouch-Tubiana *et al.* 1985, 1987) and are also recovered in broncho-alveolar lavage fluid in rabbits (Metzger *et al.* 1987).

Extravascular migration of platelets may be of particular importance because several indications exist that platelet aggregation within the pulmonary vessels *per se* is not sufficient to contribute to bronchial hyper-responsiveness. The induction of platelet aggregation by ADP or collagen does not provoke bronchial hyper-responsiveness or eosinophil infiltration (Robertson & Page, 1987; Page, 1988a).

It should be clarified that platelets are not involved in every type of experimental bronchoconstriction and neither are all the effects of PAF on the lungs mediated by platelets. The bronchospasm induced in guinea-pigs by the intravenous injection of the anaphylotoxin C5a, for instance, is not accompanied by platelet activation

(Regal, 1988) and neither is the bronchoconstriction provoked by the administration of PAF in sheep (Christman *et al.* 1986). Increase in mucus secretion produced by PAF injection into ferrets is not platelet-mediated (Hahn *et al.* 1986) and neither is the microvascular leakage in the mucosal region of the tracheobronchial tree of guinea-pigs (O'Donnell & Barnett, 1987).

The platelet in asthma: studies in man

Sporadic studies on platelet involvement in clinical allergy and asthma date back to the 1950s: for example, a 15% drop of circulating platelets was reported upon exposure of sensitive individuals to a specific allergen (Storck *et al.* 1955). Old studies also suggested an increased tendency to develop thrombo-embolic phenomena in patients with asthma (Hartman, 1963) possibly due to hyperactive platelets; contrasting reports have also appeared (Szczeklik *et al.* 1977).

A new impetus to the studies of platelets in asthma came with the introduction of the technique of platelet aggregometry (Born & Cross, 1963). Lately, a reprise of interest started after the discovery of PAF and the appearance of the first reports on the participation of platelets in experimental bronchoconstriction in animals.

The quite conspicuous number of papers on platelet involvement in asthma can be grouped into five categories: studies on platelet aggregation *in vitro*; studies on other aspects of *in vitro* platelet function; studies aimed at detecting *in vivo* platelet activation; studies testing drugs effective on platelet function in patients with asthma; and, most recently, studies on the direct effects of PAF in humans.

Platelet aggregation *in vitro*

The first group of studies is the most numerous: at least 12 publications have analysed platelet aggregation in asthma. Platelet aggregation was induced by ADP, adrenaline, collagen, thrombin, streptococcal M protein, arachidonic acid, PAF, PAF plus collagen (Table 6.1). The results of the studies are rather conflicting, with substantially normal data (Harwell *et al.* 1973; McDonald *et al.* 1974; Greer *et al.* 1984; Hemmendinger *et al.* 1989) as opposed to strikingly abnormal behaviour of platelets (Fischel & Zwemer, 1970; Solinger *et al.* 1973; Maccia *et al.* 1977; Szczeklik *et al.* 1986).

The most carefully performed studies have tried to differentiate within the patient populations those with an immunological basis of their disease, non-atopic asthmatics or aspirin-sensitive asthmatics (Maccia *et al.* 1977; Palma-Carlos *et al.* 1988). It was evident that not all the patients presented the same degree of abnormality of *in vitro* platelet function. The frequency of pathological results was higher among patients with immunologically mediated asthma in the study of Maccia and co-workers (1977); interestingly, these authors reported that the abnormality of platelet function was not consistent when studied in the same patients several months after the end of the allergy season.

Table 6.1 *In vitro* platelet aggregation in human asthma

Patients (no.)	Aggregating agent	Results	Reference
n.s.	ADP	Abnormal (2nd phase)	Fishel *et al.* (1970)
26	Adrenaline	Abnormal (2nd phase)	Solinger *et al.* (1973)
10	Adrenaline ADP Streptococcal M protein	Normal	Harwell *et al.* (1973)
15	Collagen	↑ sensitivity to aspirin	Schwartz & Bennett (1973)
41	Adrenaline	Normal	McDonald *et al.* (1974)
33	Adrenaline ADP Thrombin Collagen	Abnormal Abnormal Abnormal (±) Abnormal (±)	Maccia *et al.* (1977)
12	PAF Collagen	Abnormal Normal	Thompson *et al.* (1984)
6	ADP	Normal	Greer *et al.* (1984)
31	Collagen ADP PAF	Abnormal Abnormal Normal	Szczeklik *et al.* (1986)
10	PAF + collagen	Normal	Menz *et al.* (1987)
73	ADP Adrenaline Collagen AA	Abnormal (±) Abnormal (±) Abnormal (±) Abnormal (±)	Palma-Carlos *et al.* (1988)
10	Adrenaline AA PAF	Normal Normal Normal	Hemmendinger *et al.* (1989)

n.s. = not specified.

Platelet aggregometry, although widely used, is a technique with an inherent variability and a rather low sensitivity and one which requires an elevated degree of standardization to give reliable results. It is quite obvious, for instance, that a slight deficiency of platelet aggregation can be missed when using fixed, supra-threshold concentrations of the stimulus; none of the published studies have tried to compare the minimal concentrations of different inducers needed to give platelet aggregation in patients and controls. Differences in the methodology used may thus explain the conflicting results appearing in the literature; in addition, different patient populations studied or different degrees of activity of the disease at the moment of the study can also explain the contrasting findings.

Most of the abnormalities reported (absence of second wave of platelet aggregation induced by ADP or adrenaline, increase of collagen lag time) are similar to those observed in conditions of platelet 'exhaustion' due to overstimulation *in vivo* (Harker *et al.* 1980; Pareti *et al.* 1980).

By analogy with the observations in the rabbit described above (Henson & Pinckard, 1977) it has been reported that platelets develop specific desensitization to PAF in asthmatics after bronchial allergen challenge (Thompson *et al.* 1984).

Other parameters of platelet function *in vitro*

A second group of reports has dealt with other *in vitro* aspects of platelet function different from platelet aggregability (Table 6.2).

Table 6.2 Various parameters of *in vitro* platelet function in human asthma

Patients (no.)	Parameter studied	Results	Reference
33	Release of 5-HT, PF4 (by collagen, adrenaline, ADP)	↓	Maccia *et al.* (1977)
2	Intraplatelet nucleotides	↓	D'Souza and Glueck, (1977)
18	uptake of 5-HT	↓	Malmgren *et al.* (1982)
n.s.	Platelet β-adrenergic response	↓	Fishel and Zwemer (1970)
40	Platelet β-adrenergic response	↓	Coffey and Middleton (1975)
10	Platelet α_2-adrenergic response	N	Davis and Lieberman (1982)
9	Resting cytoplasmic Ca^{2+} and IP_3	↑	Block *et al.* (1988)
n.s.	Oxygen generation by platelets challenged with antigen	↑	Capron *et al.* (1985)
19	Platelet lipo/cyclooxygenase	↑	Yen and Morris (1981)
11	Platelet lipo/cyclooxygenase	↓	Audera *et al.* (1988)
10	PAF production	N	Lurie *et al.* (1987)

n.s. = not specified.
N = normal.

A defective *in vitro* release of platelet 5-HT and PF4 after stimulation with collagen, adrenaline or ADP was described (Maccia *et al.* 1977). Similarly, a defect of liberation of platelet nucleotides was later reported (D'Souza & Glueck, 1977). These data are perfectly compatible with the absence of the second wave of ADP or adrenaline-induced aggregation previously described.

A reduction of nucleotide levels in resting platelets of patients with asthma has also been reported (D'Souza & Glueck, 1977). Similar decreases are observed in so-called exhausted platelets, i.e. in platelets that have undergone an *in vivo* release reaction due to previous stimulation (Harker *et al.* 1980; Pareti *et al.* 1980).

The uptake of 5-HT by platelets from asthmatic patients has been found to be inhibited (Malmgren *et al.* 1982); such an impaired mechanism of uptake may be caused by a previous exposure of platelets to an increased concentration of 5-HT (Malmgren *et al.* 1982). Increased blood levels of 5-HT have been reported in asthma (Bakulin & Joffe, 1979). These findings might be compatible with a previous *in vivo* platelet activation with release of the amine; indeed, platelets transport most of the circulating 5-HT in blood.

A group of studies have discussed the possible derangement of adrenergic receptors of human platelets in view of the adrenergic-receptor dysregulation reported in asthma (Middleton, 1972; Henderson *et al.* 1979). Already in the study of Fishel and Zwemer (1970) on *in vitro* platelet aggregation in allergic asthma the authors suggested a β-adrenergic malfunction of platelets from asthmatics because the disaggregation pattern was similar to that observed in normal platelets pretreated with propranolol. Later, other authors proposed a derangement of platelet β-adrenergic receptors as an explanation of their finding of an increased ATPase activity in platelets of asthmatic children (Coffey & Middleton, 1975). More recently, a careful assessment of the platelet α_2-adrenergic responses in asthmatics did not reveal any abnormality (Davis & Lieberman 1982).

In view of the latter findings and of the unclear role of platelet β-adrenergic receptors (Kerry & Scrutton, 1985) it is at present rather doubtful that adrenergic derangement plays a role in the platelet dysfunction of patients with asthma.

Recent, and still preliminary, studies have revealed alterations of some signal transduction mechanisms in platelets from patients with asthma: an elevation of resting cytoplasmic Ca^{2+} levels and a higher basal inositol-triphosphate (IP_3) production were described in patients with asthma (Block *et al.* 1988). Increases of Ca^{2+} and IP_3 are typically produced by platelet stimulation (Haslam, 1987), suggesting a possible previous *in vivo* activation of platelets in asthma.

Attempts to demonstrate an imbalance of platelet arachidonic acid metabolism in asthmatics have given conflicting results. An initial report of an imbalance of arachidonic acid metabolism in favour of lipoxygenase products in platelets (Yen & Morris, 1981) was not confirmed in a more recent study which even suggested a higher production of cyclooxygenase metabolites (Audera *et al.* 1988).

The production of PAF by stimulated platelets has also been analysed in patients with asthma and found to be normal (Lurie *et al.* 1987).

Finally, an interesting *in vitro* observation is represented by the activation of platelets from asthmatic patients after *in vitro* challenge with the specific allergen or with anti-IgE antibodies; platelets from healthy donors did not react to the above-mentioned stimuli but their prior incubation with IgE from allergic patients rendered them reactive. Interestingly, platelet activation here takes the form of the liberation of a burst of oxygen and cytotoxic activity and not of platelet aggregation or release (Capron *et al.* 1985).

Detection of *in vivo* platelet activation

Several authors have approached the problem of the possible participation of platelets in asthma by trying to detect *in vivo* platelet activation (Table 6.3).

The measurement of plasmatic levels of platelet-specific proteins, either β-thromboglobulin (β-TG) or PF4, has been carried out in at least eight different studies on a total of 94 patients with asthma. Conflicting results were reported, with significant elevations detected concomitantly to allergen-induced bronchoconstriction (Knauer *et al.* 1981; Gresele *et al.* 1982, 1985; Metzger *et al.* 1985; Johnson *et al.* 1986) as opposed to no changes (Greer *et al.* 1984; Durham *et al.* 1985; Shephard *et al.* 1985; Hemmendinger *et al.* 1989). Possible explanations for these contrasting data may be: the small number of patients studied in the individual series associated with the variability of the parameters analysed; possible differences in the patient populations studied; disparate techniques used to challenge the patients with the allergen; poor methodology adopted for the sampling or processing of blood for β-TG/PF4 measurement.

Increased plasma levels of platelet-specific proteins is a reliable parameter of *in vivo* platelet activation. However, special precautions must be taken to obtain meaningful results. The best information can be obtained through the simultaneous measurement of the two proteins: an increase of the β-TG:PF4 ratio indicates *in vivo* platelet activation (Kaplan & Owen, 1981). Such an approach has been adopted in four studies: in the two studies showing *in vivo* platelet activation a significant increase in β-TG was associated with no change (Metzger *et al.* 1985) or only a small rise (Johnson *et al.* 1986) of PF4. In the other two studies no modification of either parameter was detected (Durham *et al.* 1985; Hemmendinger *et al.* 1989).

In vivo platelet activation following allergic bronchoconstriction has also been detected on the basis of microscopic studies: an increased number of circulating platelet aggregates (Gresele *et al.* 1982), evaluated by the technique of Wu and Hoak (1974), or the morphological demonstration of activated platelets in the circulation (Traietti *et al.* 1984), were described. These techniques have been disputed because it can not be excluded that they detect an *in vitro* and not an *in vivo* activation of platelets (Kohanna *et al.* 1984).

Reports claiming the detection of *in vivo* platelet activation in asthma by the measurement of plasma levels of thromboxane (TX) B_2 (Morris *et al.* 1980;

Shephard *et al.* 1985), the stable metabolite of TXA_2, are invalidated by the unavoidability of artefacts when measuring TXB_2 in plasma (FitzGerald *et al.* 1983). Recently, however, it has been convincingly demonstrated that TxA_2-release accompanies the exposure of allergic asthmatics to inhaled antigen by the measurement of the urinary excretion of TxB_2-metabolites (Lupinetti *et al.* 1989).

At least four groups have attempted to evaluate *in vivo* platelet behaviour in asthma by studying platelet turnover. A shortened platelet life-span is considered as a sensitive index of *in vivo* platelet activation leading to accelerated platelet consumption (Harker, 1978).

Ind and co-workers (1985) injected ^{111}In-labelled platelets and ^{99}Tc-red blood cells into three atopic asthmatics and three non-asthmatic volunteers with the aim of measuring the pulmonary platelet transit time. This was found to be normal both in basal conditions and during bronchoconstriction provoked by allergen challenge; no evidence of an increased ^{111}In-signal in the lung was observed. Platelet survival was normal in the three asthmatics; no details are given on the respiratory condition of the patients during the platelet survival studies. This study was based on the theory that activated platelets might get trapped in the lungs, as already observed in animals (Page *et al.* 1982). In the animal experiments, however, a striking intravascular aggregation was induced by intravenous injection of platelet stimuli: it is unlikely that the platelet activation accompanying allergic bronchoconstriction can attain levels such as to allow the entrapment of a sufficient number of platelets to be detected by surface counting.

Another study using ^{111}In-labelled platelets has revealed a significantly shortened platelet survival in 10 patients with allergic asthma in asymptomatic phase as compared to healthy controls; corticosteroid-treated patients ($n = 10$) had a longer platelet survival than untreated patients. The decay curve of circulating radioactivity was biexponential in asthmatics indicating that 30–50% of the patients' platelets suffered an accelerated destruction (Taytard & Vuillemin, 1987). In this study, too, no platelet sequestration into the lungs could be observed.

In a third study (Gresele *et al.* 1987) platelet life-span was evaluated with a non-radioisotopic technique (Stuart *et al.* 1975). Seven asthmatic patients studied during a period of symptomatic spontaneous bronchoconstriction (forced expiratory volume in one second (FEV_1) reduction = 40%) (pollination season) had a significantly shorter platelet regeneration time than six age- and sex-matched controls. When studied again in an asymptomatic period (FEV_1 reduction $\approx$ 15%) the platelet regeneration time was normal (Gresele *et al.* 1987).

Finally, ^{111}In-platelet survival was reported to be normal by Hemmendinger and coworkers (1989) in five patients undergoing allergen inhalation test. However, platelet recovery 30 minutes after injection was significantly lower in asthmatics than in controls (Hemmendinger *et al.* 1989).

Bleeding time is also a sensitive parameter which assesses the *in vivo* platelet function. In the presence of a normal platelet number a prolongation of the bleeding time is an expression of defective platelet function (Harker & Slichter, 1972). Although earlier studies, using less sensitive methods, did not show any

Table 6.3 *In vivo* platelet function in human asthma

Patients (no.)	Clinical condition	Parameter studied	Results	References
13	Antigen challenge	PF4	↑	Knauer *et al.* (1981)
15	Antigen challenge	β-TG	↑	Gresele *et al.* (1982) Gresele *et al.* (1985)
20	Antigen challenge	β-TG PF4	↑ =	Metzger *et al.* (1985)
9	Exercise challenge	β-TG PF4	↑ ↑ (±)	Johnson *et al.* (1986)
6	Antigen challenge	β-TG	=	Greer *et al.* (1984)
13	Antigen challenge	β-TG PF4	= =	Durham *et al.* (1985)
8	Antigen challenge	β-TG	=	Shephard *et al.* (1985)
10	Antigen challenge	β-TG PF4	= =	Hemmendinger *et al.* (1989)
15	Antigen challenge	Circulating platelet aggregate	↑	Gresele *et al.* (1982) Gresele *et al.* (1985)
8	Spontaneous attack	Circulating activated platelets	↑	Traietti *et al.* (1984)
19	Exercise challenge	TXB_2	↑	Morris *et al.* (1980)
8	Antigen challenge	TXB_2	↑	Shephard *et al.* (1985)
3	Antigen challenge	Platelet survival (^{111}In)	=	Ind *et al.* (1985)
10	Antigen challenge	Platelet survival (^{111}In)	↓	Taytard and Vuillemin (1987)
7	Spontaneous attack	Platelet regeneration time (MDA)	↓	Gresele *et al.* (1987)
5	Antigen challenge	Platelet survival (^{111}In)	=	Hemmendinger *et al.* (1989)
33	Asymptomatic	Bleeding time	=	Maccia *et al.* (1977)

Table 6.3 Continued

Patients (no.)	Clinical condition	Parameter studied	Results	References
31	Asymptomatic	Bleeding time	↑	Szczeklik *et al.* (1986)
12	Antigen challenge	Platelets in BAL	↑	Metzger *et al.* (1985)
3	Status asthmaticus	Megakaryo-cytes in lung	↑	Slater *et al.* (1985)

BAL = broncho-alveolar lavage; MDA = malondialdehyde.

alteration of bleeding time in asthma (Maccia *et al.* 1977), more recently a significant prolongation of the bleeding time in patients with asthma has been reported (Szczeklik *et al.* 1986). An impairment of platelet function, of the type of that acquired by platelets activated in the bloodstream (Harker *et al.* 1980), can lead to a prolongation of the bleeding time.

Platelet size (Audera *et al.* 1988), platelet count and platelet mass (Szczeklik *et al.* 1986) have been found to be increased in asthma.

Particularly interesting approaches to the *in vivo* involvement of platelets in human asthma are those tending to put in evidence the presence of platelets in the asthmatic lung.

Large numbers of megakaryocytes have been found at autopsy in the lungs of three patients dying from status asthmaticus whereas control lungs only contain rare megakaryocytes (Slater *et al.* 1985). In addition, platelets have been detected by electron microscopy in the broncho-alveolar lavage fluid of asthmatic patients after allergen bronchoprovocation; some platelets were degranulated and granules free in the lavage were also observed (Metzger *et al.* 1985). Platelets were often found in approximation to macrophages in broncho-alveolar lavage also after local antigen challenge into a subsegmental airway (Metzger *et al.* 1987).

Antiplatelet agents in asthma

A limited number of reports discussed the effects of antiplatelet treatments in allergic bronchoconstriction. Aspirin or sulphinpyrazone were given to four asthmatic patients before allergen challenge: the increase in β-TG induced by antigen inhalation was not inhibited by either antiplatelet drug; no effects were seen on bronchoconstriction (Gresele *et al.* 1985). The activation of platelets and the bronchospasm induced *in vivo* by PAF in animals is not inhibited by aspirin or sulphinpyrazone at doses similar to those clinically administered (Vargaftig *et al.* 1982; Ambler & Wallis, 1983).

Prostacyclin, a potent inhibitor of platelet activation, has been given to healthy volunteers undergoing PAF inhalation. The drug was unable to affect the bronchoconstrictor response to the phospholipid despite *ex vivo* inhibition of platelet aggregation (Lammers *et al.* 1988).

Finally, PAF-receptor antagonists have been administered to asthmatic patients undergoing allergen-challenge: a significant depression of early bronchoconstriction was obtained. No studies on platelets were carried out (Guinot *et al.* 1987).

Effects of PAF administration

As already mentioned, the most likely mediator that links platelets and asthma is PAF. After the first demonstration that PAF-inhalation in healthy volunteers provokes acute bronchoconstriction and protracted bronchial hyper-reactivity (Cuss *et al.* 1986) several other studies have analysed the effects of PAF in humans. A detailed analysis of these studies goes beyond the scope of the present paper; the reader is referred to several recent good reviews (Benveniste, 1987; Chung & Barnes, 1988; Page, 1988b; Mencia-Huerta *et al.* 1989; Pretolani *et al.* 1989).

Conclusions

There is now overwhelming evidence that platelets are involved, and play an active role, in allergic bronchoconstriction in experimental animals. This appears to be true not only for the acute bronchospasm but also, and more interestingly, for the inflammatory alterations that are the basis for bronchial hyper-responsiveness.

Although the role of platelets in human asthma has not been conclusively demonstrated, a large number of observations are accumulating on the participation of these cells in clinical asthma, too. Despite the sometimes conflicting results it is indeed very likely that platelets are in some way involved in human asthma. One limitation of the studies on platelets in asthma is represented by the fact that most of them have examined the acute effects of bronchial challenges on circulating platelets. Allergen provocation procedures are rather dramatic and do not necessarily reflect the natural history and the sequence of events following spontaneous exposure to antigens. More interesting information might be obtained by the study of the inter-relationships between platelets and the clinical expressions of airway inflammation in asthma, such as late asthmatic reactions or bronchial hyper-reactivity. Initial studies showing a correlation between platelet activation and nocturnal asthma, a typical bronchospastic condition associated with inflammatory changes, look promising (Morrison *et al.* 1988).

There is little doubt that platelets are involved in a number of pathophysiological phenomena not directly linked to haemostasis (Gordon & Milner, 1976; de Gaetano *et al.* 1987; Page, 1988a; see Chapters 5 and 8). It is, however, evident that their participation in non-haemostatic processes does not necessarily imply the same functional responses as those operating in haemostasis or thrombosis.

Adhesion, aggregation or release may not be of primary importance for platelet participation in asthma. Platelet diapedesis or liberation of oxygen radicals upon appropriate stimulation (Lowenhaupt *et al.* 1973; Coeugnet 1979; Capron *et al.* 1985) are two examples of non-haemostatic functions of platelets. It is possible that more definitive evidence for platelet involvement in human asthma will come from the application of unconventional approaches to the study of platelets in this clinical condition.

Acknowledgements

The help of Dr C. Corona with the preparation of the manuscript and of Dr K. Tonato with typing is gratefully acknowledged.

References

Ambler, J. & Wallis, R.B. (1983) A comparison between platelet aggregation and ATP secretion induced by collagen and by PAF acether and their inhibition by phenylbutazone, sulphinpyrazone and its metabolites. *Thromb Res* **31**, 577–589.

Ameisen, J.C., Capron, A., Joseph, M., Maclouf, J., Vorng, H., Pancrè, V., Fournier, E., Wallaert, B. & Tonnel, A.B. (1985) Aspirin-sensitive asthma: abnormal platelet response to drugs inducing asthmatic attacks. Diagnostic and physiopathological implications. *Int Arch Allergy Appl Immunol* **78**, 438–448.

Arnoux, B., Grimfeld, A., Duroux, P. & Denjean, A. (1983) Alveolar macrophages Paf-acether. A new association in the pathogenesis of human asthma. In Benveniste, J. & Arnoux, B. (eds) *Platelet Activating Factor*, pp. 335–41. Elsevier/North Holland Biomedical Press, Amsterdam.

Audera, C., Rocklin, R., Vaillancourt, R., Jakubowski, J.A. & Deykin, D. (1988) Altered arachidonic acid metabolism and platelet size in atopic subjects. *Clinical Immunol Immunopathol* **46**, 352–359.

Bakulin, M.P. & Joffe, E.J. (1979) Content of biologically active substances, histamine and serotonin in patients with bronchial asthma. *Teraputicheskii Arkhiv (Moskva)* **51**, 45–49.

Barnes, P.J. (1988) Inflammatory mechanisms and nocturnal asthma. *Am J Med* **85** (Suppl 1B), 64–70.

Benveniste, J. (1987) A role for PAF-acether (platelet-activating factor) in bronchial hyperreactivity. *Am Rev Respir Dis* **195**, 52–54.

Berk, B.C., Alexander, R.W., Brock, T.A., Gimbrone, M.A. & Webb, R.C. (1986) Vasoconstriction: a new activity for platelet-derived growth factor. *Science* **232**, 87–90.

Block, L.H., Imhof, E. & Perruchoud, A.P. (1988) Platelets of asthmatics show increased phosphatidylinositol turnover in response to PAF. *Am Rev Respir Dis* **137**, 235 (Abstr).

Born, G.V.R. & Cross, M.J. (1963) The aggregation of blood platelets. *J Physiol* **168**, 178–195.

Boucek, R.J. & Alvarez, T.R. (1970) 5-Hydroxytryptamine: A cytospecific growth stimulator of cultured fibroblasts. *Science* **167**, 898–899.

Braquet, P., Etienne, A., Touvay, C., Bourgain, R.H., Lefort, J. & Vargaftig, B.B. (1985) Involvement of platelet activating factor in respiratory anaphylaxis, demonstrated by PAF-acether inhibitor BN 52021. *Lancet* **i**, 1501.

Braunstein, P.W., Cuénoud, H.F., Joris, I. & Majno, G. (1980) Platelets, fibroblasts, and inflammation. *Am J Pathol* **99**, 53–66.

Brindley, L.L., Sweet, J.M. & Goetzl, E.J. (1983) Stimulation of histamine release from human basophils by human platelet factor 4. *J Clin Invest* **72**, 1218–1223.

Butler, K.D. & Smith, J.R. (1981) Mechanisms of Forssman-induced bronchospasm and their inhibition. *Br J Pharmacol* **73**, 25–32.

Canoso, R.T., Rodvien, R., Scoon, K., Levin, P.H. (1974) Hydrogen peroxide and platelet function. *Blood* **43**, 645–656.

Capron, A., Ameisen, J.C., Joseph, M., Auriault, C., Tonnel, A.B. & Caen, J. (1985) New functions for platelets and their pathological implications. *Int Arch Allergy Appl Immunol* **77**, 107–114.

Capron, A., Joseph, M., Ameisen, J.C., Capron, M., Pancrè, V. & Auriault, C. (1987) Platelets as effectors in immune and hypersensitivity reactions. *Int Arch Allergy Appl Immunol* **82**, 307–312.

Cheng, C.M. & Hawiger, J. (1979) Affinity isolation and characterization of immunoglobulin G Fc fragment-binding glycoprotein from human blood platelets. *J Biol Chem* **254**, 2165–2167.

Chignard, M., Wal, F., Lefort, J. & Vargaftig, B.B. (1982) Inhibition by sulphinpyrazone of the platelet-dependent bronchoconstriction due to platelet-activating factor (PAF-acether) in the guinea pig. *Eur J Pharmacol* **78**, 71–79.

Chignard, M., Selak, M.A. & Smith, J.B. (1986) Direct evidence for the existence of a neutrophil-derived platelet activator (neutrophilin). *Proc Natl Acad Sci USA* **83**, 8609–8613.

Chignard, M., Lalau Keraly, C., Nunez, D., Coëffier, E. & Benveniste, J. (1987) PAF-acether and platelets. In MacIntyre, D.E. & Gordon, J.L. (eds) *Platelets in Biology and Pathology III*, pp. 289–315. Elsevier/North Holland Biomedical Press, Amsterdam.

Chihara, J., Fukuda, K., Yasuba, H., Kishigami, N., Sugihara, R., Kubo, H. & Nakajima, S. (1988) Platelet factor 4 enhances eosinophil IgG and IgE Fc receptor and has eosinophil chemotactic activity. *Am Rev. Respir Dis* **137**, 421.

Chihara, J., Uenishi, H., Sugihara, R., Hakano, N., Kubo, H. & Nakajima, S. (1989) Interactions among PAF, platelet, eosinophil and endothelial cells in allergic reactions. *3rd Int Conf on PAF*, May 8–12, Tokyo, (abstr).

Christman, B.W., Portes, D.K., King, G.A., Leffects, P.L. & Snapper, J.R. (1986) Synthetic platelet-activating factor alters pulmonary haemodynamics, lung mechanics, and lung fluid/solute exchange in awake sheep: role of platelets and granulocytes and effects of synthetic platelet-activating factor on airway reactivity. *Am Rev Respir Dis* **133**, 174–181.

Chung, K.F., Evans, T.W., Graf, P.D. & Nadel, J.A. (1985) Modulation of cholinergic neurotransmission in canine airways by thromboxane mimetic U46616. *Eur J Pharmacol* **117**, 373–375.

Chung, K.F., Aizawa, H., Leikauf, G., Ueki, I.F., Evans, T.W. & Nadel, J.A. (1986) Airway hyperresponsiveness induced by platelet activating factor: role of thromboxane generation. *J Pharmacol Exp Ther* **236**, 580–584.

Chung, K.F. & Barnes, P.J. (1988) PAF antagonists. Their potential therapeutic role in asthma. *Drugs* **35**, 93–103.

Coeffier, E., Chignard, M., Delautier, D. & Benveniste, J. (1984) Cooperation between platelets (P) and neutrophils (N) for PAF-acether formation. *Fed Proc* **43**, 781 (abstr).

Coeugniet, E. (1979) Thrombocyte migration inhibitory activity of concanavalin by dipyridamole and acetylsalicylic acid. *Thromb Res* **15**, 297–307.

Coffey, R.G., & Middleton, E. (1975) Increased adenosine triphosphatase activity in platelets of asthmatic children. *Int Arch Allergy Appl Immunol* **48**, 171–181.

Cotran, R.S. (1965) The delayed and prolonged vascular leakage in inflammation. II. An electron microscopic study of the vascular response after thermal injury. *Am J Pathol* **46**, 589–620.

Coyle, A.J., Urwin, S.C., Page C.P., Touvay, C., Villain, B. & Braquet, P. (1988) The effect of the selective PAF antagonist BN 52021 on PAF-and antigen-induced bronchial hyper-reactivity and eosinophil accumulation. *Eur J Pharmacol* **148**, 51–58.

Cuss, F.M., Dixon, C.M.S. & Barnes, P.J. (1986) Effects of inhaled platelet activating factor on pulmonary function and bronchial responsiveness in man. *Lancet* **ii**, 189–191.

Daffonchio, L., Lees, I., Payne, A.N. & Whittle B.J.R. (1987) Non-specific airway hyper-reactivity following bronchial anaphylaxis in anaesthetised guinea-pigs. *Br J Pharmacol* **90**, 114P.

Da Prada, M., Richards, J.G. & Kettler, R. (1981) Amine storage organelles in platelets. In Gordon, J.L. (ed.) *Platelets in Biology and Pathology-2*, pp. 107–45. Elsevier/North Holland Biomedical Press, Amsterdam.

Davis, P.B. & Lieberman, P. (1982) Normal alpha$_2$-adrenergic responses in platelets from patients with asthma. *J Allergy Clin Immunol* **69**, 35–38.

Day, R.P., Behrmann, S., Dolovich, J. & Hargreave, F.E. (1975) Inflammatory effects of leukocytes and platelets. *J Allergy Clin Immunol* **55**, 87–92.

Defreyn, G., Deckmyn, H. & Vermylen, J. (1982) A thromboxane synthetase inhibitor reorients endoperoxide metabolism in whole blood towards prostacyclin and prostaglandin E2. *Thromb Res* **26**, 389–400.

de Gaetano, G., Cerletti, C., Nanni-Costa, M.P. & Poggi, A. (1987) Blood platelets as inflammatory cells. In Born, G.V.R. & Neri Serneri, G.G. (eds) *Antiplatelet Therapy: Twenty Years' Experience*, pp. 52–62. Excerpta Medica, Amsterdam.

De Monchy, J.G.R., Kaufman, H.P., Venge, P., Koeter, G.H., Jansen, H.M., Sluiter, H.J. & DeVries K. (1985) Bronchoalveolar eosinophilia during allergen-induced late asthmatic reactions. *Am Rev Respir Dis* **131**, 373–376.

Deuel, T.F., Senior, R.M., Chang, D., Griffin, G.L., Heinrickson, R.L. & Kaiser, E.T. (1981) Platelet factor 4 is chemotactic for neutrophils and monocytes. *Proc Natl Acad Sci USA* **78**, 4584–4587.

Deuel, T.F., Senior, R.M., Huang, J.S. & Griffin, G.L. (1982) Chemotaxis of monocytes and neutrophils to platelet-derived growth factor. *J Clin Invest* **69**, 1046–1049.

D'Souza, L. & Glueck, H.I. (1977) Measurement of nucleotide pools in platelets using high pressure liquid chromatography. *Thromb Haemost* **38**, 990–1001.

Durham, S.R., Dawes, J. & Kay, A.B. (1985) Platelets in asthma. *Lancet* **ii**, 36.

Fishel, C.W. & Zwemer, R.L. (1970) Aggregation of platelets form *B. Pertussi*-injected mice and atopically sensitive human individuals. *Fed Proc* **29**, 640 (abstr).

FitzGerald, G.A., Pedersen, A.K. & Patrono, C. (1983) Analysis of prostacyclin and thromboxane A2 biosynthesis in cardiovascular disease. *Circulation* **67**, 1174–1177.

Fitzgerald, M.F., Moncada, S. & Parente, L. (1986) The anaphylactic release of platelet-activating factor from perfused guinea-pig lungs. *Br J Pharmacol* **88**, 149–153.

Frigas, E. & Gleich, G.J. (1986) The eosinophil and the pathology of asthma. *J Allergy Clin Immunol* **77**, 527–537.

Goetzl, E.J., Woods, J.M. & Gorman, R.R. (1977) Stimulation of human eosinophil and neutrophil polymorphonuclear leukocyte chemotaxis and random migration by 12-L-hydroxy-5,8,10,14-eicosatetraenoic acid. *J Clin Invest* **59**, 179–183.

Goldberg, I.D., Stemerman, M.B. & Handin, R.I. (1980) Vascular permeation of platelet factor 4 after endothelial injury. *Science* **209**, 611–612.

Gordon, J.L. & Milner, A.J. (1976) Blood platelets as multifunctional cells. In Gordon, J.L. (ed) *Platelets in Biology and Pathology*, pp. 3–22. Elsevier/North Holland Biomedical Press, Oxford.

Greer, I.A., Winter, J.H., Gaffney, D., McLoughlin, K., Belch, J.J.F., Boyd, G. & Forbes, C.D. (1984) Platelets in asthma. *Lancet* **ii**, 1479.

Gresele, P., Todisco, T., Merante, F. & Nenci, G.G. (1982) Platelet activation and allergic asthma. *New Engl J Med* **306**, 549.

Gresele, P., Grasselli, S., Todisco, T. & Nenci, G.G. (1985) Platelets and asthma. *Lancet* **i**, 347.

Gresele, P., Arnout, J., Coene, M.C., Deckmyn, H. & Vermylen, J. (1986) Leukotriene B4 production by stimulated whole blood: comparative studies with isolated polymorphonuclear cells. *Biochem Biophys Res Commun* **137**, 334–342.

Gresele, P., Ribaldi, E., Grasselli, S., Todisco, T. & Nenci, G.G. (1987) Evidence for platelet activation in allergic asthma. *Agents and Actions Suppl* **21**, 119–128.

Grotendorst, G.R., Seppa, H.E.J., Kleinman, H.K. & Martin, G.R. (1981) Attachment of smooth muscle cells to collagen and their migration toward platelet-derived growth factor. *Proc Natl Acad Sci USA* **78**, 3669–3672.

Guinot, P., Brambilla, C., Duchier, J., Braquet, P., Bonvoisin, B. & Cournot, A. (1987) Effect of BN 52063, a specific PAF-acether antagonist, on bronchial provocation test to allergens in asthmatic patients. A preliminary study. *Prostaglandins* **34**, 723–731.

Hahn, H.-L., Purnama, I., Lang, M. & Sannwald, U. (1986) Effects of platelet activating factor on tracheal mucus secretion, on airway mechanics and on circulating blood cells in live ferrets. *Eur J Respir Dis* **69**, 277–284.

Hallberg, T., Dohlsten, M. & Baldetorp, B. (1984) Demonstration of histamine receptors on human platelets by flow cytometry. *Scand J Haematol* **32**, 113–118.

Halonen, M., Palmer, J.D., Lohman, C., McManus, L.M. & Pinckard, R.N. (1981) Differential effects of platelet depletion on the physiologic alterations of IgE anaphylaxis and acetyl ether phosphorylcoline infusion in the rabbit. *Am Rev Respir Dis* **124**, 416–419.

Hanahan, D.J. (1986) Platelet activating factor: a biologically active phosphoglyceride. *Annu Rev Biochem* **55**, 483–509.

Harker, L.A. (1978) Platelet survival time: its measurement and use. *Prog Haemost Thromb* **4**, 321–347.

Harker, L. & Slichter, S. (1972) The bleeding time as a screening test for evaluation of platelet function. *New Engl J Med* **287**, 155–159.

Harker, L.A., Malpass, T.W., Branson, H.E., Hessel, E.A. & Slichter, S.J. (1980) Mechanism of abnormal bleeding in patients undergoing cardiopulmonary bypass: acquired transient platelet dysfunction associated with selective alpha granule release. *Blood* **56**, 824–834.

Hartman, M.M. (1963) Thrombo-embolic phenomenon in severe asthma. Use of heparin for prevention and treatment in patients receiving ACTH or glucosteroids. *Calif Med* **98**, 27–31.

Harwell, W.B., Patterson, J.T., Lieberman, P. & Beachey, E. (1973) Platelet aggregation in atopic and normal patients. *J Allergy Clin Immunol* **51**, 274–284.

Haslam, R.J. (1987) Signal transduction in platelet activation. In Verstraete, M., Vermylen, J., Lijnen, R. & Arnout, J. (eds) *Thrombosis and Haemostasis 1987*, pp. 147–174. Leuven University Press, Leuven.

Hemmendinger, S., Pauli, G., Tenabene, A., Pujol, J.L., Bessot, J.C., Eber, M. & Cazenave J.P. (1989) Platelet function: aggregation by PAF or sequestration in lung is not modified during immediate or late allergen-induced bronchospasm in man. *J Allergy Clin Immunol* **83**, 990–996.

Henderson, W.R., Shelhamer, J.H., Reingold, D.B., Smith, L.J., Evans, R. & Kaliner, M. (1979) Alpha-adrenergic hyper-responsiveness in asthma. *New Engl J Med* **300**, 642–647.

Henson, P.M. & Ginsberg, M.H. (1981) Immunological reactions of platelets. In Gordon, J.L. (ed.) *Platelets in Biology and Patholgy-2*, pp. 265–308. Elsevier/North Holland Biomedical Press, Oxford.

Henson, P.M. & Pinckard, R.N. (1977) Basophil-derived platelet-activating factor (PAF) as an *in vivo* mediator of acute allergic reactions: demonstration of specific desensitization of platelets to PAF during IgE-induced anaphylaxis in the rabbit. *J Immunol* **119**, 2179–2184.

Hiti-Harper, J., Wohl, H. & Harper, E. (1978) Platelet factor 4: an inhibitor of collagenase. *Science* **199**, 991–992.

Holmsen, H. & Weiss, H.J. (1979) Secretable storage pools in platelets. *Annu Rev Med* **30**, 119–134.

Humphrey, J.H. & Jaques, R. (1954) The histamine and 5-hydroxytryptamine content of platelets and leucocytes in various species. *J Physiol* **124**, 305–310.

Humphrey, J.H. & Jaques, R. (1955) The release of histamine and 5-hydroxy-tryptamine (serotonin) from platelets by antigen-antibody reactions (*in vitro*). *J Physiol* **128**, 9–27.

Ind, P.W., Peters, A.M., Malik, F., Lavender, J.P. & Dollery, C.T. (1985) Pulmonary platelet kinetics in asthma. *Thorax* **40**, 412–417.

Johnson, C.E., Belfield, P.W., Davis, S., Cooke, N.J., Spencer, A. & Davies J.A. (1986) Platelet activation during exercise induced asthma: effect of prophylaxis with cromoglycate and salbutamol. *Thorax* **41**, 290–294.

Jorgensen, L., Hovig, T., Roswell, H.C. & Mustard, J.F. (1970) Adenosine diphosphate-induced platelet aggregation and vascular injury in swine and rabbits.

Am J Pathol **61**, 161–176.

Kaplan, K.L. & Owen, J. (1981) Plasma levels of β-thromboglobulin and platelet factor 4 as indices of platelet activation *in vivo*. *Blood* **57**, 199–202.

Kerry, R. & Scrutton, M.C. (1985) Platelet adrenoceptors: In Longenecker, G.L. (ed.) *The Platelets. Physiology and Pharmacology*, pp. 113–157. Academic Press Inc., Orlando.

Klysner, R., Geiseer, A., Hansen, K.W., Stahl Skov, P. & Norn, S. (1980) Histamine H2 receptors-mediated cyclic AMP formation in human platelets. *Acta Pharmacol Toxicol* **47**, 1–4.

Knauer, K.A., Lichtenstein, L.M., Adkinson, N.F. & Fish J.E. (1981) Platelet activation during antigen-induced airway reactions in asthmatic subjects. *New Engl J Med* **304**, 1404–1407.

Knauer, K.A., Kagey-Sobotka, A., Adkinson, N.F. & Lichtenstein, L.M. (1984) Platelet augmentation of IgE-dependent histamine release from human basophils and mast cells. *Int Arch Allergy Appl Immunol* **74**, 29–35.

Kohanna, F.H., Smith, M.H. & Salzman, E.W. (1984) Do patients with thromboembolic disease have circulating platelet aggregates? *Blood* **64**, 205–207.

Kravis, T. & Henson, P.M. (1977) Accumulation of platelets at sites of antigen-antibody-mediated injury. *J Immunol* **118**, 1569–1573.

Kulka, J.P., Bocking, D., Ropes, M.W. & Bauer, W. (1955) Early joint lesions of rheumatoid arthritis. *Arch Pathol* **59**, 129–150.

Lammers, J.W., Kioumis, I., McCusker, M., Chung, K.F. & Barnes, P.J. (1988) Effect of prostacyclin (PGI2) on bronchoconstriction induced by platelet-activating factor (PAF) in man. *Am Rev Respir Dis* **137** (suppl): A373.

Lavell, K.J., Ransdell, B.A. & Trygstad, C.W. (1975) Identification of a new platelet aggregating factor released by sensitized leukocytes. *Clin Immunol Immunopathol* **3**, 492–502.

Lee, T.C., Lenihan, D.J., Malone, B., Roddy, L.L. & Wasserman, S.I. (1984) Increased biosynthesis of platelet-activating factor in activated human eosinophils. *J Biol Chem* **259**, 5526–5530.

Lefort, J. & Vargaftig, B.B. (1978) Mechanism of collagen-induced bronchoconstriction and thrombocytopenia in the guinea-pig. *Eur J Pharmacol* **62**, 422 p.

Lellouch-Tubiana, A., Lefort, J., Pirotzky, E., Vargaftig, B.B. & Pfister, A. (1985) Ultrastructural evidence for extra-vascular platelet recruitment in the lung upon intravenous injection of platelet-activating factor (PAF-acether) to guinea-pigs. *Br J Exp Pathol* **66**, 345–355.

Lellouch-Tubiana, A., Lefort, J., Pfister, A. & Vargaftig, B.B. (1987) Interactions between granulocytes and platelets with guinea-pig lung in passive anaphylactic shock. Correlations with PAF-acether-induced lesions. *Int Arch Allergy Appl Immunol* **83**, 198–205.

Lellouch-Tubiana, A., Lefort, J., Simon, M.-T., Pfister, A. & Vargaftig, B.B. (1988) Eosinophil recruitment into guinea pig lungs after PAF-acether and allergen administration. Modulation by prostacyclin, platelet depletion, and selective antagonists. *Am Rev Respir Dis* **137**, 948–954.

Lin, A.H., Morton, D.R. & Gorman, R.R. (1982) Acetyl glyceryl ether phosphorylcholine stimulates leukotriene B4 synthesis in human polymorphonuclear leukocytes. *J Clin Invest* **70**, 1058–1065.

Lonky, S.A. & Wohl, H. (1981) Stimulation of human leucocyte elastase by platelet factor 4. Physiologic, morphologic and biomedical effects on hamster lungs *in vitro*. *J. Clin Invest* **67**, 817–826.

Lowenhaupt, R., Miller, M. Glueck, H.I. (1973) Platelet migration and chemotaxis demonstrated *in vitro*. *Thromb Res* **3**, 477–486.

Lupinetti, M.D., Sheller, J.R., Catella, F., Fitzgerald, S.A. (1989) Thromboxane biosynthesis in allergen-induced bronchospasm. *Am Rev Resp Dis* **142**, 932–935.

Lurie, A., Dessanges, J.F., Delautier, D., Coëffier, E., Chignard, M., Crémer, G.A., Benveniste, J., Marsac, J. & Lockhart, A. (1987) Exercise-and allergen-induced asthma do not change the production of PAF-acether by neutrophils and platelets. *Bull Eur Physiopatol Respir* **23**, 347–351.

McDonald, J.R., Tan, E.M., Stevenson, D.D. & Vaughan, J.H. (1974) Platelet aggregation in asthmatic and normal subjects. *J Allergy Clin Immunol* **54**, 200–208.

McManus, L.M., Morley, C.A., Levine, S.P. & Pinckard, R.N. (1979) Platelet activating factor (PAF) induced release of platelet factor 4 (PF4) *in vitro* and during IgE anaphylaxis in the rabbit. *J Immunol* **123**, 2835–2841.

Maccia, C.A., Gallagher, J.S., Ataman, G., Glueck, H.I., Brooks, S.M. & Bernstein, I.L. (1977) Platelet thrombopathy in asthmatic patients with elevated immunoglobulin E. *J Allergy Clin Immunol* **59**, 101–108.

Maclouf, J., Fruteau de Laclos, B. & Borgeat, P. (1982) Stimulation of leukotriene biosynthesis in human blood leukocytes by platelet-derived 12-hydroperoxy-icosatetraenoic acid. *Proc Natl Acad Sci USA* **79**, 6042–6046.

Maclouf, J., Henson, P.M. & Murphy, R.C. (1987) Platelet–neutrophil interactions: formation of leukotriene C4 by transcellular metabolism. *Blood* **70**, 354a.

Majno, G. & Palade, G.E. (1961) Studies on inflammation-I-the effect of histamine and serotonin on vascular permeability: an electron microscope study *J Biophys Biochem Cytol* **11**, 571–605.

Malmgren, R., Grubbström, J., Olsson, P., Theorell, H., Tornling, G. & Unge, G. (1982) Defective serotonin (5-HT) transport mechanism in platelets from patients with endogenous and allergic asthma. *Allergy* **37**, 29–39.

Marcus, A.J., Weksler, B.B., Jaffe, E.A. & Broekman, M.J. (1980) Synthesis of prostacyclin from platelet-derived endoperoxides by cultured human endothelial cells. *J Clin Invest* **66**, 979–986.

Marcus, A.J., Broekman, M.J., Safier, L.B., Ullman, H.L., Islam, N., Serhan, C.N., Rutherford, L.E., Korchak, H.M. & Weissmann, G. (1982) Formation of leukotrienes and other hydroxy acids during platelet-neutrophil interactions *in vitro*. *Biochem Biophys Res Commun* **109**, 130–137.

Marcus, A.J., Safier, L.B., Ullman, H.L., Broekman, M.J., Islam, N., Oglesby, T.D., Gorman, R.R. & von Schacky, C. (1986) Platelet neutrophil interactions in the eicosanoid pathway. In Oppenheim, J.J. & Jacobs, D.M. (eds) *Leukocytes and Host Defense*, pp. 365–371. Alan R. Liss, New York.

Mazza, J.J., Gatlin, P.F., & Marx, J.J. (1980) Inhibition of platelet aggregation with histamine. *Am J Haematol* **8**, 257–263.

Mehta, J., Mehta, P., Lawson, D.L., Ostrowski, N. & Brigmon, L. (1985) Influence of a selective thromboxane synthetase blocker CGS-13080 on thromboxane and prostacyclin synthesis in whole blood: evidence for synthesis of prostacyclin by leukocytes from platelet derived endoperoxides. *J Lab Clin Med* **106**, 246–252.

Mehta, P., Mehta, J., Lawson, D., Krop, I. & Letts, L.G. (1986) Leukotrienes potentiate the effects of epinephrine and thrombin on human platelet aggregation. *Thromb Res* **41**, 731–738.

Mencia-Huerta, J.M., Hadji, L. & Benveniste, J. (1981) Release of a slow-reacting substance of anaphylaxis from rabbit platelets. *J Clin Invest* **6**, 1586–1591.

Mencia-Huerta, J.M., Hosford, D. & Braquet, P. (1989) Acute and long-term pulmonary effects of platelet-activating factor. *J. Clin Exp Immunol* **19**, 125–142.

Menz, G., Schmitz-Schumann, M., Böttiger, J. & Virchow, C. (1987) Lack of PAF release in extrinsic asthma. *Agents and Actions Suppl* **21**, 139–144.

Metzger, W.J., Hunninghake, H.B. & Richerson, H.B. (1985) Late asthmatic responses: inquiry into mechanisms and significance. *Clin Rev Allergy* **3**, 145–165.

Metzger, W.J., Sjoerdsma, K., Richerson, H.B., Moseley, P., Zavala, D., Monick, M. & Hunninghake, G.W. (1987) Platelets in bronchoalveolar lavage from asthmatic patients and allergic rabbits with allergen-induced late phase responses. *Agents and Actions* Suppl **21**, 151–159.

Middleton, E. (1972) Autonomic imbalance in asthma with special reference to beta adrenergic blockade. *Adv Int Med* **18**, 177–197.

Morris, H.G., Sherman, N.A., Shepperdson, F.T. & Selner, J.C. (1980) Radioimmunoassay of thromboxane B2 in plasma of normal and asthmatic subjects. *Adv. Prostaglandin Thromboxane Res* **8**, 1759–1764.

Morrison, J.F.J., Bramley, P.B., Craig, I.R., Pearson, S.B. & Dean, H.G. (1988) Platelet activation and nocturnal asthma. *Clin Sci* **74**, 4P (abstr).

Nachman, R.L., Weksler, B. & Fabris, B. (1972) Characterization of human platelet vascular permeability-enhancing activity. *J Clin Invest* **51**, 549–556.

Niewiarówski, J.F. (1977) Proteins secreted by the platelets. *Thromb Haemost* **38**, 924–938.

O'Byrne, P.M. (1988) Leukotrienes, airway hyperresponsiveness, and asthma. *Ann NY Acad Sci* **254**, 282–288.

Oda, M., Satouchi, K., Yasunago, K. & Saito, K. (1986) Polymorphonuclear leukocyte-platelet interactions: acetylglyceryl ether phosphocholine-induced platelet activation under stimulation with chemotactic peptide. *J Biochem* **100**, 1117–1123.

O'Donnell, S.R. & Barnett, C.J.K. (1987) Microvascular leakage to platelet activating factor in guinea-pig trachea and bronchi. *Eur J Pharmacol* **138**, 385–396.

Orchard, M.A., Kagey-Sobotka, D., Proud, D. & Lichtenstein, L.M. (1985) A platelet derived supernatant (PDS) releases histamine from human basophils: evidence for interaction with IgE. *Thromb Haemost* **54**, 232 (abstr).

Oxholm, P. & Winther, K. (1986) Thrombocyte involvement in immune inflammatory reactions. *Allergy* **41**, 1–10.

Page, C.P. (1987) A role for platelet-activating factor and platelets in the induction of bronchial hyperreactivity. *Int J Tissue React* **9**, 27–32.

Page, C.P. (1988a) The involvement of platelets in non-thrombotic processes. *Trends Pharmacol Sci* **9**, 66–71.

Page, C.P., (1988b) The role of platelet-activating factor in asthma. *J Allergy Clin Immunol* **81**, 144–152.

Page, C.P., Paul, W., & Morley, J. (1982) An *in vivo* model for studying platelet aggregation and disaggregation. *Thromb Haemost* **47**, 210–213.

Page, C.P., Paul, W., Douglas, G.J., Casals-Stentel, J. & Morley, J. (1983) PAF-acether, platelets and bronchospasm. In Benveniste, J. & Arnoux, B. (eds) *Platelet-Activating Factor and Structurally Related Ether-Lipids*, pp. 327–334. Elsevier/North Holland Biomedical Press, Amsterdam.

Page, C.P., Paul, W. & Morley, J. (1984) Platelets and bronchospasm. *Int Arch Allergy Appl Immunol* **74**, 347–350.

Page, C.P., Archer, C.B., Guerreiro, D. & Morley, J. (1985) Properties of PAF-acether appropriate to a mediator of the inflammatory aspects of asthma. *Int J Tissue React* **7**, 351–354.

Palma-Carlos, A.G., Palma-Carlos, M.L., Santos, M.C. & Santos, E. (1988) Platelet aggregation in asthma. *Prostaglandins* **35**, 801 (abstr).

Pareti, F.I., Capitanio, A., Mannucci, L., Ponticelli, C. & Mannucci, P.M. (1980) Acquired dysfunction due to the circulation of 'exhausted' platelets. *Am J Med* **69**, 235–240.

Pinckard, R.N., Halonen, M., Palmer, J.D., Butler, C., Shaw, J.O. & Henson, P.M. (1977) Intravascular aggregation and pulmonary sequestration of platelets during IgE-induced systemic anaphylaxis in the rabbit: abrogation of lethal anaphylactic shock by platelet depletion. *J Immunol* **119**, 2185–2193.

Polley, M.J. & Nachman, R.L. (1979) Human complement in thrombin-mediated platelet function. Uptake of the C56-9 complex. *J Exp Med* **150**, 633–645.

Polley, M.J. & Nachman, R.L. (1981) The human complement system in thrombin-mediated platelet function. In Gordon, J.L. (ed.) *Platelets in Biology and Pathology–2*, pp. 309–319. Elsevier/North Holland Biomedical Press, Oxford.

Polley, M.J. & Nachman, R.L. (1983) Human platelet activation by C3a and C3a des-arg. *J Exp Med* **158**, 603–615.

Pretolani, M., Ferrer-Lopez, P. & Vargaftig, B.B. (1989) From anti-asthma drugs to PAF-acether antagonism and back. *Biochem Pharmacol* **38**, 1373–1384.

Regal, J.F. (1988) C5a-induced bronchoconstriction: absence of a role of circulating white blood cells and platelets. *Int Arch Allergy Appl Immunol* **86**, 196–200.

Robertson, D.N. & Page, C.P. (1987) Effect of platelet agonist on airway reactivity and intrathoracic platelet accumulation. *Br J Pharmacol* **92**, 105–111.

Samuelsson, B., Goldyne, M., Granström, E., Hamberg, M., Hammarström, S. & Malmsten, C. (1978) Prostaglandin and thromboxanes. *Annu Rev Biochem* **47**, 997–1029.

Saxena, S.P., Brandes, L.J., Becker, A.B., Simons, K.J., LaBella, F.S. & Gerrard J.M. (1989) Histamine is an intracellular messenger mediating platelet aggregation. *Science* **243**, 1596–1599.

Schellenberg, R.R., Walker, B. & Pul, U.B.C. (1983) Platelet-dependent contraction of human bronchus by platelet-activating factor. *J Allergy Clin Immunol* **71**, 145.

Schumacher, H.R. (1975) Synovial membrane and fluid morphologic alterations in early rheumatoid arthritis: microvascular injury and virus-like particles. *Ann NY Acad Sci* **256**, 39–64.

Schwartz, H.J. & Bennett, B. (1973) The differential effect of acetylsalicytic acid on *in vitro* aggregation of platelets from normal, asthmatic and aspirin-sensitive subjects. *Int Arch Allergy* **45**, 899–904.

Shephard, E.G., Malan, L., Macfarlane, C.M., Mouton, W. & Joubert, J.R. (1985) Lung function and plasma levels of thromboxane B2, 6-ketoprostaglandin F1α and β-thromboglobulin in antigen-induced asthma before and after indomethacin pretreatment. *Br J Clin Pharmacol* **19**, 459–470.

Slater, D.N., Martin, J.F. & Trowbridge, E.A. (1985) The platelet in asthma. *Lancet* **i**, 110.

Solinger, A., Bernstein, I.L. & Glueck, H.I. (1973) The effect of epinephrine on platelet aggregation in normal and atopic subjects. *J Allergy Clin Immunol* **51**, 29–34.

Storck, H., Hoigné, R. & Koller, F. (1955) Thrombocytes in allergic reactions. *Int Arch Allergy* **6**, 372–384.

Stuart, M.J., Murphy, S. & Oski, F.A. (1975) A simple nonradioisotope technique for the determination of platelet life span. *New Engl J Med* **292**, 1310–1313.

Sundsmo, J.S. & Fair, D.S. (1983) Relationship among the complement, kinin, coagulation and fibrinolytic systems in the inflammatory reaction. *Clin Physiol Biochem* **1**, 225–284.

Szczeklik, A., Nizankowski, R. & Mruk, J. (1977) Myocardial infarction in status asthmaticus. *Lancet* **i**, 658–659.

Szczeklik, A., Milner, P.C., Birch, J., Watkins, J. & Martin, J.F. (1986) Prolonged bleeding time, reduced platelet aggregation, altered PAF-acether sensitivity and increased platelet mass are a trait of asthma and hay fever. *Thromb Haemost* **56**, 283–287.

Taytard, A. & Vuillemin, L. (1987) Platelet kinetics in stable asthmatic patients. *Agents and Actions Suppl* **21**, 161.

Thompson, P.J., Hanson, J.M., Bilani, H., Turner-Warwick, M. & Morley, J. (1984) Platelets, platelet activator factor and asthma. *Am Rev Respir Dis* **129**, A3 (abstr).

Traietti, P., Marmaggi, S., Dardes, N., Moscatelli, B., Bologna, E. & Vulterini, S. (1984) Circulating platelet activation in respiratory diseases: differences between arterial and venous blood in COLD and asthmatic patients. *Respiration* **46**, (suppl 1), 62–63.

Tvedten, H.W., Till, G.O. & Ward, P.A. (1985) Mediators of lung injury in mice following systemic activation of complement. *Am J Pathol* **119**, 92–100.

Tzeng, D.Y., Deuel, T.F., Huang, J.S. & Boehner, R.L. (1985) Platelet-derived growth factor promotes human peripheral monocyte activation. *Blood* **66**, 179–183.

Vaage, J. & Hauge, A. (1977) Small airway constriction and closure after induced intravascular platelet aggregation. *Acta Physiol Scand* **100**, 221–230.

Valone, F.H. (1986) Synergistic platelet activation by aggregates of IgG and the phospholipid platelet-activating factor 1-O-alkyl-2-acetyl-sn-glycero-3-phosphorylcholine. *J Clin Immunol* **6**, 57–64.

Vargaftig, B.B. & Benveniste, J. (1983) Platelet activating factor today. *Trends Pharmacol Sci* **4**, 341–343.

Vargaftig, B.B. & Lefort, J. (1979) Differential effects of prostacyclin and prostaglandin E1 on bronchoconstriction and thrombocytopenia during collagen and arachidonate infusions and anaphylactic shock in the guinea pig. *Prostaglandins* **18**, 519–528.

Vargaftig, B.B., Lefort, J., Chignard, M. & Benveniste, J. (1980) Platelet-activating factor induces a platelet-dependent bronchoconstriction unrelated to the formation of prostaglandin derivatives. *Eur J Pharmacol* **65**, 185–192.

Vargaftig, B.B., Lefort, J., Wal, F., Chignard, M. & Medeiros, M.C. (1982) Interference of non-steroidal anti-inflammatory drugs associated to anti-histamine and anti-serotonin agents with the bronchial and platelet effects of "platelet-activating factor" (PAF-acether). *Eur J Pharmacol* **82**, 121–130.

Wahl, S.M., Hunt, D.A., Wakefield, L.M., McCartney-Francis, N., Wahl, L.M., Roberts, A.B. & Sporn, M.B. (1987) Transforming growth factor type beta induces monocyte chemotaxis and growth factor production. *Proc Natl Acad Sci USA* **84**, 5788–5792.

Ward, P.A., Till, G.O. & Johnson, K.J. (1986) Role of platelets in neutrophil dependent, oxygen radical mediated lung injury. *Fed Proc* **45**, 380 (abstr).

Weksler, B. & Coupal, C.E. (1973) Platelet dependent generation of chemotactic activity in serum. *J Exp Med* **137**, 1419–1430.

Wu, K.K. & Hoak, J.C. (1974) A new method for the quantitative detection of platelet aggregates in patients with arterial insufficiency. *Lancet* **ii**, 924–926.

Yaron, M. & Djaldetti, M. (1978) Platelets in synovial fluid. *Arthritis Rheum* **21**, 607–608.

Yen, S.S. & Morris, H.G. (1981) An imbalance of arachidonic acid metabolism in asthma. *Biochem Biophys Res Commun* **103**, 774–779.

Zawilska, K., Giroud, J.P., Timsit, S. & Caen, J.P. (1973) Plaquettes et inflammation. *Pathol Biol (Paris)* **21**, (Suppl). 51–56.

7: Interactions of Platelets with the Blood Vessel Wall

Philip K. Moore

Introduction

The symbiotic relationship which exists between platelets and the vascular endothelium is complex. The biochemical basis of what can only be described as a very intimate co-operation between these two cell types has begun to be appreciated only within the last decade. It is now clear that platelets are necessary for endothelial viability while a healthy and undamaged endothelial cell layer is a prerequisite to prevent inappropriate platelet activation and thereby to maintain the fluidity of blood in the circulation.

The physiological sequelae of damage to the vascular endothelium which include platelet adhesion to subendothelial elements in the blood vessel wall, localized vasoconstriction, recruitment of circulating platelets to form a haemostatic plug and its subsequent consolidation with strands of fibrin are now well established. Furthermore, it is a simple matter to envisage how an exaggeration of this physiological process may trigger intravascular thrombus formation which, superimposed upon existing atherosclerotic damage to blood vessels, may be the cause of potentially life-threatening conditions such as myocardial infarction, stroke and pulmonary embolism (reviewed elsewhere in this volume, see Chapter 10). However, such a straightforward description of the platelet–blood vessel interaction leaves hidden a number of more complicated events including the molecular mechanism of platelet adhesion to endothelial cells and subendothelial elements, the role of platelets in triggering blood coagulation and vascular smooth muscle repair and importantly the haemostatic processes which control these functions.

The principal aim of this chapter is to review the literature concerning the mechanisms which initiate and provide the 'fine tuning' of platelet adhesion and intravascular aggregation. The role of platelets in the initiation of blood coagulation and as providers of mitogenic substances for vascular smooth muscle are discussed elsewhere in this volume.

Platelet adhesion to the blood vessel wall

The adhesion of platelets to the blood vessel wall is a little understood process particularly when compared with the wealth of information which has accumulated about the mechanism of platelet–platelet interaction (i.e. aggregation). One reason for this discrepancy is likely to be that platelet adhesion is less readily examined *in vitro* than platelet aggregation. This situation has been improved considerably with the development of an annular chamber technique in which sections of inverted rabbit aorta are exposed to blood either from normal, healthy subjects or from patients with platelet disorders (Baumgartner, 1983). Subsequently, this technique has been modified by Sakariassen and co-workers (1983) and the flow dynamics of the annular chamber assessed in detail and shown to approximate closely to the situation *in vivo*. The application of such methods, as well as techniques to investigate the adhesion of platelets to endothelial cells in culture, has allowed a more detailed examination of this process enabling a better understanding of the molecular mechanisms involved.

Platelet adhesion involves a number of separate, identifiable steps:

1 attachment of the platelet to exposed subendothelium of a damaged blood vessel;

2 flattening of the platelet on to the substratum;

3 transformation of the gross structure of the platelet from a relatively smooth outline to one exhibiting numerous cytoplasmic protrusions which make intimate contact with the subendothelium.

Very little information is available concerning the final two mechanisms. However, it has recently become clear, primarily from the kind of studies outlined above, that the platelet–blood vessel attachment process involves both haemodynamic effects and a chemical interaction between collagens in the vessel wall and platelet glycoprotein acceptor molecules (e.g. glycoprotein Ib, glycoprotein IIa–IIIb). The latter process is either accelerated (von Willebrand factor, fibronectin) or retarded (prostacyclin, endothelium derived nitric oxide) by products released from vascular endothelial cells. The part played by haemodynamic as well as the numerous chemical components of the platelet–vessel–wall interaction is discussed in the following sections.

Haemodynamic influences

The flow rate in blood vessels affects the interaction between platelets and the vascular wall in a number of ways involving a combination of shear rate and red blood cell count (i.e. haematocrit). For example, at low shear rates similar to those encountered in large veins, platelet adhesion to the subendothelium increases as the haematocrit rises to 40%. Increases in haematocrit above this value (up to 70%) produce no further increase in platelet adhesiveness. In contrast, at the high shear rates which occur in the microcirculation, platelet adhesion increases in a graded manner as the haematocrit is elevated from 10% through to 70% (Turrito & Weiss, 1980). The effect of haematocrit is presumably related to the ability of red blood cells to deflect platelets laterally thereby increasing the frequency of platelet–vessel wall collisions. As is clear from the above the influence of haematocrit is dependent upon both flow and shear rate.

Role of the subendothelium

The biochemical composition of the subendothelium is of great importance in determining the thrombogenicity of the blood vessel wall. The subendothelium is synthesized both by the overlaying endothelial cells and by the underlying smooth muscle cells. It is reasonable to suppose that endothelial cells manufacture the outer parts of the subendothelial wall while smooth muscle cells make a proportionately greater contribution to the inner subendothelium. Consequently, the biochemical composition of the subendothelium may vary not only from one blood vessel to the next but also between healthy and atherosclerotic blood vessels. Thus, platelet adhesion to a healthy blood vessel wall is not necessarily identical with adhesion to diseased vessels. Unfortunately, this possibility is often overlooked by experimenters.

Connective tissue of the subendothelium comprises collagen fibres, elastic fibres, sulphated proteoglycans and non-collagenous proteins secreted by endothelial cells such as von Willebrand factor (vWF), fibronectin, thrombospondin, laminin and nidogen (e.g. Jaffe & Mosher, 1978; Gospodarowicz *et al.*, 1981; Oohira *et al.* 1983). Of these, neither elastic fibres (Barnes & MacIntyre, 1979) nor thrombospondin play a significant part in platelet adhesion to the vessel wall. Indeed, thrombospondin, like fibrinogen, is probably more important for platelet – platelet interaction (i.e. aggregation). In contrast, purified laminin (I11 *et al.* 1984) and nidogen (de Groot *et al.* 1985) support the adhesion of platelets but do not cause them to spread, elicit secretion of platelet contents or indeed trigger further platelet aggregation (Tryggvason *et al.* 1981). Thus, laminin and nidogen probably have only a minor role in the platelet adhesion mechanism. The part played by vWF and fibronectin in facilitating platelet adhesion is discussed in detail later in this chapter.

Of all the component parts of the subendothelium it is the various types of collagen proteins which are most important for initiating and controlling platelet adhesion to the blood vessel wall. At least seven different types of collagen occur naturally in the vessel wall and will be exposed to flowing blood and hence platelets following perturbation of the endothelial layer. The two most important and abundant collagen molecules involved in platelet adhesion are probably the interstitial collagens I and III (Barnes, 1985) which occur in the medial region of the vessel wall (Madri *et al.* 1980). In addition, other collagens occur naturally in the vessel wall including collagen type IV in the basement membrane of cultured cells and vascular tissue sections (Barnes, 1985), type V associated with the surfaces of smooth muscle cells, and type VI found throughout the vessel wall. Although less well established, blood vessel walls may contain in addition collagens type VIII and X (Majack & Bornstein, 1985) the precise locations and functions of which are not clear.

That blood vessel walls contain such a plethora of different collagen types is clearly of biochemical interest but it is the effect of these collagen subtypes on platelet function which is of physiological importance. Numerous researchers have provided evidence that assuming the collagen in question maintains an appropriate tertiary and quaternary structure all the collagens type I–IV have the ability to trigger platelet adhesion and aggregation *in vitro* (Santoro & Cunningham, 1977; Barnes, 1985). Collagen types I and II are the most potent in this respect. Collagen type V does not form fibrils in solution and fails to aggregate or adhere to platelets *in vitro* although its position on the luminal aspect of endothelial cells and thus in contact with flowing blood implies some, as yet, unknown function in the control of platelet adhesiveness.

The adhesion of platelets to subendothelial collagen fibrils is not a direct process but requires the participation of one or more intermediate, so-called adhesive proteins (reviewed by Packham & Mustard, 1984; Plow *et al.*, 1987). A number of plasma proteins are candidates for mediators of platelet adhesion to collagen. The most important of these are undoubtedly vWF and fibronectin.

Role of the adhesive proteins

Patients with von Willebrand's disease exhibit prolonged bleeding, abnormal platelet agglutination and reduced platelet adhesion (Zimmerman & Ruggeri, 1983). Addition of purified vWF to blood obtained from patients with this disease corrected the platelet adhesion deficiency thereby implying that a lack of this factor causes the haemostatic problems associated with the disease (Moroose & Hoyer, 1987). It is now established that vWF is essential for platelet adhesion to the subendothelium that is exposed by tissue damage (Stel *et al.* 1985).

Von Willebrand factor is a glycoprotein synthesized by endothelial cells and deposited both into the subendothelium and into the plasma (Sussman & Rand, 1982). It may be taken up from the plasma into platelet α-granules and released during secretion (Bloom, 1979). Like other endothelial products such as tissue plasminogen activator (tPA), vWF is released by a variety of stimuli including adrenaline, vasopressin, exercise and venous occlusion. Indeed, von Willebrand's disease has been treated successfully with desmopressin, a synthetic analogue of vasopressin (de la Fuente *et al.* 1985).

Von Willebrand factor has a multimeric structure composed of a number of protomers each with molecular weight approximately 250 000. Within its complex structure vWF exhibits at least four binding 'sites' or 'domains'. One such domain which has been identified by the use of selective monoclonal antibodies interacts with the platelet glycoprotein Ib (GpIb) acceptor site (reviewed by Marguerie *et al.* 1987). This domain (a 55 000 molecular weight subunit at the amino terminal end of the vWF subunit) is probably involved in platelet adhesion and functions in accord with a second such binding domain which interacts directly with collagen types I, II and III (Santoro, 1981). In this way vWF facilitates the interaction between platelets and the subendothelium by binding both collagen and the platelet GpIb site and thereby allowing platelets to 'stick' and subsequently spread along the collagen fibrils. Such a mechanism explains the bleeding defect associated with von Willebrand's disease as described above and also of Bernard–Soulier syndrome which is correlated with a deficiency of platelet GpIb (Hardisty & Caen, 1981).

The effect of vWF on platelet adhesion depends upon the wall shear rate. At low shear rates which occur in arteries and veins platelet adhesion to the blood vessel wall is independent of vWF. In contrast, at the high shear rates which occur in, for example, resistance blood vessels platelet adhesion appears to require vWF (Turitto & Baumgartner, 1983). It seems likely that at high shear rates the amount of time spent by an individual platelet at the vessel wall is short and in this circumstance vWF is a necessity for successful adhesion.

Under appropriate conditions, e.g. following exposure to thrombin, vWF also binds to a GpIIb–IIIa complex on the platelet membrane surface. This binding site is probably important for platelet aggregation since, among other reasons, vWF competes with fibrinogen for this glycoprotein. However, since little or no vWF binding occurs at physiological concentrations of fibrinogen (Schullek *et al.* 1984) the precise role of vWF in platelet aggregation remains unclear.

In addition to vWF the second major adhesive protein which is of physiological importance in initiating platelet adhesion to the vessel wall is fibronectin (Plow *et al.* 1987). Like vWF, fibronectin occurs in at least three sites: endothelial cell basement membranes, platelet α-granules and plasma. The structure of fibronectin determined from recombinant DNA and protein sequence studies is known. This substance is a glycoprotein with a molecular weight in excess of 340 000 and is composed of two chains linked by two disulphide bonds (Petersen *et al.*, 1983; Hynes, 1986). Fibronectin does not bind to resting platelets but will bind to platelets exposed to thrombin or collagen (Plow & Ginsberg, 1981). Although fibronectin does interact with the platelet GpIIb–IIIa site (Plow *et al.* 1985) this combination is probably only of importance in platelet aggregation. A second as yet unknown platelet binding site presumably accounts for the interaction with fibronectin. Fibronectin also binds avidly to collagen fibrils and thus presumably has a similar haemostatic function to vWF linking platelets with the subendothelium and promoting platelet adhesion and spreading. If anything, the effect of fibronectin on platelet adhesion may be even more complex than the corresponding effect of vWF, since antibodies raised against fibronectin reportedly do not prevent platelet–collagen binding (Santoro & Cunningham, 1977). however, the possibility that fibronectin may exist in multiple forms, not all of which react with the antibodies generated for this study should also be considered. That fibronectin is a physiologically relevant adhesive protein is strongly suggested by clinical experience with patients suffering Ehlers–Danlos syndrome. This condition is associated with defective platelet function which may be corrected by fibronectin infusion (Arneson *et al.* 1980) thereby suggesting that deficient fibronectin activity may underly the bleeding deficiency.

Arachidonic acid metabolites

Isolated blood vessels synthesize large amounts of prostacyclin (PGI_2) (Moncada *et al.* 1976). Very early experiments revealed that endothelial cells are the principal site of vascular PGI_2 formation (Moncada *et al.* 1977; MacIntyre *et al.* 1978) although later work has revealed significant generation of this prostanoid by vascular smooth muscle cells (Larrue *et al.* 1980).

Endothelial cells also form small amounts of PGI_2 when challenged with arachidonic acid (Weksler *et al.* 1977) or much larger amounts of PGI_2 when provided with prostaglandin endoperoxides (i.e. PGG_2 or PGH_2) (Moncada *et al.* 1976). Production of PGI_2 persists even after numerous subcultures of these endothelial cells (Christofinis *et al.* 1979). The finding that cultured endothelial cells and fresh vascular tissue make better use of prostaglandin endoperoxides than arachidonic acid has led to the suggestion that these cells are relatively deficient in the cyclooxygenase enzyme but are replete with prostacyclin synthetase.

Endothelial cells do not only produce PGI_2 (Gerritsen, 1987). Cultured aortic endothelial cells also synthesize small amounts of other prostaglandins such as PGE_2, $PGF_{2\alpha}$ and thromboxane A_2 (TXA_2) (Ingerman-Wojenski *et al.* 1981; Miller *et al.* 1985). In this respect, studies have revealed that some smaller blood vessels in particular convert arachidonic acid principally to prostanoids other than PGI_2. Thus, PGE_2 is the most abundant prostanoid produced by small coronary (Gerritsen & Choli, 1983), cerebral (Koide *et al.* 1985) and foreskin capillaries (Charo *et al.* 1984). Unlike PGI_2, the importance of PGE_2 in platelet adhesion and aggregation is not clear.

It should, perhaps, be pointed out that the above experiments may be the exceptions which prove the rule since other microvessels, e.g. in the rat brain, do convert endogenous arachidonic acid mainly into PGI_2 (Goehlert *et al.* 1981). Weighing the available evidence it still seems more than likely that PGI_2 quantitatively is the principal prostanoid manufactured by endothelial cells in most types of blood vessels from the majority of vascular beds and in the majority of species. Interestingly, endothelial cells also contain 11- and 15-lipoxygenase enzymes (Buchanan *et al.* 1985). Again the significance of these enzyme pathways for the control of platelet function *in vivo* is not known.

In contrast to the situation in blood vessels, platelets appear to generate large amounts of prostaglandin endoperoxides by virtue of high cyclooxygenase activity, which are avidly converted by platelet thromboxane synthetase into TXA_2. These findings led to the proposal that aggregating platelets approaching the blood vessel wall 'feed' prostaglandin endoperoxides to the endothelium for conversion into PGI_2. According to this proposal, platelet cyclooxygenase enzyme synthesizes prostaglandin endoperoxides from endogenous arachidonic acid for conversion into TXA_2 which then initiates platelet aggregation. However, if the platelet is in close contact or even simply approaching the blood vessel wall then some of the prostaglandin endoperoxides are 'stolen' by endothelial cells and converted to

PGI_2 which repulse the approaching platelet (Bunting *et al.* 1976). In this way, PGI_2 formation by the vascular endothelium would clearly be pulsatile occurring only when required to prevent platelet adhesion. Obviously if the vascular endothelial cells do steal prostaglandin endoperoxides in the manner described then it represents a very intimate biochemical co-operation between the two different cell types.

No matter how attractive such a mechanism may appear, and the obvious haemostatic advantages it might confer, the theory remains controversial. For example, Aiken *et al.* (1981) have provided evidence that platelets only provide prostaglandin endoperoxides to the vascular endothelium when thromboxane synthetase activity is blocked suggesting that aggregating platelets have little or no 'spare' prostaglandin endoperoxides for utilization by endothelial cells.

Platelet aggregation is inhibited by PGI_2 (see later) as is adhesion by a mechanism which involves stimulation of platelet adenylate cyclase leading to accumulation of cyclic 3′,5′ adenosine monophosphate (cAMP) (Gorman *et al.* 1977). In this respect, PGI_2 is considerably more potent than other antiplatelet prostanoids such as PGE_1, PGD_2 and 6 oxo PGE_1. Within the platelet cytoplasm accumulated cAMP inhibits platelet activation most probably by inhibiting calcium influx from the extracellular plasma or by promoting calcium uptake into platelet α-granules (Kaser-Glanzmann *et al.* 1977).

It is not yet clear whether the principal function of PGI_2 is to limit platelet adhesion to the subendothelium or to prevent platelet aggregation and the subsequent formation of a haemostatic plug. Interestingly, very much higher concentrations of PGI_2 are required to prevent platelet adhesion than are required to prevent platelet aggregation (Higgs *et al.* 1978) suggesting a proportionately greater influence of this prostanoid on the aggregation process. Furthermore, PGI_2 appears unable to prevent adhesion of thrombin-stimulated platelets while aspirin treatment of cultured endothelial cells to inhibit PGI_2 biosynthesis does not stimulate platelet adhesion *in vitro* (Fry *et al.* 1980). In addition, Curwen and co-workers (1980) have observed that the increased adhesiveness of platelets to virally transformed endothelial cells is incompletely reduced by addition of exogenous PGI_2. On the other hand, rabbit aorta segments rubbed to remove the vascular endothelium avidly bind platelets which is completely prevented by PGI_2.

In conclusion, there seems little doubt that PGI_2 released by endothelial cells plays an important part in regulating intravascular platelet activation. In this way it may provide the 'fine tuning' for the platelet–collagen–vWF/fibronectin interaction which underpins the ability of platelets to adhere to damaged blood vessel walls as described above.

Endothelium derived nitric oxide (EDNO)

The existence of an additional, chemically labile vasodilator released from vascular endothelial cells was first suggested by the experiments of Furchgott and Zawadzki

(1980). This labile substance originally named endothelium derived relaxing factor (EDRF) has recently been identified as nitric oxide (Palmer *et al.* 1987) and is now sometimes referred to as endothelium derived nitric oxide (EDNO). Although the complete pathway for EDNO biosynthesis has yet to be elucidated evidence has been presented that its physiological precursor within the endothelium is either L-arginine (Palmer *et al.* 1988) or an L-arginine containing peptide (Thomas & Ramwell, 1988).

Endothelium derived nitric oxide is released from isolated arteries and veins as well as from resistance arterioles of a number of perfused vascular beds (Furchgott, 1983). Substances which release EDNO from these sources include acetylcholine, histamine, bradykinin and tachykinins such as substance P (Vane *et al.* 1988). Of particular relevance to this chapter is the finding that substances released from aggregating platelets (e.g. adenosine diphosphate (ADP) and adenosine triphosphate (ATP) as well as thrombin which is generated during blood coagulation also trigger efflux of EDNO from vascular endothelial cells (Furchgott, 1983).

With this in mind it is perhaps not surprising that EDNO has been reported to influence platelet activation. Thus, biologically generated EDNO prevents the adhesion of platelets to segments of endothelium-denuded rabbit aorta (Sneddon & Vane, 1988) while chemically prepared nitric oxide similarly reduces platelet adhesion to cultured bovine aortic endothelial cells (Radomski *et al.* 1987a,b). The mechanism of the antiplatelet activity of EDNO probably depends upon activation of platelet guanylate cyclase activity leading to a build up of cyclic 3′,5′ guanosine monophosphate (cGMP) within the platelet cytoplasm (Waldman & Murad, 1987).

It is presumed, although as yet not proved, that cGMP accumulation inside the platelet has a similar effect to that of cAMP in reducing calcium influx or utilization. Thus, EDNO and PGI_2 retard platelet adhesion by similar processes operating via cGMP and cAMP, respectively. With such molecular mechanisms of action it is likely that these two endogenous endothelial products synergize in their ability to inhibit platelet adhesion to the vessel wall. That EDNO influences platelet function may help to explain the failure of PGI_2 to prevent thrombin-induced platelet adhesion (Fry *et al.* 1980). Similarly, the inability of PGI_2 to reverse the increased adhesion of platelets to virally transformed endothelial cells which was reported by Curwen and co-workers (1980) as described previously may be explained at least in part by an inability of these cells to synthesize not only PGI_2 but also EDNO. The effect of EDNO on platelet aggregation is discussed in a subsequent section.

Effect of heparin/heparans

Heparin, first used clinically in 1937, is a mixture of highly sulphated, linear glucosaminoglycans with a strong negative charge. Chemically, heparin is structurally related (approximately 20% homology) (Atkins & Neiduszyski, 1977) to the endogenous heparans which line the intimal surface of vascular endothelial cells (Marcum & Rosenberg, 1985). Heparans and heparin exhibit sufficiently similar biological effects (but see Gamse *et al.* 1978) to make the difference between them 'moot from the functional viewpoint' (Engelberg, 1984).

In vitro tests in intact blood have revealed that heparin/heparans are anticoagulants agents by interacting with, and accelerating, the inhibition by antithrombin III of thrombin and Factor Xa activity. However, it has been realized for many years that the clinical antithrombotic effect of heparin is probably unrelated to prevention of blood coagulation and relies in large part upon inhibition of platelet adhesion to the subendothelium.

It now seems clear that part of the antithrombotic effect of clinically administered heparin is to mimic the effect of endogenous, endothelial heparans. A similar mechanism reduces leucocyte adhesion to endothelial cells in culture (Hoover *et al.* 1978). This effect is related to prevention of platelet adhesion most probably by promoting the electronegativity of the endothelium. Direct electrophysiological measurements have demonstrated that the endothelial cell is electronegative ($-160\,\text{mV}$) and that a thrombus forms only when the surface becomes electropositive ($+260\,\text{mV}$) (Engelberg, 1985). Endothelial electronegativity is maintained primarily by the presence of heparan anionic groups and can be abolished by vascular damage either physical or induced by a number of other stimuli including viruses (Gordon & Pearson, 1982). Similarly, administration of cationic substances such as protamine to neutralize endothelial electronegativity also initiates thrombosis (Pelikan *et al.* 1979; Jacques, 1982). Heparin administration reduces the adhesion of platelets to injured arterial walls (Gregorious & Rand, 1976).

Heparin/heparans also exhibit a number of other effects which promote their antithrombotic effect. These include reducing intrinsic blood coagulation by antithrombin III binding (Engelberg, 1985), stimulation of tissue plasminogen activator release (Marckwardt & Klocking, 1977), neutralization of lysosomal cationic proteins released from leucocytes (Saba *et al.* 1968), prevention of increase of vascular permeability due to histamine and bradykinin (Engelberg, 1984) and enhanced absorption of α-acid-glycoprotein.

Aggregation of platelets: role of the blood vessel wall

Pro-aggregatory effect of blood vessel components

Platelet adhesion to the subendothelium is believed to be followed by the release reaction whereby contents of the platelet α- and dense granules are released (Holmsen, 1975). The release reaction was first defined *in vitro* and subsequently confirmed *in vivo* by radioimmunoassay of plasma β-thromboglobulin and platelet factor 4 (PF4) (Pepper, 1979). Platelet constituents released during this process trigger many haemostatic events including further platelet recruitment (ADP, prostaglandin endoperoxides, TXA_2, fibronectin), blood coagulation (PF4), proliferation of vascular smooth muscle (platelet derived growth factor) and localized vasoconstriction (5-hydroxytrytamine, TXA_2). Of these processes only platelet aggregation triggered by blood vessel wall elements such as collagen is considered relevant in the context of the present chapter. The reader is referred to specialized reviews for more detailed information about the mechanism of platelet aggregation (e.g. de Gaetano, 1981; Leung & Nachman, 1986; Mackie & Neal, 1987).

Collagen exposed by damage to the blood vessel wall causes not only platelet adhesion but also platelet aggregation, i.e. types I and III, are the same forms which initiate platelet adhesion. Collagen types IV and V are also pro-aggregatory but are considerably less potent. Interestingly, a specific nonapeptide sequence within the collagen molecule has been observed to prevent collagen binding to platelets (Legrand *et al.* 1980).

The molecular mechanism of action of collagen in this respect is complex and involves three distinct pathways (Kinlough-Rathbone *et al.* 1977). At low doses collagen causes de-esterification of membrane phospholipids by activation of phospholipase enzymes (i.e. phospholipase A_2 or phospholipase C followed by diglyceride lipase) causing liberation of free arachidonic acid which is subsequently converted into pro-aggregatory prostaglandin endoperoxides and TXA_2. These prostanoids cause further platelet recruitment followed by the release of ADP which in turn triggers additional platelet aggregation. Thus, aspirin inhibits collagen-induced platelet aggregation *in vitro*. Higher doses of collagen are able to 'break through' such aspirin inhibition most probably by promoting the biosynthesis of platelet activating factor (PAF) which amongst other pharmacological effects also produces powerful platelet aggregation (Chignard *et al.* 1980; Marcus *et al.* 1981). The molecular mechanism of collagen-induced platelet aggregation *in vitro* and *in vivo* is probably associated with a decrease in platelet intracellular cAMP concentration causing release of calcium ions from intracellular granules and activation of platelet contractile proteins (de Gaetano, 1981).

Anti-aggregatory effect of arachidonic acid metabolites

Numerous prostanoids synthesized by vascular endothelial cells inhibit platelet aggregation *in vitro*. Of these the most potent is undoubtedly PGI_2 which exhibits an EC_{50} (50% effective concentration) in human platelet rich plasma using ADP as an aggregating agent of between 0.1 and 0.5 ng/ml. Interaction of PGI_2 occurs with specific platelet prostoglandin (IP) receptor 6 oxo PGE_1 which is formed from PGI_2 by a prostaglandin 9-hydroxydehydrogenase enzyme found in platelets (Griffiths & Moore, 1983), is also a potent inhibitor of platelet aggregation as are PGD_2 and PGE_1. In each case the mechanism of effect is likely to be via stimulation of platelet adenylate cyclase activity and increased intracellular accumulation of cAMP. In addition, prostanoids inhibit thoracic platelet aggregation in the anaesthetized rat following ADP administration *in vivo* (Oyekan & Botting, 1986) and reduce or prevent laser induced thrombosis in the microcirculation of rat mesenteric vessels (Weichert & Breddin, 1986).

The prostacyclin PGI_2 as well as drugs which promote its biosynthesis or effect have been employed clinically with varying degrees of success in a number of thrombotic conditions including vasospastic arterial disease, coronary artery disease, pulmonary hypertension, thrombotic thrombocytopaenic purpura and haemolytic uraemic syndrome, adult respiratory distress syndrome and retinal vein thrombosis (Yardumian & Machin, 1987). Similarly, the therapeutic benefits of prostacyclin are well established for extracoporeal circulation procedures such as cardiopulmonary bypass, renal dialysis and charcoal haemoperfusion for liver failure (e.g. Aren *et al.* 1983). Finally, certain antithrombotic drugs such as nafazotrom are believed to exert their clinical effect *in vivo* by virtue of stimulating endothelial cell PGI_2 biosynthesis (Vermeylen *et al.* 1979).

Anti-aggregatory effect of EDNO

Since EDRF stimulates vascular smooth muscle guanylate cyclase it was suggested that EDRF might inhibit platelet aggregation by a similar mechanism of action. This hypothesis gained further support by the observation that bovine retractor penis extract, which shares many of the pharmacological effects of EDRF, was also a potent inhibitor of platelet aggregation.

The first direct evidence that EDRF influenced platelet function came from the experiments of Azuma and co-workers in (1986). In this study the effluent from a length of rabbit aorta perfused with Krebs solution containing acetylcholine (ACh) was demonstrated to inhibit arachidonic acid-induced rabbit platelet aggregation. This effect was dose-related and prevented by pretreatment of the aorta with nordihydroguaiaretic acid (NDGA) or mepacrine, which promote EDRF catabolism, or by removal of the vascular endothelium. However, these authors failed to control adequately for the possible synthesis and release of PGI_2 since no attempts were made to inhibit vascular cyclooxygenase activity.

Since this first experiment other more detailed and carefully controlled studies demonstrating EDRF-mediated inhibition of platelet aggregation have been reported. In such experiments EDRF has been released from rabbit aortic strips (Furlong *et al.* 1987) or from cultured endothelial cells (Alheid *et al.* 1987; Radomski *et al.* 1987c) and inhibits the aggregation of platelets suspended either in platelet-rich plasma or in physiological salt solution. Endothelium derived relaxing factor generated by carbachol challenge of rat aortic rings also inhibits ADP-induced aggregation of human platelets suspended in intact blood (Bhardwaj *et al.* 1988).

Authentic, chemically prepared nitric oxide (NO) also inhibits both human platelet aggregation and adhesion *in vitro* (Radomski *et al.* 1987c; MacDonald *et al.* 1988). The anti-aggregatory effect of NO was potentiated by M&B 22948, a selective inhibitor of cyclic GMP phosphodiesterase, and by superoxide dismutase and was inhibited by haemoglobin (Radomski *et al.* 1987c). These results suggest that NO-induced inhibition of platelet aggregation is related to activation of guanylate cyclase enzyme and accumulation intracellularly of cGMP.

That biologically generated EDRF and authentic NO inhibit platelet aggregation *in vitro* is clearly of interest. However, if this mechanism is to be of physiological significance then it is necessary to demonstrate a similar effect of EDRF/NO in the intact animal *in vivo*. To date there have been no such studies in man. However, Hogan and co-workers (1988) have recently reported that intravenous injection of carbachol into anaesthetized rats to trigger endogenous EDRF efflux inhibited ADP-induced platelet aggregation in whole blood removed at timed intervals thereafter. This effect was abolished by haemoglobin infusion. Similarly, administration of carbachol to anaesthetized rats reduced ADP-induced accumulation of ^{111}indium-labelled rat platelets in the pulmonary vascular bed (Bhardwaj *et al.* 1988). Administration of methylene blue, an inhibitor of soluble guanylate cyclase, reduced the platelet inhibitor effect of released EDRF. The experimental procedure used in the latter study allows platelet aggregation to be initiated and measured *in vivo* (Oyekan & Botting, 1986) and is thus a considerable advance over previously reported techniques.

Effect of heparin/heparans

In addition to an effect on platelet adhesion to the blood vessel wall heparin also exhibits complex effects on platelet aggregation. Surprisingly, heparin has been reported to potentiate ADP-induced aggregation of platelets suspended in citrated platelet-rich plasma (Michalski *et al.* 1977). The mechanism of this *in vitro* effect is not clear but may be related to enhanced fibrinogen binding to ADP-treated platelets. In contrast, heparin reduced platelet aggregation triggered by collagen (Bestermann & Gillet, 1973). The pro-aggregatory effect of heparin in response to challenge with ADP may be prevented by treatment with antithrombin III but only in the presence of citrate. For this reason it seems most likely that heparin augments platelet aggregation indirectly by promoting the activity of endogenous thrombin. Thus, these effects of heparin on platelet aggregation are probably *in vitro* phenomena which have little or no relevance to the effect of injected heparin or that of endogenous heparans on platelet function *in vivo*.

Similar *in vitro* experimets have suggested an interaction between heparin and platelet anti-aggregatory PGI_2. As detailed previously PGI_2 is probably the most potent naturally occurring inhibitor of platelet aggregation discovered to date. At high concentrations, heparin reversed the inhibitory effect of PGI_2 on ADP-induced platelet aggregation *in vitro* (Bertele *et al.* 1983). However, whether this action represents non-specific potentiation of platelet aggregation as described above or a direct interaction with PGI_2 is not entirely clear. Certainly, heparin does not influence PGI_2 biosynthesis by fresh vascular tissue (Ronsanglione *et al.*

1980) unless stimulated by thrombin (Buchanan *et al.* 1979) and does not antagonize the coronary vasodilator effect of this prostanoid (Eldor *et al.* 1980). In complete contrast heparin administration to man *in vivo* increased PGI_2 concentration in coronary sinus blood (Wallis *et al.* 1982) which, as opposed to the above results, would suggest a beneficial effect of heparin on platelet aggregation, i.e. synergism with released PGI_2.

Although heparin exerts varied and complex effects on platelet aggregation *in vitro* many of these actions are likely to be artefacts related to the stimulation of thrombin activity by heparin–antithrombin II binding. Whether heparin has a significant effect on platelet aggregation *in vivo* remains to be determined.

Contribution of platelets to endothelial integrity

Evidence has also been accumulated that platelets release substances which are vital for normal endothelial cell function. Thus, endothelial thinning is characteristic of blood vessels removed from thrombocytopaenic rabbits (Kitchens & Weiss, 1975). In addition, platelets augment DNA synthesis in cultured endothelial cells (Maca *et al.* 1977), most probably consequent upon the release of a platelet-derived endothelial mitogen. Attempts to purify this mitogen have resulted in the identification of numerous substances with different molecular weights each of which exhibits mitogenic activity (Miyazono *et al.* 1985). These considerations may well explain the inability to culture vascular endothelial cells in medium lacking serum (de Groot *et al.* 1983).

Conclusion

The interaction between platelets and the vascular endothelium is complex and only partially understood. That the endothelial cell regulates the function of platelets and vice versa is now becoming clear. A fuller understanding of the mechanisms involved will undoubtedly lead to a deeper insight into the process of thrombosis and potentially to the development of powerful antithrombotic drugs with novel mechanisms of action.

References

Aiken, J.W., Shebuski, R.J., Miller, O.V. & Gorman, R.R. (1981) Endogenous PGI_2 contributes to the efficacy of a thromboxane synthetase inhibitor for preventing coronary artery thrombosis. *J Pharmacol Exp Ther* **219**, 299–308.

Alheid, U., Frölich, J.C. & Forstermann, U. (1987) Endothelium derived relaxing factor from cultured human endothelial cells inhibits aggregation of human platelets. *Thromb Res* **47**, 561–569.

Aren, C., Fedderson, K. & Radegran, K. (1983) Effects of prostacyclin infusion on platelet activation and post-operative blood loss in coronary bypass. *Ann Thorac Surg* **36**, 49–54.

Arneson, M.A., Hammerschmidt, D.E., Furch, L.T. & King, R.A. (1980) A new form of Ehlers–Danlos syndrome. Fibronectin corrects defective platelet function. *J Am Med Assoc* **244**, 144–147.

Atkins, E.D.T. & Neiduszyski, I.A. (1977) Effect of alpha-L-iduronate conformation on the molecular shape of heparin. *Fed Proc* **36**, 78–83,.

Azuma, H., Ishikawa, M. & Sekizaki, S. (1986) Endothelial dependent inhibition of platelet aggregation.

Br J Pharmacol **88**, 411–415.

Barnes, M.J. (1985) Collagens in atherosclerosis. *Coll Relat Res* **5**, 65–97.

Barnes, M.J. (1986) Blood vessel wall matrix components involved in vessel wall thrombogenicity. In Jolles, G., Legrand, Y.J. & Nurden, A. (eds) *Biology and Pathology of Platelet Vessel Wall Interactions*, pp. 21–38. Academic press, New York.

Barnes, M.J. & MacIntyre, D.E. (1979) Platelet reactivity of isolated constituents of the blood vessel wall. *Haemostasis* **8**, 158–170.

Baumgartner, H.R. (1983) The role of blood flow in platelet adhesion, fibrin deposition and formation of mural thrombi. *Microvasc Res* **5**, 167–179.

Bertele, V. Roncanglione, M.C., Donati, M.B. & de Gaetano, G. (1983) Heparin counteracts the anti-aggregating effect of prostacyclin by potentiating platelet aggregation. *Thromb Haemost* **49**, 81–83.

Bestermann, E.M.M. & Gillet, M.P.I. (1973) Heparin effects on plasma lysolecithin formation and platelet aggregation. *Atherosclerosis* **17**, 503–513.

Bhardwaj, R., May, G., Page, C.P. & Moore, P.K. (1988) Endothelium derived relaxing factor inhibits platelet aggregation in human whole blood *in vitro* and the rat *in vivo*. *Eur J Pharmacol* **157**, 83–92.

Bloom, A.L. (1979) Biosynthesis of factor VIII. *Clin Haematol* **8**, 53–77.

Buchanan, M.R., De Jana, E., Cazenave, J.P., Mustard, J.F. & Hirsch, J. (1979) Uncontrolled PGI_2 production by whole vessel wall segments due to thrombin generation in vivo and its prevention by heparin. *Thromb Res* **16**, 551–555.

Buchanan, M.R., Butt, R.W., Magas, Z., Van Ryn, J., Hirsch, J. & Nazir, D.J. (1985) Endothelial cells produce a lipoxygenase-derived chemorepellant which influences platelet/endothelial cell interactions — effect of aspirin and salicylate. *Thromb Haemost* **53**, 306–311.

Bunting, S., Gryglewski, R.J., Moncada, S. & Vane, J.R. (1976) Arterial walls generate from prostaglandin endoperoxides a substance (PGX) which relaxes strips of mesenteric and coeliac artery and inhibits platelet aggregation. *Prostaglandins* **12**, 897–913.

Charo, I., Shak, S., Karasek, M.A., Davidson, P.A. & Goldstein, I.M. (1984) Prostaglandin I_2 is not a major metabolite of arachidonic acid in cultured endothelial cells from human foreskin microvessels. *J Clin Invest* **74**, 914–919.

Chignard, M., LeCoudec, J.P., Tence, M., Vargaftig, B.B. & Benveniste, J. (1980) The role of platelet activating factor in platelet aggregation. *Nature* **279**, 799–800.

Christofinis, G.J., Moncada, S., Bunting, S. & Vane, J.R. (1979) Prostacyclin release by rabbit aortic and human umbilical vein endothelial cells after prolonged subculture. In Vane, J.R. & Bergstrom, S. (eds) *Prostacyclin*, pp. 77–79. Raven Press, New York.

Curwen, K.D., Gimbrone, M.A. & Handin, R.I. (1980) *In vitro* studies of thromboresistance: the role of prostacyclin (PGI_2) in platelet adhesion to cultured normal and virally transformed human endothelial cells. *Lab Invest* **42**, 366–374.

de Gaetano, G. (1981) Platelets, prostaglandins and thrombotic disorders. In Prentice, C.R.M. (ed.) *Thrombosis*, pp. 297–326. W.B. Saunders, London.

de Groot, Ph. G., Willems, C., Gonsalves, M.D., van Aken, W.G. & van Mourik, J.A. (1983) The proliferation of human umbilical endothelial cells in serum-free medium. *Thromb Res* **31**, 623–634.

de Groot, Ph. G., Ottenhof-Rovers, M., Dziadek, M., Timpl, R. & Sixma, J.J. (1985) Nidogen is present in the extracellular matrix of human endothelial cells and is involved in platelet adhesion to this matrix. *Thromb haemost* **54**, 231.

de la Fuente, B., Kaspar, C.K., Rickles, F.R. & Hoyer, L.W. (1985) The responses of patients with mild and moderate haemophilia A and von Willebrand's disease to treatment with desmopressin (DDAVP). *Ann Intern Med* **103**, 6–14.

Eldor, A., Allan, G. & Weksler, B.B. (1980) Heparin-prostacyclin interaction: Heparin does not modify the prostacyclin-induced relaxation of coronary vasculature. *Thromb Res* **19**, 719–723.

Engelberg, H. (1984) Heparin and the atherosclerotic process. *Pharmacol Rev* **36**, 91–110.

Engelberg, H. (1985) Heparin, heparin fractions and the atherosclerotic process. *Sem Thromb. Haematol* **11**, 45–55.

Fry, G.L., Czervionke, R.L., Hoak, J.C., Smith, J.B. & Haycraft, D.L. (1980) Platelet adhesion to cultured vascular cells: influence of prostacyclin (PGI_2). *Blood* **55**, 271–275.

Furchgott, R.F. (1983) Role of the endothelium in responses of vascular smooth muscle. *Circ Res* **53**, 557–573.

Furchgott, R.F. & Zawadzki, J.V. (1980) The obligatory role of endothelial cells in the relaxation of arterial smooth muscle by acetylcholine. *Nature* **288**, 373–376.

Furlong, B., Henderson, A.H., Lewis, M.J. & Smith, J.A. (1987) Endothelium derived relaxing factor inhibits *in vitro* platelet aggregation. *Br J Pharmacol* **90**, 687–692.

Gamse, G., Fromme, H.G. & Kresse, H. (1978) Metabolism of sulphated glycosaminoglycans in cultured endothelial and smooth muscle cells from bovine aorta. *Biochim Biophys Acta* **544**, 514–528.

Gerritsen, M.E. (1987) Functional heterogeneity of vascular endothelial cells. *Biochem Pharmacol* **36**, 2701–2711.

Gerritsen, M.E & Choli, C.D. (1983) Arachidonic acid and prostaglandin endoperoxide metabolism in isolated rabbit coronary microvessels and cultured coronary microvessel endothelial cells. *J Clin Invest* **72**, 1658–1671.

Goehlert, U.G., Ng Ying Kin, N.M.K. & Wolfe, L.S. (1981) Biosynthesis of prostacyclin in rat cerebral microvessels and the choroid plexus. *J Neurochem* **36**, 1192–1201.

Gordon, J.L. & Pearson, J.D. (1982) Response of endothelial cells to injury. In Nossel, H.J. & Vogel, H.L. (eds) *Pathology of the Endothelial Cell*, pp. 433–454. Academic Press, New York.

Gorman, R.R., Bunting, S. & Moncada, S. (1977) Modulation of human platelet adenylate cyclase by prostacyclin (PGX). *Prostaglandins* **13**, 377–388.

Gospdarowicz, D., Greenberg, D., Foidart, J.M. & Savison, N. (1981) The production and localisation of laminin in cultured vascular and corneal endothelial cells. *J Cell Physiol* **107**, 171–183.

Gregorious, F.K. & Rand, R.W. (1976) Scanning electron microscopy of the rat common carotid artery. III. Heparin effect on platelets. *Surgery* **79**, 583–589.

Griffiths, R.J. & Moore, P.K. (1983) Conversion of prostacyclin to 6 keto prostaglandin E_1 by rat, rabbit, guinea pig and human platelets. *Br J Pharmacol* **80**, 395–402.

Hardisty, R.M. & Caen, P. (1981) Disorders of platelet function. In Bloom, A.L. & Thomas, D.P. (eds) *Haemostasis and Thrombosis*, pp. 301–302. Churchill Livingstone, Edinburgh.

Higgs, E.A., Moncada, S., Vane, J.R., Caen, J.P., Michel, H., & Tobelem G. (1978) Effect of prostacyclin (PGI_2) on platelet adhesion to rabbit arterial subendothelium. *Prostaglandins* **16**, 17–22.

Hogan, J.C., Lewis, M.J. & Henderson, A.H. (1988) *In vivo* EDRF activity influences platelet function. *Br J Pharmacol* **94**, 1020–1022.

Holmsen, H. (1975) Biochemistry of the platelet release reaction. In *Biochemistry and Pharmacology of Platelets*, Ciba Foundation Symp 35 (new series) pp. 175–205. Elsevier, Amsterdam.

Hoover, R.L., Briggs, R.T. & Karnovsky, M.J. (1978) The adhesive interaction between polymorphonuclear leucocytes and endothelial cells *in vitro*. *Cell* **14**, 423–428.

Hynes, R.O. (1986) The interaction of fibronectin with platelets. In Jolles, G., Legrand, Y.J. & Nurdern, C. (eds) *Biology and Pathology of Platelet-Vessel Wall Interactions* pp. 75–94. Academic Press, New York.

Ill, C.R., Engvall, E. & Ruoslahti, E. (1984) Adhesion of platelets to laminin in the absence of activation. *J Cell Biol* **99**, 2140–2145.

Ingerman-Wojenski, C., Silver, M.J., Smith, J.B. & Macarak, E. (1981) Bovine endothelial cells in culture produce thromboxanes as well as prostacyclin. *J Clin Invest* **67**, 1292–1296.

Jacques, L.B. (1982) Heparin: a unique misunderstood drug. *Trends Pharmacol Sci* **3**, 289–291.

Jaffe, E.A. & Mosher, D.F. (1978) Synthesis of fibronectin by cultured endothelial cells. *J Exp Med* **147**, 1779–1791.

Kaser-Glanzmann, R., Jakaboua, M., George, J.N. & Luscher, E.F. (1977) Stimulation of calcium uptake in platelet membrane vesicles by adenosine 3′,5′ monophosphate and protein kinase. *Biochim Biophys Acta* **466**, 429–440.

Kinlough-Rathbone, R.L., Packham, M.A. & Mustard, J.F. (1977) Synergism between platelet aggregating agents: the role of the arachidonate pathway. *Thromb Res* **11**, 567–580.

Kitchens, C.S. & Weiss, L. (1975) Ultrastructural changes to endothelium associated with throbocytopaenia. *Blood* **46**, 567–578.

Koide, T., Gotoh, O., Asano, T. & Takamura, K. (1985) Alteration of the eicosanoid synthesis capacity of rat brain microvessels following ischaemia: relevance to ischaemic brain edema. *J Neurochem* **44**, 85–93.

Larrue, J., Rigaud, M., Daret, D., Demond, J., Durand, J. & Bricaud, H. (1980) Prostacyclin production by cultured smooth muscle cells from atherosclerotic rabbit aorta. *Nature* **285**, 480–482.

Legrand, Y.J., Karniguian, A., Lefrancier, P., Fauvel, F. & Caen, P. (1980) Evidence that a collagen-derived nona-peptide is a specific inhibitor of platelet-collagen interaction. *Biochem Biophys Res Commun* **96**, 1579–1585.

Leung, L.L.K. & Nachman, R.L. (1986) Complex formation of platelet thrombospondin with fibrinogen. *J Clin Invest* **70**, 542–549.

Maca, R.D., Fry, G.L., Hoak, J.C. & Loh, P.T. (1977) The effect of intact platelets on cultured endothelial cells. *Thromb Res* **11**, 715–727.

MacDonald, P.B., Read, M.A. & Dusting, G.J. (1988) Synergistic inhibition of platelet aggregation by endothelium derived relaxing factor and prostacyclin. *Thromb Res* **49**, 437–449.

MacIntyre, D.E., Pearson, J.D. & Gordon, J.L. (1978) Localisation and stimulation of prostacyclin production in vascular cells. *Nature* **271**, 549–551.

Mackie, I.J. & Neal, C.R. (1987) The platelet. In Pittilo, R. & Machin, S.J. (eds) *Platelet Vessel Wall Interactions*, pp. 1–32. Springer-Verlag, Berlin.

Madri, J.A., Dreyer, B., Pitlick, F.A. & Furthmayr, H. (1980) The collagenous components of the subendothelium: correlation of structure and function. *Lab Invest* **43**, 305–315.

Majack, R.A. & Bornstein, P. (1985) Heparin regulates the collagen phenotype of vascular smooth muscle cells. Induced synthesis of a Mr 60,000 collagen. *J Cell Biol* **100**, 613–619.

Marckwardt, F. & Klocking, H.P. (1977) Heparin-induced release of plasminogen activator. *Fed Proc* **22**, 619–624.

Marcum, J.A. & Rosenberg, R.D. (1985) Heparin-like molecules with anticoagulant activity are synthesised by cultured endothelial cells. *Biochem Biophys Res Commun* **126**, 365–372.

Marcus, A.J., Safier, L.B. & Ullman, H.L. (1981) Effects of acety glyceryl phosphorylcholine on human platelet function *in vitro*. *Blood* **58**, 1027–1031.

Marguerie, G., Ginsberg, M.H. & Plow, E.F. (1987) Fibrinogen and platelet adhesion. In Holmsen, H. (ed.) *Platelet Responses and Metabolism*, pp. 285–296. CRC Press, Orlando.

Michalski, R., Lane, D.A. & Kakkar, V.J. (1977) Comparison of heparin and a semi-synthetic heparin analogue. II. Some effects on platelet function. *Br J*

Haematol **37**, 247–256.

Miller, D.K., Sadowski, S., Soderman, D. & Kuehl, F.A. (1985) Endothelial cell prostacyclin production induced by activated neutrophils. *J Biol Chem* **260**, 1006–1014.

Miyazono, K., Tetsuro, O., Ishibashi, S., Urabe, A. & Takaku, F. (1985) A platelet factor stimulating the proliferation of vascular endothelial cells. Partial purification and characterisation. *Exp Cell Res* **159**, 487–494.

Moncada, S., Gryglewski, R.J., Bunting, S. & Vane, J.R. (1976) An enzyme isolated from arteries transforms prostaglandin endoperoxides to an unstable substance that inhibits platelet aggregation. *Nature* **263**, 663–665.

Moncada, S., Herman, A.G., Higgs, E.A. & Vane, J.R. (1977) Differential formation of prostacyclin (PGX or PGI_2) by layers of the arterial wall: an explanation for the anti-thrombotic properties of vascular endothelium. *Thromb Res* **11**, 323–344.

Moroose, R. Hoyer, L.W. (1987) Von Willebrand factor and platelet function. *Ann Rev Med* **37**, 157–163.

Oohira, A., Wight, T.N. & Bornstein, P. (1983) Sulphated proteoglycan synthesised by vascular endothelial cells in culture. *J Biol Chem* **258**, 2014–2021.

Oyekan, A.O. & Botting, J.H. (1986) A minimally invasive technique for the study of intravascular platelet aggregation in anaesthetised rats. *J Pharmacol Meth* **15**, 271–276.

Packham, M.A. & Mustard, J.F. (1984) Platelet adhesion. In Spaet, T.H. (ed.) *Progress in Haemostasis and Thrombosis*, Vol. 7, pp. 211–228. Grune & Stratton, New York.

Palmer, R.M.J., Ferrige, A.G. & Moncada, S. (1987) Release of nitric oxide accounts for the biological activity of endothelium derived relaxing factor. *Nature* **327**, 524–526.

Palmer, R.M.J., Ashton, D.S. & Moncada, S. (1988). Vascular endothelial cells synthesise nitric oxide from L-arginine. *Nature* **333**, 664–666.

Pelikan, D., Gimbrone, M.A. & Cotran, R.S. (1979) Distribution and movement of anionic surface sites in cultured human vascular endothelial cells. *Atherosclerosis* **32**, 69–80.

Pepper, D.S. (1979) Macromolecules released from platelet storage organelles. *Thromb Haemost* **42**, 1667–1672.

Petersen, T.E., Thogersen, H.C., Skorstengaard, K., Vibe-Pedersen, K., Sahl, P., Sottrup-Jensen, L. & Magnusson, S. (1983) Partial primary structure of bovine plasma fibronectin. Three types of internal homology. *Proc Natl Acad Sci USA* **80**, 137–141.

Plow, E.F. & Ginsberg, M.H. (1981) Specific and saturable binding of plasma fibronectin to thrombin-stimulated platelets. *J Biol Chem* **256**, 9477.

Plow, E.F., Marguerie, G.A. & Ginsberg, M.H. (1985) Fibronectin binding to thrombin-stimulated platelets: evidence for fibrin(ogen) independent and dependent pathways. *Blood* **66**, 26–32.

Plow, E.F., Marguerie, G. & Ginsberg, M. (1987) Fibrinogen, fibrinogen receptors, and their peptides that inhibit these interactions. *Biochem Pharmacol* **36**, 4035–4040.

Radomski, M.W., Palmer, R.M.J. & Moncada, S. (1987a) Endogenous nitric oxide inhibits human platelet adhesion to vascular endothelium. *Lancet* **ii**, 1057–1058.

Radomski, M.W., Palmer, R.M.J. & Moncada, S. (1987b) The role of nitric oxide and cGMP in platelet adhesion to vascular endothelium. *Biochem Biophys Res Commun* **148**, 1482–1489.

Radomski, M.W., Palmer, R.M.J. & Moncada, S. (1987c) The anti-aggregating properties of vascular endothelium interactions between prostacyclin and nitric oxide. *Br J Pharmacol* **92**, 639–646.

Ronsanglione, M.C., Mirino, G.D. & de Gaetano, G. (1980) Increased PGI_2 activity in venous tissue from rats on oral contraceptives is not prevented by heparin administration. *Thromb Res* **18**, 895–896.

Saba, H.I., Roberts, H.R. & Herion, J.C. (1968) Antiheparin activity of lysosomal cationic proteins from polymorphonuclear leucocytes. *Blood* **31**, 369–380.

Sakariasson, K.S., Aarts, P.A.M.M., de Groot, P.G., Houdijk, W.P.M. & Sixma, J.J. (1983) A perfusion chamber developed to investigate interaction in flowing blood with human vessel wall cells, their extracellular matrix and purified components. *J Lab Clin Med* **102**, 522–535.

Santoro, S.A. (1981) Adsorption of von Willebrand factor/factor VIII by the genetically distinct interstitial collagens. *Thromb Res* **21**, 689–693.

Santoro, S.A. & Cunningham, L.W. (1977) Collagen-mediated platelet aggregation. Evidence for multivalent interactions of intermediate specificity between collagen and platelets. *J Clin Invest* **60**, 1054–1060.

Schullek, J., Jordan, J. & Montgomery, R.R. (1984) Interaction of von Willebrand factor with human platelets in the plasma milieu *J Clin Invest* **73**, 421–428.

Sneddon, J.M. & Vane, J.R. (1988) Endothelium-derived relaxing factor reduces platelet adhesion to bovine endothelial cells. *Proc Natl Acad Sci USA* **85**, 2800–2804.

Stel, H.V., Sakariassen, K.S., de Groot, P.G., van Mourik, J.A. & Sixma, J.J. (1985) von Willebrand factor in the vessel wall mediates platelet adhesion. *Blood* **65**, 85–90.

Sussman, I.I. & Rand, J.R. (1982) Subendothelial deposition of von Willebrand factor requires the presence of subendothelial cells. *J Lab Clin Med* **100**, 526–532.

Thomas, G. & Ramwell, P.W. (1988) Peptidyl arginine deiminase and endothelium dependent relaxation. *Eur J Pharmacol* **153**, 147–148.

Tryggvason, K., Oikarinen, J., Viinikka, L. & Ylikorkala, O. (1981) Effects of laminin proteoglycan and type IV collagen, components of basement membranes, on platelet aggregation. *Biochem Biophys Res Commun* **100**, 233–239.

Turrito, V.T. & Baumgartner, H.R. (1983) Platelet adhesion. In Harker, L.A. & Zimmerman, T.S. (eds) *Measurements of Platelet Function*, pp. 46–63. Churchill Livingston, Edinburgh.

Turrito, V.T. & Weiss, H.J. (1980) Red blood cells; their dual role in platelet function. *Science* **207**, 541–543.

Vane, J.R., Gryglewski, R.J. & Botting, R. (1988) The endothelial cell as a metabolic and endocrine organ. *Trends Pharmacol Sci* **8**, 491–496.

Vermeylen, J., Chamone, D.A.F. & Verstraete, M. (1979) Stimulation of prostacyclin release from vessel wall by BAY g 6575, an anti-thrombotic compound. *Lancet* **i**, 1073–1075.

Waldman, S.A. & Murad, F. (1987) Cyclic GMP synthesis and function. *Pharmacol Rev* **39**, 163–196.

Wallis, K., Moses, J.W., Borer, J.S., Weksler, B.B., Goldberg, H.L., Fisher, J., Kase, M., Talk-Goldman, K., Carter, J. & Calle, S. (1982) Coronary blood flow in coronary artery disease. Heparin-induced potentiation caused by prostacyclin release. *Circulation* **66**, (suppl II), 263.

Weichert, W. & Breddin, H.K. (1986) Laser-induced thrombosis in the microcirculation of rat mesenteric vessels. In Jolles. G., Legrand, Y.J. & Nurden, A. (eds) *Biology and Pathology of Platelet–Vessel Wall Interaction*, pp. 321–336. Academic Press, London.

Weksler, B.B., Marcus, A.J. & Jaffe, E.A. (1977) Synthesis of prostaglandin I_2 (prostacyclin) by cultured human and bovine endothelial cells. *Proc Natl Acad Sci USA* **71**, 3922–3926.

Yardumian, A. & Machin, S.J. (1987) Newer pharmacological agents. In Pittilo, R. & Machin, S.J. (eds) *Platelet-Vessel Wall Interactions*, pp. 167–192. Springer-Verlag, Berlin.

Zimmerman, T.S. & Ruggeri, Z.M. (1983) von Willebrand's disease. *Clin Haematol* **12**, 175–200.

8: Platelets and Tumour Metastasis

Andreina Poggi and Maria B. Donati

Introduction

Metastasis formation is a multistep process, involving detachment of cells from the primary tumour, intravasation, circulation through blood or lymphatic vessels, adherence to the vascular lumen, penetration of the basement membrane, and lodging and growth in extravascular spaces (Poste & Fidler, 1980). Platelets may interfere with this process at several steps, as suggested by experimental and clinical data. Gasic and Gasic (1962) made the original observation that thrombocytopenia significantly inhibited metastasis formation and showed that treatment with aspirin would reduce the incidence of metastases in mice (Gasic *et al.* 1972). The possibility to cure metastasis with antiplatelet agents was subsequently attempted, with contrasting results, in experimental models and clinical trials (reviewed, among others, by Mehta, 1984; Zacharski *et al.* 1988). Extensive studies on the *in vitro* interactions between platelets and tumour cells were also performed on the basis of the observation that tumour cells can induce platelet aggregation *in vitro* (Gasic *et al.* 1973; Pearlstein *et al.* 1979). The discovery that platelets are the source of growth and transforming factors further stimulated these studies (Ross *et al.* 1986; Sporn *et al.* 1986). More recently, the mechanisms regulating tumour cell or platelet adhesion to endothelial cells and to the extracellular matrix have been studied. These late *in vitro* observations have led to new *in vivo* approaches to the control of metastasis formation; indeed, monoclonal antibodies to the glycoprotein (Gp) IIb–IIIa receptor complex and peptides that inhibit cellular binding to fibronectin were found to be able to inhibit lung colony formation in experimental tumour models in mice (Humphreys *et al.* 1986; Karpatkin *et al.* 1988). We shall review here briefly the main steps in the knowledge of platelet–tumour cell interactions which, during the past 20 years, have led to the development of different platelet inhibitors as possible antimetastasic agents in experimental and clinical malignancies.

Platelet–tumour cell interactions *in vitro*

Platelet–tumour cell aggregation

Morphological studies showed the presence of platelet–tumour cell emboli in tumour-bearing animals, suggesting that tumour cell–platelet microthrombi may facilitate tumour cell arrest and lodging in the vessel wall (Wood, 1958; Warren, 1981). The ability of tumour cells to induce platelet aggregation was first observed by Gasic *et al.* (1973) and subsequently by Pearlstein *et al.* (1979), who found that it was due to shedding of vesicles containing a complex of proteins, lipids, and sialic acid from the tumour cells. Two other mechanisms were suggested thereafter:

1 generation of thrombin via tumour-mediated activation of clotting factors (Pearlstein *et al.* 1981);

2 leakage of ADP (adenosine diphosphate) by tumour cells (Bastida *et al.* 1982).

The subject has been reviewed by Jamieson *et al.* (1987). More recently, a trypsin-sensitive protein, responsible for platelet aggregation, has been identified on the membrane of a murine colon adenocarcinoma with high metastatic ability (Watanabe *et al.* 1988).

A positive correlation between platelet-aggregating activity and spontaneous metastatic potential was initially found by Gasic *et al.* (1973) and by Pearlstein *et al.* (1980) in experimental tumour lines with different metastatic activity. This type of relation has been questioned in subsequent studies (Donati *et al.* 1982; Grignani *et al.* 1983; Estrada & Nicolson, 1984; Kimura *et al.* 1987; Sugimoto *et al.* 1987). It has been suggested that qualitative more than quantitative differences may be related to the metastatic potential of tumour cells. Indeed, highly metastatic tumours, such as B16 melanoma and Lewis lung carcinoma in mice, induce platelet aggregation via thrombin generation rather than via other more platelet-specific mechanisms (Lerner *et al.* 1983; Tohgo *et al.* 1986). Moreover, by comparing some murine tumour variants with different metastatic activity from B16 melanoma and MMTV mammary carcinoma, Lampugnani and Crawford (1987) observed that the greatest metastatic activity was associated with the highest thrombin-dependent aggregatory activity.

Platelet activation products and tumour cells

Platelet activation, following aggregation, is accompanied by release of several components of platelet α-granules, such as peptides with mitogenic and chemotactic activity, adhesive proteins and proteolytic enzymes (Niewiarowski & Varma, 1982). Some of these factors have been implicated in the pathogenesis of tumour and metastasis development (Gasic, 1984, for a review).

The most relevant mitogenic factors released by platelets are the 'platelet derived growth factor' (PDGF) (Ross *et al.* 1986) and the 'transforming growth factor beta' (TGF-β) (Sporn *et al.* 1986). The major growth factor for mesenchymal cells present in serum, PDGF, is a polypeptide composed of two chains (A and B). The discovery that a large structural homology was present between the B chain of PDGF and the product of the activated *v sis* gene in SSV-transformed cells prompted studies on the release of PDGF-like growth factors by tumour cells (see Goustin *et al.* 1986; Poggi *et al.* 1988 for reviews). Since then, growth factors similar to PDGF A or B have been found in the conditioned medium of several human and murine tumour cells (van Zoelen *et al.* 1985; Betsholtz *et al.* 1986). Tumour cells may modulate their own growth, via an 'autocrine' loop, through the release of these factors (Heldin & Westermark, 1984).

Very few data were available until now about the role of PDGF or PDGF-like growth factors in metastasis. We found that tumour cells from a murine fibrosarcoma with low metastatic activity were more sensitive to PDGF than cells with high metastatic activity (Poggi *et al.* 1988). Release of PDGF-like proteins in several clones of human glioma showed variations without a definite trend (Nister *et al.* 1986). Cultured cells from a human melanoma (primary tumour) and two of its metastatic nodules released similar amounts of PDGF; however, the cell line derived from the primary tumour showed a greater expression of PDGF B, as compared with PDGF A (Westermark *et al.* 1986).

TGF-β is characterized by its transforming ability, i.e. by the capacity to stimulate anchorage-independent cell growth in agar (Sporn *et al.* 1986). It is released by several human and experimental tumour cells in culture (Goustin *et al.* 1986). Besides their activity as mitogenic factors, TGF-β and PDGF are able to promote chemotaxis of polymorphonuclear cells, monocytes and fibroblasts, release of proteolytic enzymes and secretion of collagen and other components of the extracellular matrix (Sporn & Roberts, 1986). Platelet derived growth factor-like proteins or TGF-β released by tumour cells in the milieu may stimulate fibroblasts to form a granulation tissue with a protective and nutritive role for the producing cells (Dvorak, 1986).

Several tumour cells also release proteolytic enzymes (collagenase, elastase), that are able to degrade the extracellular matrix surrounding the tumours (Liotta *et al.* 1983). An increased release of endoglycosidases has also been associated with the metastatic potential of tumour cells, in a series of experimental models (Vlodavsky *et al.* 1984; Parish *et al.* 1987). It may be noticed that platelets release not only PDGF, and TGF-β but also an endoglycosidase (Oldberg *et al.* 1980), that may contribute, in addition to factors released by tumour cells, to tissue remodelling around tumours.

Other components of platelet α-granules, such as platelet factor 4 (PF4) and thrombospondin, may also play a relevant role in metastasis formation. Platelet factor 4 is a potent chemoattractant for fibroblasts and monocytes (Deuel *et al.* 1982); in addition, PF4 restores immunosuppression induced by concanavalin A in mice (Zucker *et al.* 1989). Thrombospondin, a large adhesive protein, is released primarily by platelets, but also by smooth muscle and endothelial cells (Silverstein *et al.* 1986; Frazier, 1987). Thrombospondin has also been implicated in cancer and metastasis growth, since it binds to tumour cells and promotes their adhesion (Roberts *et al.* 1987; Tuszynski *et al.* 1987a; Riser *et al.* 1988). An increase of the number of lung colonies has also been shown after the injection of T241 sarcoma cells, pre-incubated with thrombospondin, in mice (Tuszynski *et al.* 1987b).

Platelet-mediated tumour cell adhesion to endothelium

Arrest and survival of cancer cells in the microvasculature is essential for metastasis formation (Poste & Fidler, 1980; Weiss *et al.* 1989). *In vivo* and *in vitro* studies have shown that cancer cells adhere to the endothelial surface at junctions between the endothelial cells; this phenomenon is followed by endothelial retraction and by adhesion of cancer cells to the underlying basement membrane (Crissman *et al.* 1988). Surface determinants would be responsible for the specificity of the interactions between tumour cells and the endothelial lumen of different organs, as suggested by Nicolson in a long series of experiments (1988, for a review). Different adhesive properties seem to characterize tumour variants with different metastatic activity (Tao & Johnson 1982; Chung *et al.* 1988).

Activated platelets enhance the adherence of Walker 256 carcinosarcoma cells to subendothelial matrix (Menter *et al.* 1987). Platelet membranes, but not secreted platelet products, were apparently responsible for this effect. The stimulatory effect of platelets on tumour cell adhesion was confirmed by Abecassis *et al.* (1987), on a line of human breast carcinoma (MCF-7). Bastida *et al.* (1989) found that the effect of platelets on tumour cell adhesion was shear-rate dependent and was modulated by fibronectin.

A complex system of messages from platelets and leucocytes modulates tumour cell adhesion to the endothelium or to the subendothelial matrix. For instance, monocyte-derived mediators, such as interleukin 1, are potent stimulators of tumour cell adhesion (Lauri *et al.* 1989); moreover, an important role in these interactions is played by tumour and endothelial cell-derived cyclooxygenase and lipooxygenase products. Buchanan and Bastide (1987) demonstrated that endothelial cells synthesize, via the lipooxygenase pathway, a linoleic acid metabolite, 13-hydroxyoctadecadienoic acid (13-HODE), that contributes to the non-adhesive properties of endothelial cells for platelets. Bastida *et al.* (1990) found that tumour cells also synthesize 13-HODE and that the level of this metabolite was inversely related to the tumour cell ability to adhere to endothelial cells and to subendothelial matrix. Tumour cells also release 15-hydroxyeicosatetraenoic acid (15-HETE), a derivative of arachidonic acid via the lipooxygenase pathway, that has the ability to stimulate adhesion. The adhesive properties of tumour cells are apparently dependent on the ratio between 13-HODE and 15-HETE released by the cells.

Integrins, platelets and tumour cells

Integrins are a family of transmembrane glycoproteins composed of two non-covalently bound units: the alpha and beta chain (Hynes, 1987). Fibronectin receptor, vitronectin receptor and platelet membrane glycoprotein GpIIb–IIIa are representative members of this family (Philips *et al.* 1988). Receptors for adhesive proteins are present on platelets, lymphocytes, tumour and endothelial cells (Ruoslahti & Pierschbacher, 1987).

The GpIIb–IIIa receptor is a Ca^{+}-dependent, heterodymeric complex present on the surface of platelets (Phillips *et al.* 1988). Activation of the GpIIb–IIIa complex on platelet membranes mediates fibrinogen binding, which in turn is responsible for platelet aggregation (Marguerie *et al.* 1980). GpIIb–IIIa mediates also platelet adhesion to fibronectin, von Willebrand factor and vitronectin. A complex similar to GpIIb–IIIa has been found on the surface of endothelial cells and lately been identified as the vitronectin receptor (Phillips *et al.* 1988).

Glycoproteins immunologically related to the GpIIb–IIIa complex (IR–GpIIb–IIIa) have been identified on the surface of several tumour cells, such as human colon carcinoma and melanoma (Boukerche *et al.* 1989a), rat Walker 256 carcinosarcoma (Chopra *et al.* 1988), murine B16 amelanotic melanoma and Lewis lung carcinoma cells (Grossi *et al.* 1989). It is likely that IR–GpIIb–IIIa mediates the interactions between tumour cells, platelets and endothelial cells. Indeed, monoclonal antibodies to GpIIb–IIIa inhibited the adhesion of human melanoma cells to fibronectin (Knudsen *et al.* 1988a) and tumour-cell-induced platelet aggregation (Chopra *et al.* 1988). The expression of IR–GpIIb–IIIa on the surface of tumour cells is apparently stimulated by 12-HETE, a lipooxygenase metabolite of arachidonic acid, known to stimulate tumour cell adhesion to endothelium (Grossi *et al.* 1989).

Figure 8.1 summarizes in a very schematic and simplified way the interactions thought to occur *in vitro* between platelets, their activation products, vascular and tumour cells; these interactions may be particularly relevant to the extravasation step of metastasis formation.

Platelet-tumour cell interactions *in vivo*

Involvement of platelets in experimental metastases

The involvement of blood platelets during growth and dissemination of experimental tumours has been studied in different models and may greatly vary, depending on the type of tumour and the route of administration used (Donati & Poggi, 1980). In general, two models of metastasis have been developed in experimental animals:

1 The intravenous (i.v.) injection of tumour cells in mice, which leads to development of tumour nodules in the lungs, in the following weeks. This model is also termed as 'artificial' metastases, since huge amounts of tumour cells are given to a previously healthy animal in the absence of all those metabolic and biochemical changes generally associated with the growth of a solid tumour in clinical conditions.

2 The subcutaneous (s.c.) or intramuscular (i.m.) injection of tumour cells, which leads to the growth of a primary tumour at the site of implantation and to the subsequent dissemination to distant organs, where metastatic nodules may grow. This model is termed 'spontaneous' metastasis, since its development mimics more closely, than that of the 'lung colony model, the clinical evolution in patients with solid tumours from which tumour cells gradually migrate to distant organs.

When tumour cells are injected i.v. in mice ('artificial' model), a marked thrombocytopenia occurs as a part of an intravascular coagulation syndrome, characterized also by low fibrinogen levels and by high fibrinogen-degradation products. Thrombocytopenia can be detected 3 minutes after tumour cell injection and is rapidly reversible. The fall in platelet counts is presumably due to platelet aggregation in response to the release of their potent agonist, thrombin, developing from the procoagulant activities of tumour cells. Indeed, tumour cells can induce *in vivo* thrombocytopenia independently from their direct platelet aggregatory properties; moreover, *in vivo* platelet consumption can be prevented not only by antiplatelet agents, but also, and even better, by treatment of animals with the anticoagulant warfarin (Poggi *et al.* 1977; Mussoni *et al.* 1978; Donati *et al.* 1982). Tumour cell-induced thrombocytopenia does not occur in mice with a congenital deficiency of platelet functions due to defective content of their dense granules, the so-called 'beige' mice (Valori *et al.* 1983).

The above-mentioned changes are very short-lived and are reversible within 1 hour of tumour cell injection. The subsequent development of lung colonies is not accompanied by any haematological changes; indeed normal platelet and red blood cell counts and fibrinogen levels are measured during the growth of 'artificial' metastases (Poggi *et al.* 1981).

In contrast, several changes occurring during 'spontaneous' metastases have been described in the Lewis lung carcinoma, the JW sarcoma and the mFS6 fibrosarcoma in mice (Poggi *et al.* 1977; Chmielewska *et al.* 1980; Delaini *et al.* 1981). The platelet changes occurring during development of Lewis lung carcinoma implanted i.m. have been extensively studied (Poggi *et al.* 1977). Mild intravascular coagulation, with micro-angiopathic haemolytic anaemia, thrombocytopenia and raised fibrinogen levels with increased fibrinogen turnover were observed, during tumour growth. Thrombocytopenia was not accompanied by increase of platelet turnover or by changes in the splenic pool; bone marrow examination and indirect pharmacological data further confirmed that it was rather due to impaired platelet production than to enhanced intravascular consumption. Indeed, thrombocytopenia was not abolished by chronic treatment with antiplatelet or anticoagulant agents; the lack of a clear pathogenetic link to metastasis formation was suggested also by the observation that tumour-bearing animals treated with warfarin showed a marked inhibition of metastases (Poggi *et al.* 1978, 1981). In conclusion, thrombocytopenia appeared to be related to the presence of the primary tumour, as also indicated by normal platelet counts in mice whose primary tumour was surgically removed when metastatic growth had already started (Poggi *et al.* 1981). It is thus conceivable that thrombocytopenia under these conditions could be favoured by the release of some, as yet undefined, toxic factors from the primary tumour.

During the last decade new experimental systems have been used to study the biological processes related to cancer metastasis: in particular, 'metastatic variants', i.e. sublines obtained through *in vitro/in vivo* passages from the same parental line, characterized by marked differences in their metastatic potential in either spontaneous or artificial models of dissemination, have been developed. We studied the platelet involvement in mFS6 fibrosarcoma, a benzopyrene-induced tumour, and in several metastatic sublines derived from its metastatic lung nodules; the potential for spontaneous metastasis of the sublines ranged from 0 to 100% incidence of lung nodules. Gradual thrombocytopenia developed (until about 30% of starting levels) in all the sublines studied, whatever the occurrence of metastasis, thus reinforcing the concept that the observed platelet drop in murine tumours is not related to metastatic growth. Moreover, in the same model, platelet drop could not be ascribed to intravascular platelet consumption, since it was observed both with sublines able to induce *in vitro* platelet aggregation and with those devoid of such property (Delaini *et al.* 1981; Donati *et al.* 1982; Vicenzi *et al.* 1987).

Some interest is presently devoted to the blood platelet involvement during growth of human tumours implanted in athymic 'nude' mice. We studied the occurrence of haemostatic changes in mice implanted with several lines of human melanoma or colon carcinoma, but we did not find, so far, marked signs of platelet drop, in comparison with the above-mentioned changes in murine tumours (Falanga *et al.*, in preparation).

Treatment of metastases with antiplatelet agents

Thrombocytopenia, induced by injection of neuraminidase or by antiplatelet serum, inhibited lung colony formation in mice injected with TA3 carcinoma or other experimental tumours (Gasic and Gasic 1962) (Table 8.1). Pearlstein *et al.* (1984) confirmed these data, showing that a specific antibody to mouse platelets had a potent inhibitory effect on three different tumour models (CT26 colon adenocarcinoma, B16 amelanotic melanoma and Lewis lung carcinoma); the antibody was effective only when the animals were treated at least 6 hours before tumour cell injection. The antiplatelet antibody also inhibited the formation of spontaneous lung metastases in mice with Lewis lung carcinoma. The relevance of the interactions between platelets and tumour cells was further suggested by

Table 8.1 Antiplatelet agents and metastasis treatment

Treatment	Tumour	Effect	References
Thrombocytopenia induced	TA3	↓	Gasic *et al.* (1968)
by neuraminidase/	CT26, 3LL	↓	Pearlstein *et al.* (1984)
anti-platelet antibody	B16a		
Polyclonal antibody to vWF	CT26, 3LL	↓	Karpatkin *et al.* (1988)
	B16a		
Monoclonal antibody to	CT26, 3LL	↓	Karpatkin *et al.* (1988)
GpIIB–IIIA	B16a		

3LL = Lewis lung carcinoma; B16a = B16 amelanotic melanoma; CT26 = CT26 colon adenocarcinoma; TA3 = TA3 mammory adenocarcinoma.

Karpatkin *et al.* (1988), who found that 10E5, a monoclonal antibody to GpIIb–IIIa, reduced lung colonization of mouse CT26 carcinoma and human HCT8 colon carcinoma cells in mice. The same authors also found that a polyclonal specific antibody to murine von Willebrand factor (vWF) had an inhibitory effect in the same system. More recently, Boukerche *et al.* (1989b) observed that a monoclonal antibody to GpIIb–IIIa inhibited the growth of human melanoma cells implanted in nude mice.

Table 8.2 Antiplatelet drugs and metastasis treatment

Drug	Model	Effect	References
Aspirin	MCA, T241	↓	Gasic *et al.* (1972, 1973)
		→	Wood and Hilgard (1972)
		→	Hilgard *et al.* (1976)
	3LL, CT26	→	Karpatkin *et al.* (1988)
Ditazole	3LL	→	Mussoni *et al.* (1977, 1978)
Ticlopidine	3LL, CT26	→	Karpatkin *et al.* (1988)
PGI_2, Iloprost,	B16a	↓	Honn *et al.* (1981)
Nafazatrom,	B16a, CT26, 3LL	→	Honn (1983).
Dazmegrel	M4	→	Karpatkin *et al.* (1984)
	B16BL6	↓	Vicenzi *et al.* (1987)
			Costantini *et al.* (1988)
Dipyridamole,	W256	↓	Gastpar (1972)
RA 233	B16, 3LL	→	Lichtner *et al.* (1985)
Nifedipine,	B16a, W256	↓	Honn *et al.* (1983,
Nimodipine,		↓	1984, 1985)
Felodipine			

3LL = Lewis lung carcinoma, B16a = B16 amelanotic melanoma; T241 = T241 fibrosarcoma; CT26 = CT26 colon adenocarcinoma; M4 = M4 fibrosarcoma; B16BL6 = B16BL6 melanoma; W256 = Walker 256 carcinosarcoma; MCA = methylcholanthrene-induced sarcoma.

Treatment of metastases with antiplatelet agents gave contrasting results (see Gasic 1984; Mehta 1984; Rickles & Hancock 1988, for reviews). Table 8.2 briefly summarizes the most relevant data. The antimetastatic effect of aspirin was first observed by Gasic and co-workers in artificial and spontaneous models of metastasis (1972, 1973). This effect was not confirmed by other investigators, in different experimental models (Wood & Hilgard, 1972; Hilgard *et al.* 1976). More recently, Karpatkin *et al.* (1988) did not observe any protective effect, making a comparison of different schedules of administration and different dosages of aspirin in mice bearing the CT26 or Lewis lung carcinoma. In the same set of experiments, ticlopidine, an inhibitor of the first wave of platelet aggregation, was also devoid of antimetastatic activity. Another non-steroidal anti-inflammatory drug with antiplatelet activity, ditazole, was unable to reduce metastasis growth in a spontaneous model of dissemination, but potentiated metastasis formation in the artificial model (Mussoni *et al.* 1977, 1978). The effect of other anti-inflammatory agents, such as indomethacin have been the most variable until now (Rickles & Hancock, 1988).

Honn *et al.* (1981) first demonstrated that prostacyclin (PGI_2), a derivative of arachidonic acid and a potent inhibitor of platelet aggregation, was a potent antimetastatic agent in B16 amelanotic melanoma in mice. Lung colony formation in mice was inhibited also by a prostacyclin stimulatory agent (nafazatrom, Bayer), by a thromboxane (TX) synthase inhibitor and by a thromboxane A_2 (TXA_2) receptor antagonist (Honn, 1983). Similar results were obtained more recently by Costantini *et al.* (1988), with iloprost, a stable analogue of prostacyclin. On the contrary, no antimetastatic effects were observed by Karpatkin *et al.* (1984) or by Vicenzi *et al.* (1987) using similar compounds. Dipyridamole and other pyrimido-pyrimidine derivatives, such as RA 233, were found active as antimetastatic agents (Gastpar, 1972); however, their effects on artificial and spontaneous models of metastasis have been questioned (see Lichtner *et al.* 1985, for a review). Dipyridamole and pyrimido-pyrimidine derivatives stimulate PGI_2 release and inhibit tumour cell adhesion to endothelium; however, they also show several collateral effects, such as a direct cytotoxic activity and inhibition of nucleoside incorporation (Bastida *et al.* 1985).

Finally, calcium channel blockers have been suggested as potential antimetastatic agents by Honn *et al.* (1983). Felopidine, nimodipine and nifedipine were active on artificial and spontaneous models of metastasis (Honn *et al.* 1984, 1985). Their antimetastatic effect was apparently related to the ability to inhibit tumour-cell-induced platelet aggregation and tumour cell adhesion to endothelium.

To summarize, it may be schematically stated that the antimetastatic effects of the antiplatelet agents studied were rather variable in spontaneous and artificial metastasis models. The variety of collateral effects and the number of different targets (platelets, endothelial cells, tumour cells) which may be reached by these agents may justify the variety of results obtained when the drugs were used on metastasis development.

RGD-containing peptides and tumour cells

The amino acid sequence arginyl–glycyl–aspartic acid (RGD) has been identified as the common cell adhesion site of many attachment molecules, such as fibronectin, vitronectin, type I collagen, fibrinogen and vWF and may also be important in other attachment molecules, such as laminin. Peptides with RGD sequence induce adhesion of normal and tumour cells to plastic; soluble RGD peptides inhibit the attachment of cells to insolubilized fibronectin (Pierschbacher & Ruoslahti, 1984).

Humphries *et al.* (1986) showed a reduced lung colonization upon intravenous injection of cells of a highly metastatic variant of B16 melanoma (F10) incubated with a synthetic peptide GRGDS (glycyl–arginyl–glycyl–aspartyl–serine) prior to the injection. Other peptides with a modified sequence, such as GRGES (glycyl–arginyl–glycyl–glutamyl–serine), were ineffective. The antimetastatic activity of GRGDS was apparently dependent of its inhibitory effect on tumour cell adhesion and spreading *in vitro*, and on its ability to accelerate the disappearance of radiolabelled tumour cells from the lungs, *in vivo*. Treatment with RGDS or GRGDS significantly prolonged survival time of animals (Humphries *et al.* 1988). Several RGD-containing peptides have been tested on experimental tumours, mostly on the 'artificial' model of dissemination, as summarized in Table 8.3. In these models RGDS or GRGDS were consistently active (Ugen *et al.* 1988; Bretti *et al.* 1989; Saiki *et al.* 1989). A reduction of 'spontaneous' lung colonies following

Table 8.3 Effect of different RGD-containing peptides on lung colony formation in mice*

Tumour	Peptide	Effect	References
B16F10 melanoma	GRGDS	↓	Humphries *et al.* (1986, 1988)
	RGDS	↓	
	GRGES	→	
B16BL6 melanoma	RGD	↓	Saiki *et al.* (1989)
3LL carcinoma	POLY–RGD	↓ ↓	
B16BL6 melanoma (i.m. + surgery)	RGD	↓	Saiki *et al.* (1989)
	POLY–RGD	↓ ↓	
PAK 17.15 fibrosarcoma	GRGS	→	Ugen *et al.* (1988)
	GRGDS	↓	
SR–BALB fibrosarcoma	GRGESP	↓	Bretti *et al.* (1989)
	GRGDSP	→	
M4 Fibrosarcoma	RGDS	→	Poggi *et al.* (unpublished data)
	RGDW	→	
	RGGW	→	
B16BL6 Melanoma	RGDS	↓	Poggi *et al.* (unpublished data)
	RGDW	↓ ↓	
	RGGW	→	

* Tumour cells were injected i.v., if not otherwise stated.

sub-plaster administration and surgery was also observed by Saiki *et al.* (1989). We tested a new synthetic peptide, RGDW (arginyl–glycyl–aspartyl–tryptophane), a potent protective agent in a model of experimental thrombosis in mice (Poggi *et al.* 1989), as a potential antimetastatic agent. It appeared to be more potent than RGDS to prevent lung colony formation in mice following i.v. injection of B16BL6 melanoma cells, whereas it was almost ineffective in the M4 fibrosarcoma model (Poggi *et al.*, in preparation). Another peptide, RGGW (arginyl–glycyl–glycyl–tryptophan), devoid of anti-aggregatory and anti-thrombotic activity, was also ineffective in both tumour models. The use of trigramin, a RGD-containing polypeptide, extracted from snake venom, which is 500 times more potent than RGDS to inhibit tumour cell adhesion to fibronectin, appears very promising (Knudsen *et al.* 1988b).

Clinical studies with antiplatelet agents

All the above-mentioned studies on the possible role of blood platelets in metastasis formation have laid down the rationale for the possible use of antiplatelet agents in patients with different types of solid tumours. In the past 20–30 years, many 'pilot' studies were conducted, which, due to their limited number of patients or poorly controlled design, could not reach clear-cut conclusions about the efficacy of treatments. During the eighties, some controlled randomized clinical trials have been organized using non-steroidal anti-inflammatory drugs, pyrimido-pyrimidine compounds and calcium channel blockers. The studies already completed and those still in progress have been put together in a registry of clinical trials on anti-thrombotic drugs in cancer patients which has been published lately by the Sub Committee on Malignancy and Hemostasis of the International Society for Hemostasis and Thrombosis (Zacharski & Donati, 1989).

The registry includes a number of studies already completed and a group of clinical trials still in progress at the time of compilation. In the studies that have been completed, non-steroidal anti-inflammatory agents and pyrimido-pyrimidine derivatives have mainly been used as antiplatelet agents (aspirin, benorilate, aspirin plus dipyridamole and RA 233). The studies have been conducted on a variety of tumours (Duke's B and C colorectal cancer, anaplastic primary breast cancer, disseminated lung and colon cancer, limited small cell lung carcinoma). The most interesting results have been observed in the study of RA 233 treatment in non-small cell carcinoma of the lung. RA 233, a dipyridamole congener, now termed 'mopidamole', was tested for its possible additive antitumor effect — in conjunction with 'standard' chemotherapy alone as in the control arm — in a large, randomized trial involving lung and colon cancer patients. The results of this study cast some doubts on the 'antiplatelet' hypothesis, at least in the area of small cell lung cancer, whereas previous work of Zacharski *et al.* (1981) had indicated additive activity for the anticoagulant warfarin. In limited non-small cell lung cancer, however, this RA 233 study stands alone, among randomized trials

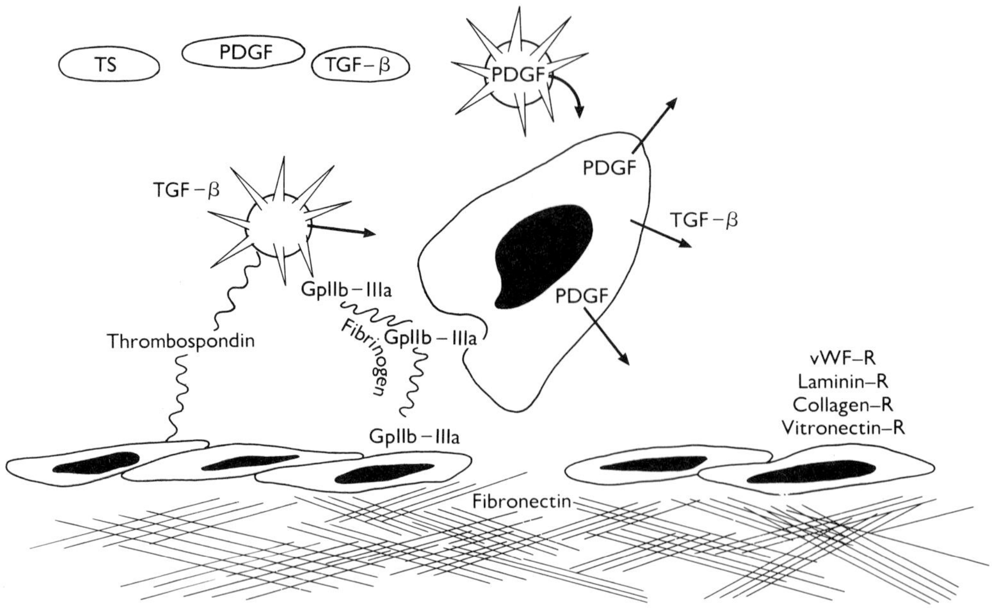

Figure 8.1 Schematic representation of tumour cell interaction with the vascular wall and of the role of activated platelets (represented as spiked spheres as opposed to discoid-shaped cells in resting conditions); of platelet activation products: TS=thrombospondin, PDGF=platelet derived growth factor, TGF-β=transforming growth factor beta; of cell membrane receptors: GP IIb–IIIa, von Willebrand factor receptor (vWF), laminin receptor, collagen receptor, vitronectin receptor; and of adhesive proteins such as fibrinogen and fibronectin. An extracellular matrix network is represented immediately under the endothelial cell layer.

reported to date, since a statistically significant survival advantage was obtained among the group who received RA 233. Several new studies are in progress both in West Germany and in the USA with RA 233 in different types of tumour, such as renal cell, breast, ovary, melanoma, disseminated small cell lung carcinoma and non-small cell carcinoma of the lung following surgery or radiation therapy. While these results are being completed, some experimental work is being undertaken to elucidate the biochemical mechanisms possibly involved in the reported effect of RA 233.

Conclusion

Platelet–tumour cell interactions may influence metastasis formation at different levels, i.e. tumour cell arrest in the microvasculature, disruption of the endothelial layer, adhesion to the extracellular matrix, migration in extravascular spaces and growth. A better understanding of the relative roles of the cell types involved (tumour cells, platelets, endothelial cells) and of the mechanisms of these interactions (aggregation, adhesion, release of growth factors, chemoattractants, enzymes) is necessary before a therapeutical approach to tumour metastasis may be more successfully attempted.

Acknowledgements

The author's studies reported in this paper have been performed with contributions of the Italian CNR (Project 'Oncologia', Contract N.88.00733.44) and of the Italian Association for Research on Cancer. The helpful assistance of Miss Sheila Flanagan, Miss Silvia Falcone and Miss Raffaella Bertazzi with the preparation of this manuscript is gratefully acknowledged.

References

Abecassis, J., Millon-Collard, R., Klein-Soyer, C. *et al.* (1987) Adhesion of human breast cancer cell line MCF-7 to human vascular endothelial cells in culture. Enhancement by activated platelets. *Int J Cancer* **40**, 525–531.

Bastida, E., Ordinas, A. *et al.* (1982) Differentiation of platelet-aggregating effects of human tumor cell lines based on inhibition studies with apyrase, hirudin, and phospholipase. *Cancer Res* **42**, 4348–4352.

Bastida, E., del Prado, J. *et al.* (1985) Inhibitory effects of dipyridamole on growth, nucleoside incorporation, and platelet-activating capability in the U87MG and SKNMC human tumor cell lines. *Cancer Res* **45**, 4048–4052.

Bastida, E., Almirall, L. *et al.* (1989) Influence of shear stress on tumor-cell adhesion to endothelial-cell extracellular matrix and its modulation by fibronectin. *Int J Cancer* **43**, 1174–1178.

Bastida, E., Bertomeu, M.C. *et al.* (1990) Regulation of tumor cell adhesion by intracellular 13-HODE:15-HETE ratio. *J Lipid Mediators* **2**, 281–293.

Bethsholtz, C. Johnsson, A., Heldin, C-H. *et al.* (1986) cDNA sequence and chromosomal localization of human platelet-derived growth factor A-chain and its expression in tumour cell lines. *Nature* **320**, 695–699.

Boukerche, H., Berthier-Vergnes, O. *et al.* (1989a) Platelet–melanoma cell interaction is mediated by the glycoprotein IIb–IIIa complex. *Blood* **74**, 658–663.

Boukerche, H., Bertheir-Vergnes, O. *et al.* (1989b) A monoclonal antibody (LYP18) directed against the blood platelet glycoprotein IIb/IIIa complex inhibits human melanoma growth *in vivo*. *Blood* **74**, 909–912.

Bretti, S., Neri, P. *et al.* (1989) Inhibition of experimental metastasis of murine fibrosarcoma cells by oligopeptide analogues to the fibronectin cell-binding site. *Int J Cancer* **43**, 102–106.

Buchanan, M.R. & Bastida, E. (1987) The role of 13-HODE and HETEs in vessel wall/circulating blood cell interaction. *Agents and Actions* **22**, 337–339.

Chmielewska, J., Poggi, A. *et al.* (1980) Blood coagulation changes in JW Sarcoma, a new metastasizing tumour in mice. *Eur J Cancer* **16**, 1399–1407.

Chopra, H., Hatfield, J.S., Chang, Y.S. *et al.* (1988) Role of tumor cell cytoskeleton and membrane glycoprotein IRGpIIb/IIIa in platelet adhesion to tumor cell membrane and tumor cell-induced platelet aggregation. *Cancer Res* **48**, 3787–3800.

Chung, D.C., Zetter, B.R. & Brodt, D.P. (1988) Lewis lung carcinoma variants with differing metastatic specificities adhere preferentially to different defined extracellular matrix molecules. *Invasion Metastasis* **8**, 103–117.

Costantini, V., Fuschiotti, P. *et al.* (1988) Platelet–tumor cell interaction: effect of prostacyclin and a synthetic analog on metastasis formation. *Cancer Chemother Pharmacol* **22**, 289–293.

Crissman, J.D., Hatfield, J.S. *et al.* (1988) Morphological study of the interaction of intravascular tumor cells with endothelial cell and subendothelial matrix. *Cancer Res* **48**, 4065–4072.

Delaini, F., Giavazzi, R. *et al.* (1981) Tumor sublines with different metastatic capacity induce similar blood coagulation changes in the host. *Br J Cancer* **43**, 100–104.

Deuel, T.F., Senior, R.M. *et al.* (1982) Chemotaxis of monocytes and neutrofils to platelet derived growth factor. *J Clin Invest* **69**, 1046–1049.

Donati, M.B. & Poggi, A. (1980) Malignancy and haemostasis. *Br J Haematol* **44**, 173–182.

Donati, M.B., Rotilio, D. *et al.* (1982) Animal models for the study of platelet-tumor cell interactions. In Jamieson, G.A. (ed.) *Interaction of platelets and tumor cells*, pp. 159–174. A.R. Liss, New York.

Dvorak, H.F. (1986) Tumors: wounds that do not heal. Similarities between tumor stroma generation and wound healing. *New Engl J Med* **315**, 1650–1659.

Estrada, J. & Nicolson, G.L. (1984) Tumor–cell–platelet aggregation does not correlate with metastatic potential of rat 13762NF mammary adenocarcinoma tumor cell clones. *Int J Cancer* **34**, 101–105.

Frazier, W.A. (1987) Thrombospondin: a modular adhesive glycoprotein of platelets and nucleated cells.

J Cell Biol **105**, 625–632.

Gasic, G.J. (1984) Role of plasma, platelets, and endothelial cells in tumor metastasis. *Cancer Metastasis Rev* **3**, 99–116.

Gasic, G. & Gasic, T. (1962) Removal of sialic acid from the cell coat in tumor cells and vascular endothelium and its effects on metastasis. *Proc Natl Acad Sci USA* **48**, 1172–1177.

Gasic, G.J., Gasic, T. & Stewart, C.C. (1968) Antimetastatic effects associated with platelet reduction. *Proc Natl Acad Sci USA* **61**, 45–52.

Gasic, G.J., Gasic, T.B. & Murphy, S. (1972) Antimetastatic effect of aspirin. *Lancet* **ii**, 713.

Gasic, G.J., Gasic, T.B. *et al.* (1973) Platelet–tumor–cell interactions in mice: the role of platelets in the spread of malignant disease. *Int J Cancer* **11**, 704–718.

Gastpar, H. (1972) The inhibition of the cancer cell stickiness by pyrimido-pyrimidine derivatives induced by inhibition of platelet aggregation. *Acta Med Scand Suppl* **525**, 269–271.

Goustin, A.S., Leof, E.B. *et al.* (1986) Growth factors and cancer. *Cancer Res* **46**, 1015–1029.

Grignani, G., Almasio, P. *et al.* (1983) Interactions between neoplastic cell with different metastasizing capacity and platelet function. *Eur J Cancer Clin Oncol* **19**, 519–525.

Grossi, I.M., Fitzgerald, L.A. *et al.* (1989) Bidirectional control of membrane expression and/or activation of the tumor cell IRGpIIb/IIIa receptor and tumor cell adhesion by lipoxygenase products of arachidonic acid and linoleic acid. *Cancer Res* **49**, 1029–1037.

Heldin, C.-H. & Westermark, B. (1984) Growth factors: mechanism of action and relation to oncogenes. *Cell* **37**, 9–20.

Hilgard, P., Heller, H. & Schmidt, C.G. (1976) The influence of platelet aggregation inhibitors on metastasis formation in mice (3LL). *Zeit Krebsforsch* **86**, 243–250.

Honn, K.V. (1983) Inhibition of tumor cell metastasis by modulation of the vascular prostacyclin thromboxane A_2 system. *Clin Exp Metastasis* **I**, 103–114.

Honn, K.V., Cicone, B. & Skoff, A. (1981) Prostacyclin: a potent antimetastatic agent. *Science* **212**, 1270–1272.

Honn, K.V., Onoda, J.M. *et al.* (1983) Calcium channel blockers: potential antimetastatic agents. *Proc Soc Exp Biol Med* **174**, 16–19.

Honn, K.V., Onoda, J.M. *et al.* (1984) Inhibition of tumor cell–platelet interactions and tumor metastasis by the calcium channel blocker, nimodipine. *Clin Expl Metastasis* **2**, 61–72.

Honn, K.V., Onoda, J.M., Pampalona, K. *et al.* (1985) Inhibition by dihydropyridine class calcium channel blockers of tumor cell–platelet–endothelial cell interactions *in vitro* and metastasis *in vivo*. *Biochem Pharmacol* **34**, 235–241.

Humphries, M.J., Olden, K. & Yamada, K.M. (1986) A synthetic peptide from fibronectin inhibits experimental metastasis of murine melanoma cells. *Science* **233**, 467–470.

Humphries, M.J., Yamada, K.M. & Olden, K. (1988) Investigation of the biological effects of anti-cell adhesive synthetic peptides that inhibit experimental metastasis of B16–F10 murine melanoma cells. *J Clin Invest* **81**, 782–790.

Hynes, R.O. (1987) Integrins: a family of cell surface receptors. *Cell* **48**, 549–554.

Jamieson, G.A., Bastida, E. & Ordinas, A. (1987) Interaction of platelets and tumour cells. In MacIntyre D.E. & Gordon J.L. (eds) *Platelets in Biology and Pathology III*, pp. 161–189. Elsevier Science Publisher, Amsterdam.

Karpatkin, S., Ambrogio, C. & Pearlstein, E. (1984) Lack of effect of *in vivo* prostacyclin on the development of pulmonary metastases in mice following intravenous injection of CT26 colon carcinoma, Lewis lung carcinoma, or B16 amelanotic melanoma cells. *Cancer Res* **44**, 3880–3883.

Karpatkin, S., Pearlstein, E. *et al.* (1988) Role of adhesive proteins in platelet tumor interaction *in vitro* and metastasis formation *in vivo*. *J Clin Invest* **81**, 1012–1019.

Kimura, A.K., Mehta, P. *et al.* (1987) The lack of correlation between experimental metastatic potential and platelet aggregating activity of B16 melanoma clones viewed in relation to tumor cell heterogeneity. *Clin Exp Metastasis* **5**, 125–133.

Knudsen, K.A., Smith, L. *et al.* (1988a) Role of IIb–IIIa-like glycoproteins in cell–substratum adhesion of human melanoma cells. *J Cell Physiol* **136**, 471–478.

Knudsen, K.A., Tuszynski, G.P. *et al.* (1988b) Trigramin, an RGD-containing peptide from snake venom, inhibits cell–substratum adhesion of human melanoma cells. *Exp Cell* Res **179**, 42–49.

Lampugnani, M.G. & Crawford, N. (1987) Tumor cell induced platelet aggregation: studies with cloned metastatic and non metastatic variants. *Invasion Metastasis* **7**, 311–324.

Lauri, D., Bertomeu, M.C. *et al.* (1989) Differential effects of interleukin-1 and formylmethionylleucylphenylalanine on chemotaxis and human endothelium adhesivity for A549 tumor cells. *Lab Invest* **60**, 161–164.

Lerner, W.A., Pearlstein, E. *et al.* (1983) A new mechanism for tumor-induced platelet aggregation. Comparison with mechanisms shared by other tumors with possible pharmacologic strategy toward prevention of metastases. *Int J Cancer* **31**, 463–469.

Lichtner, R.B., Hutchinson, G. *et al.* (1985) Antiplatelet pyrimido-pyrimidines and metastasis. *Cancer Treat Rev* **12**, 221–234.

Liotta, L.A., Rao, C.N. & Barsky, S.H. (1983) Tumor invasion and the extracellular matrix. *Lab Invest* **49**, 636–649.

Marguerie, G.A., Edgington, T.S. & Plow, E.F. (1980) Interaction of fibrinogen with its platelet receptor as part of a multistep reaction in ADP-induced platelet aggregation. *J Biol Chem* **255**, 154–161.

Mehta, P. (1984) Potential role of platelets in the pathogenesis of tumor metastasis. *Blood* **63**, 55–63.

Menter, D.G., Steinert, B.W., Sloane, B.F. *et al.* (1987) Role of platelet membrane in enhancement of tumor cell adhesion to endothelial cell extracellular matrix. *Cancer Res* **47**, 6751–6762.

Mussoni, L., Poggi, A. *et al.* (1977) Ditazole and platelets. III. Effect of ditazole on tumor-cell induced thrombocytopenia and on bleeding time in mice. *Haemostasis* **6**, 260–265.

Mussoni, L., Poggi, A. *et al.* (1978) Effect of ditazole, an inhibitor of platelet aggregation, on a metastasizing tumour in mice. *Br J Cancer* **37**, 126–129.

Nicolson, G.L. (1988) Organ specificity of tumor metastasis: role of preferential adhesion, invasion and growth of malignant cells at specific secondary sites. *Cancer Metastasis Rev* **7**, 143–188.

Niewiarowski, S. & Varma K.G. (1982) Biochemistry and physiology of secreted platelet proteins. In: Colman, R.W., Hirsh, J., Marder, V.J. & Salzman, E.W. (eds) *Hemostasis and thrombosis*, Lippincott, Philadelphia. pp. 421–430.

Nistér, M., Heldin, C.H. & Westermark, B. (1986) Clonal variation in the production of a platelet-derived growth factor-like protein and expression of corresponding receptors in a human malignant glioma. *Cancer Res* **46**, 332–340.

Oldberg, A., Heldin, C.-H. *et al.* (1980) Characterization of a platelet endoglycosidase degrading heparin-like polysaccharides. *Biochemistry* **19**, 5755–5762.

Parish, C.R., Coombe, D.R. *et al.* (1987) Evidence that sulphated polysaccharides inhibit tumour metastasis by blocking tumour-cell-derived heparanases. *Int J Cancer* **40**, 511–518.

Pearlstein, E., Cooper, L.B. & Karpatkin, S. (1979) Extraction and characterization of a platelet-aggregating material from SV40-transformed mouse 3T3 fibroblasts. *J Lab Clin Med* **93**, pp. 332–344.

Pearlstein, E., Salk, P.L. *et al.* (1980) Correlation between spontaneous metastatic potential, platelet-aggregating activity of cell surface extracts, and cell surface sialylation in 10 metastatic-variant derivatives of a rat renal sarcoma cell line. *Proc Natl Acad Sci USA* **77**, 4336–4339.

Pearlstein, E., Ambrogio, C. *et al.* (1981) Inhibition of the platelet aggregating activity of two human adenocarcinomas of the colon and an anaplastic murine tumor with a specific thrombin inhibitor: dansylarginine N-(3-ethyl-1,5-pentanediyl) amide. *Cancer Res* **41**, 4535–4539.

Pearlstein, E., Ambrogio, C. & Karpatkin, S. (1984) Effect of antiplatelet antibody on the development of pulmonary metastases following injection of CT26 colon adenocarcinoma, Lewis lung carcinoma and B16 amelanotic melanoma tumor cells into mice. *Cancer Res* **44**, 3884–3887.

Phillips, D.R., Charo, I.F., *et al.* (1988) The platelet membrane glycoprotein II–IIIa complex. *Blood* **71**, 831–843.

Pierschbacher, M.D. & Ruoslahti, E. (1984) Cell attachment activity of fibronectin can be duplicated by small synthetic fragments of the molecule. *Nature* **309**, 30–33.

Poggi, A., Polentarutti, N. *et al.* (1977) Blood coagulation changes in mice bearing Lewis lung carcinoma, a metastasizing tumor. *Cancer Res* **37**, 272–277.

Poggi, A., Mussoni, L. *et al.* (1978) Warfarin enantiomers anticoagulation and experimental tumour metastases. *Lancet* **i**, 163–164.

Poggi, A., Donati, M.B. & Garattini, S. (1981) Fibrin and cancer cell growth: Problems in the evaluation of experimental models. In Donati, M.B., Davidson, J.F. & Garattini, S. (eds), *Malignancy and the Hemostatic System*, pp. 89–101. Raven Press, New York.

Poggi, A., Vicenzi, E. *et al.* (1988) Platelet contribution to cancer cell growth and migration: the role of platelet growth factors. *Haemostasis* **18**, 18–28.

Poggi, A., Charon, M.H. *et al.* (1989) Reduced mortality following thrombotic pulmonary embolism in mice treated with a new synthetic RGD-peptide. *Thromb Haemost* **62**, 496.

Poste, G. & Fidler, I.J. (1980) The pathogenis of cancer metastasis. *Nature* **283**, 139–146.

Rickles, F.R. & Hancock, W.W. (1988) Antimetastatic Agents. II. Summary of the interactions of tumor cells with blood coagulation factors, platelets, fibrinolytic factors, and inflammatory cells and their soluble mediators: potential for therapeutic interventions. *Semin Thromb Hemost* **14**, 126–132.

Riser, B.L., Varani, J. *et al.* (1988) Thrombospondin binding by human squamous carcinoma and melanoma cells: relationship to biological activity. *Exp Cell Res* **174**, 319–329.

Roberts, D.D., Sherwood, J.A. & Ginsburg, V. (1987) Platelet thrombospondin mediates attachment and spreading of human melanoma cells. *J Cell Biol* **104**, 131–139.

Ross, R., Raines, E.W. & Bowen-Pope, D.F. (1986) The biology of platelet-derived growth factor. *Cell* **46**, 155–169.

Ruoslahti, E. & Pierschbacher, M.D. (1987) New perspectives in cell adhesion: RGD and integrins. *Science* **238**, 491–497.

Saiki, I., Murata, J. *et al.* (1989) The inhibition of murine lung metastasis by synthetic polypeptides [poly(arg–gly–asp) and poly(tyr–ile–gly–ser–arg)] with a core sequence of cell adhesion molecules. *Br J Cancer* **59**, 194–197.

Silverstein, R.L., Leung, L.K., Nachman, R.L. *et al.* (1986) Thrombospondin: a versatile multifunctional glycoprotein. *Arterio sclerosis* **6**, 245–253.

Sporn, M.B. & Roberts, A.B. (1986) Peptide growth factors and inflammation, tissue repair, and cancer. *J Clin Invest* **78**, 329–332.

Sporn, M.B., Roberts, A.B. *et al.* (1986) Transforming

growth factor-β: biological function and chemical structure. *Science* **233**, 532–534.

Sugimoto, Y., Oh-hara, T. *et al.* (1987) Acquisition of metastatic ability in hybridomas between two low metastatic clones of murine colon adenocarcinoma 26 defective in either platelet-aggregating activity or *in vivo* growth potential. *Cancer Res* **47**, 4396–4401.

Tao, T.-W. & Johnsson, L.K. (1982) Altered adhesiveness of tumor cell surface variants with reduced metastasizing capacity-reduced adhesiveness to vascular wall components in culture. *Int J Cancer* **30**, 763–766.

Tohgo, A., Tanaka, N.G., Ogawa, H. *et al.* (1986) Platelet-aggregating activities of metastasizing tumor cells. IV. Effects of cell surface modification on thrombin generation, platelet aggregation and subsequent lung colonization. *Invasion Metastasis* **6**, 58–68.

Tuszynski, G.P., Rothman, V., Murphy, A. *et al.* (1987a) Thrombospondin promotes cell-substratum adhesion. *Science* **236**, 1570–1573.

Tuszynski, G.P., Gasic, T.B. *et al.* (1987b) Thrombospondin, a potentiator of tumor cell metastasis. *Cancer Res* **47**, 4130–4133.

Ugen, K.E., Mahalingam, M. *et al.* (1988) Inhibition of tumor cell-induced platelet aggregation and experimental tumor metastasis by the synthetic gly–arg–gly–asp–ser peptide. *J Natl Cancer Inst* **80**, 1461–1466.

Valori, V.M., Buczko, W. *et al.* (1983) Mice with congenital storage pool defect are protected from cancer cell-induced intravascular platelet aggregation. *Thromb Haemost* **50**, 214.

van Zoelen, E.J.J., van de Ven, W.J.M. *et al.* (1985) Neuroblastoma cells express c-sis and produce a transforming growth factor antigenically related to the platelet-derived growth factor. *Mol Cell Biol* **5**, 2289–2297.

Vicenzi, E., Lampugnani, M.G. *et al.* (1987) Dissociation between thromboxane generation and metastatic potential in cells from a murine fibrosarcoma. Studies with a selective thromboxane synthase inhibitor. *Int J Cancer* **39**, 488–491.

Vlodavsky, I., Futrs, Z. *et al.* (1984) Lymphoma cell-mediated degradation of sulfated proteoglycans in the subendothelial extracellular matrix: relationship to tumor cell metastasis. *Cancer Res* **43**, 2704–2711.

Warren, B.A. (1981) Cancer cell-endothelial reactions: the microinjury hypothesis and localized thrombosis in the formation of micrometastases. In Donati, M.B.. Davidson, J.E. & Garattini S. (eds) *Malignancy and the Hemostasic System*, pp. 5–26. Raven Press, New York.

Watanabe, M., Okochi, E. *et al.* (1988) Identification of a platelet-aggregating factor of murine colon adenocarcinoma 26: M_r 44 000 membrane protein as determined by monoclonal antibodies. *Cancer Res* **48**, 6411–6416.

Weiss, L., Orr, W.F. & Honn, K.V. (1989) Interactions between cancer cells and the microvasculature: a rate-regulator for metastasis. *Clin Exp Metastasis* **7**, 127–167.

Westermark, B., Johnsson, A., Paulsson, Y. *et al.* (1986) Human melanoma cell lines of primary and metastatic origin express the genes encoding the chains of platelet-derived growth factor (PDGF) and produce a PDGF-like growth factor. *Proc Natl Acad Sci USA* **83**, 7197–7200.

Wood, S. (1958) Pathogenesis of metastasis formation observed *in vivo* in the rabbit ear chamber. *AMA Archives of Pathology* **66**, 550–568.

Wood, S. & Hilgard, P. (1972) Aspirin and tumour metastasis. *Lancet* **ii**, 1416–1417.

Zacharski, L.R., Henderson, W.G. *et al.* (1981) Effect of warfarin on survival in small cell carcinoma of the lung. Veterans Administration Study n. 75, *J Am Med Assoc* **245**; 831–835.

Zacharski, L.R., Moritz, T.E., Baczek, C.A. *et al.* (1988) Effect of mopidamol on survival in carcinoma of the lung and colon: final report of Veterans Administration co-operative study No. 188. *J Natl Cancer Inst* **80**, 90–97.

Zacharski, L.R. & Donati, M.B. (1989) Registry of clinical trials of antithrombotic drugs in cancer. *Thromb Haemost* **61**, 526–528.

Zucker, M.B., Katz, I.R. *et al.* (1989) Immuno-regulatory activity of peptides related to platelet factor 4. *Proc Natl Acad Sci USA* **86**, 7571–7574.

9: Platelets and Pregnancy

G. Burton, Chris O'Neill and D. M. Saunders

Introduction

Pregnancy in eutherian mammals is a physiological event which places a stress on the female haemostatic system. Intuitively, the process of placentation is ideally suited for promoting thrombosis. Yet, as we are all evidence, most pregnancies proceed without serious thrombotic events. The platelet, being the 'hair-trigger' of the thrombotic system, has therefore received considerable attention during pregnancy, particularly in the latter stages.

There are many conflicting reports of the platelet concentration in normal pregnancy. In general, the platelet count and function does not change enough to affect clinical management of normal pregnancies. There are many claims that the count either increases, decreases or has little change (Romero & Duffy, 1980). During the third trimester there is haemodilution and possible trapping (Horger & Keane, 1979), so the relative platelet count falls slightly, but the absolute numbers are still within the normal range. There is little change during normal labour unless there is a lot of bleeding associated with the labour. Despite this picture of normality, problems with platelet number and function are still a major cause of pathology in pregnancy.

This concentration of attention on the pathological role of platelets in pregnancy has directed attention away from possible physiological roles. In particular it has recently been reported that platelet activation, and a resulting mild thrombocytopenia is the earliest recognizable maternal response to conception, occurring immediately after fertilization and persisting at least to the time of implantation of the embryo into the uterus and the initiation of placentation. This phenomenon has been shown to be essential for the successful establishment of pregnancy and directs our attention to the role platelets may play as a circulating 'endocrine organ'.

In this review we will consider:

1 the role of platelets and platelet activation in the establishment and maintenance of pregnancy (virtually all of the data for this discussion are derived from studies in experimental animals); and

2 the role of platelets in the pathologies of human pregnancy and current trends in the treatment of such diseases.

Platelets in early pregnancy

Our current understanding of a role for platelets in early pregnancy has a risen almost entirely from studies in mice. In the fetal life of most species the spleen acts as the main haematopoietic and thrombopoietic organ; this is lost after birth with the bone marrow taking over this role, but in mice the spleen continues to have important haematopoietic (Brodsky *et al.* 1966) and thrombopoietic (Layendecker & McDonald, 1982) functions. During haemostatic stress the spleen has a major thrombopoietic role. Indeed, following ablation of the bone marrow the spleen can totally maintain circulating platelet numbers (Layendecker & McDonald, 1982). In mice, the spleen is a relatively small ribbon-like organ which lies along the greater curvature of the stomach. This accessible organ makes the study of platelet production during pregnancy in mice much easier compared with other species.

A well-defined function of the spleen is that of blood storage. This was first suggested after the observation of splenic contraction following haemorrhage (Grayson & Mendel, 1965). The real importance of splenic contraction as a response to stress is still debated. In animals with relatively small spleens (e.g. man, rabbits, rodents) the contribution of blood cells to the circulation following stress is relatively small. In species with large spleens, such as many of the carnivores, the contribution is greater, and may cause an increase in the haematocrit by up to 4%.

Apart from the erythrocytes provided by splenic contraction, the supply of blood platelets is also an important consequence. The spleen contains up to one-third of the body's platelets (Aster, 1966). Following haemorrhage, the rapid provision of platelets to maintain circulating numbers is an important homeostatic mechanism. Control of splenic contraction appears to be mediated by sympathetic innervation. Release of norepinephrine by the adrenal gland augments this control (Grayson & Mendel, 1965).

There have been a number of studies of the effects of pregnancy on spleen size and cellular composition. Invariably, these have looked at the spleen following implantation. It has been found that there is an increase in spleen size from day 6 of pregnancy, reaching a maximum on day 12 (approximately 50% increase compared with the non-pregnant weight) (Sasaki *et al.* 1981) (mice have a 21-day gestation period).

An increase in the volume of both the red and white pulp accounts for this change in spleen size (Sasaki *et al.* 1981). There are more plasma cells in the white pulp during pregnancy, suggesting an elevated production of maternal immunoglobulin at this time. This is considered to represent an immune response. Enlargement of the red pulp has been shown to be due to an enhancement of the haemopoietic activity of the spleen (Sasaki & Ito, 1981) and is probably accompanied by enhanced thrombopoiesis. Since pregnancy results in an increment in the blood volume (Sejeny *et al.* 1975), an increased production of cells is required to prevent dilution anaemia. The elevated level of haematopoietic activity during pregnancy can be mimicked by the administration of oestrogen (Sasaki & Ito, 1981).

However, dramatic changes in the spleen occur much earlier in pregnancy (O'Neill, 1985). While the increment in spleen weight induced by the sex steroids in mice occurred within 24 hours of ovulation in non-pregnant animals, this did not occur for 4 days in pregnant mice. This retardation of the gain in the spleen weight was due to an approximate 50% reduction in splenic platelet pool, while the splenic erythrocyte and leucocyte count were only moderately affected. This was accompanied by a reduction in the megakaryocyte population of the red pulp of the spleen (O'Neill, 1985a). This loss of megakaryocytes was accompanied by a recruitment of these cells to the reproduction tract. These observations, in view of the role the murine spleen plays in thrombopoiesis and as a platelet reserve suggested that the reduction in the splenic platelet pool was a response to a dramatic vascular demand for platelets.

Early-pregnancy-associated thrombocytopenia

Normally, the blood platelet count for an individual remains reasonably stable (Frojmovic & Milton, 1982). The observation of splenic contraction and depletion of platelets in the spleen during the pre-implantation stage of pregnancy suggested that the spleen was responding to a demand by the circulation for platelets (Guyton, 1976).

An investigation of the platelet peripheral platelet during this early stage of pregnancy was carried out (O'Neill, 1985a). The peripheral blood count of non-pregnant, virgin female mice was $1526 \times 10^3/mm^3$ (range $1330-1800 \times 10^3/mm^3$, $n = 18$). The platelet count of pseudopregnant animals was in the same range. A decrease occurred in pregnant animals, being significant ($P < 0.05$) by 10:30 hours on the first day of pregnancy, with a further reduction by 14:30 hours ($P < 0.01$) to reach about 70% of the level found in pseudopregnant animals. This reduction persisted for the first week of pregnancy. On day 7 the platelet count had returned to the value obtained in pseudopregnant animals. This phenomenon was also examined in other species.

The marmoset is a laboratory primate which has an ovarian cycle of 28 days with ovulation occurring on about day 10 and embryo implantation occurring 11–12 days thereafter. Twenty-five female monkeys were studied in three groups. The controls ($n = 7$) were not mated. A second group ($n = 9$) was mated with fertile males and on day 8 after ovulation the uterus was flushed to collect the embryos. The third group ($n = 9$) was allowed to continue pregnancy which was confirmed by chorionic gonadotrophin determinations. Peripheral blood platelet counts were performed on all animals throughout the experimental period. Four of six non-pregnant control animals showed no changes in the platelet count over the study period while two showed a transient (1–2 days) but significant drop in the platelet count. For the mated animals in group two, six animals showed a significant drop (>15%) throughout the pre-implantation period and normal embryos were recovered from the uterus. The remaining three animals showed no significant change to the platelet count. Two of these had degenerating (abnormal) embryos while the third had an apparently normal embryo recovered from the uterus. In animals allowed to continue pregnancy, there was a significant drop in the blood platelet concentration for the days after ovulation. The platelet concentration returned to pre-ovulatory levels or greater by the expected time of implantation. There was again some individual variation in the response with some animals showing a large drop while changes in the platelet count were undetectable in others.

Preliminary data showed that early-pregnancy-associated thrombocytopenia also occurred in women following *in vitro* fertilization (IVF) and embryo transfer (O'Neill, *et al.* 1985a,b). Analysis of results from a larger group of pregnant women (O'Neill, *et al.* 1988), however, showed that the data were beset with variability. While some patients displayed thrombocytopenia throughout the pre-implantation phase and returned to pre-ovulatory levels at the time of implantation, many showed only a transient decrease or no decrease at all. Of interest was the observation that those women who failed to show thrombocytopenia generally displayed a significant increase to the platelet count. It was found that a considerable degree of the variability in response could be related to the thrombocrit (blood platelet volume) prior to embryo transfer. Thus, if an individual had a low pre-transfer thrombocrit ($1.4 \times 10^6\,\mu m^3$), thrombocytopenia was generally not observed, rather there was a consistent and significant elevation in the platelet count. By contrast, where patients had a high pre-transfer thrombocrit ($2.8 \times 10^6\,\mu m^3$) then significant thrombocytopenia was likely to occur. A possible interpretation of this observation was that activation of the thrombopoietic system occurred rapidly for those women with a low thrombocrit, but was delayed (and some degree of thrombocytopenia tolerated) in those with a high pre-transfer thrombocrit.

Thrombopoiesis in experimental animals has been shown to relate to the degree of platelet consumption (O'Dell & Murphy, 1974; Pennington *et al.* 1976). Severe consumption resulted in over-compensation of the platelet count, with the result that the platelet count rose above the initial count. It is likely that the variation in the thrombocrit aggravates this situation such that in the case of a low thrombocrit, even mild platelet consumption results in over compensation. In the case of a relatively high thrombocrit in women, considerably more platelet consumption appears to be tolerated before the thrombopoietic system is activated. As with the marmoset, the results from human IVF patients are consistent with the consumption of blood platelets as a maternal response to early pregnancy. The considerable individual variation in response means that the use of peripheral blood platelet counts on an individual basis is likely to be of little clinical benefit in the assessment of early pregnancy. Thrombocytopenia also occurred in diary cows between days 6 and 17 of pregnancy (Battista *et al.* 1989).

In mice, this decrease in the peripheral platelet count appeared to be due to platelet activation. Ultrastructural examination of the vasculature in early-pregnant mice revealed significant changes in both the platelet and the endothelial cells (O'Neill *et al.* 1986) (Fig. 9.1). Platelets were seen to be clearly undergoing activation, and endothelial cells were extensively vacuolated, in day 2 pregnant compared with pseudopregnant females. This activation was not due to intravascular coagulation since neither the bleeding time nor clotting time was altered and the activity of both the intrinsic and extrinsic pathways of coagulation cascade was identical (O'Neill, 1985).

Although the reduction in platelet numbers is such that the count would be considered to still fall within the normal range, and as such would not be considered clinically relevant, it is nevertheless, statistically significant. The thrombocytopenia was dependent on the presence of the embryo, however, as it did not occur in females in which bilateral fallopian tube ligation had occurred prior to mating, nor did it occur following mating with vasectomized mice (O'Neill, 1985a). It did occur, however, within hours of embryotransfer, and it was subsequently shown that the activation was caused by the production of 1-*o*-alkyl-2-acetyl-sn-glyceryl-3-phosphocholine (platelet activating factor) (PAF) by the pre-implantation embryo (O'Neill, 1985c; Collier *et al.* 1988).

Role of platelet activation in early pregnancy

Intravascular activation of platelets results in the formation of small aggregates which are subsequently trapped by the microvasculature resulting in thrombocytopenia (Camussi *et al.* 1983). Upon activation, platelets release a vast range of biologically active molecules, these include;

1 the biogenic amines, including serotonin;

2 derivatives of arachidonic acid, including the prostaglandins;

3 growth factors which stimulate growth of a variety of cell and tissue types and transformed cell lines;

4 factors which have an important role in the cellular attachment and adhesion; and

5 a number of factors of ill-defined function.

The release of these factors as a consequence of early-pregnancy-associated thrombocytopenia presumably has significant local and systemic effects. It is conceivable that they may act on the reproductive tract to provide a more suitable environment for embryonic growth and development and/or have a role in uterine preparation for implantation. There is some preliminary evidence to suggest that platelets have a role in the establishment of early pregnancy.

Metcalf and Metcalf (1972) showed that phytohaemagglutinin (PHA) stimulation of leucocytes was significantly different in blood collected from early-pregnant women when compared with that collected from non-pregnant women

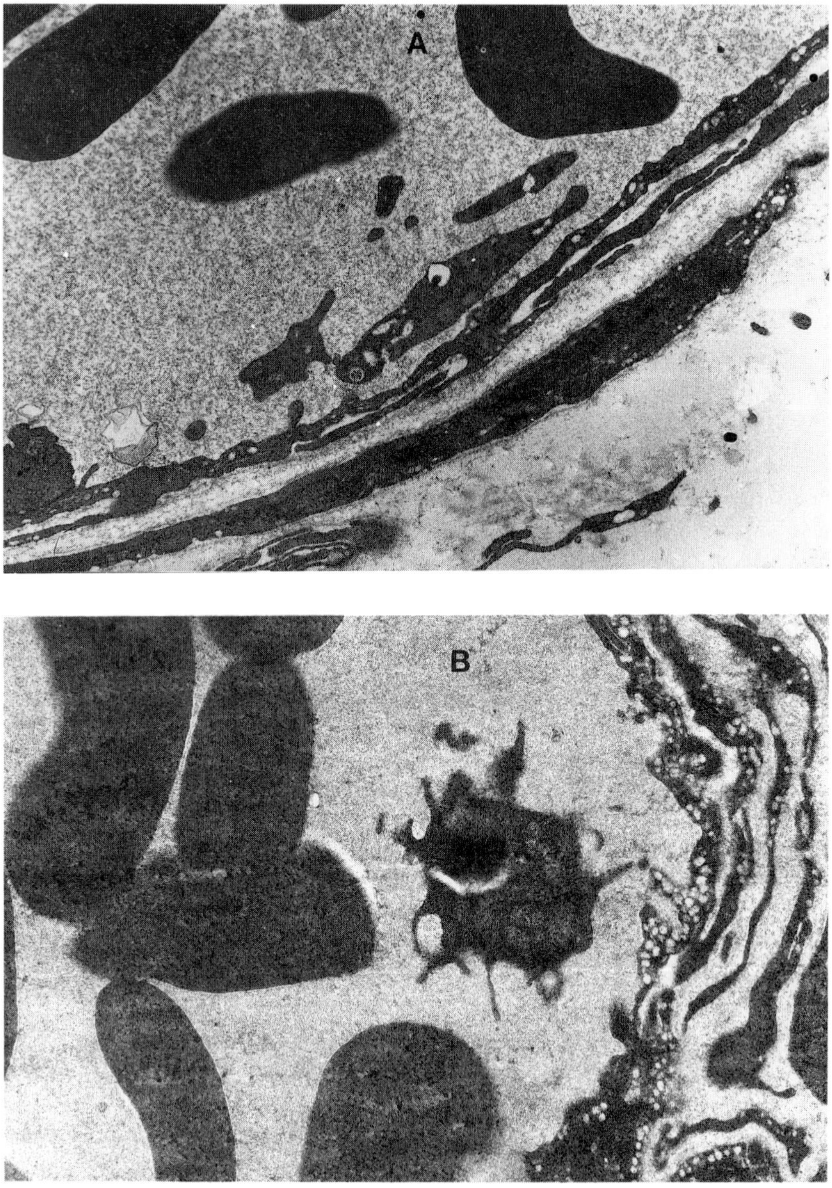

Figure 9.1 The photographs show blood vessels from the microvascular bed of the oviduct of mice on (A) day 2 of pseudopregnancy and (B) day 2 of pregnancy. On this day the embryo is at the two-cell stage, is located in the oviduct and is actively secreting PAF. The differences in the two samples is clearly apparent. In the tissue from pregnant mice the platelet is activated, showing shape change and degranulation and the endothelial cells are highly vacuolated. By contrast the platelets in the tissue from the pseudopregnant mouse are normal, discoid in shape, and the endothelium shows normal morphology.

and men. They showed that the difference in leucocyte activity was dependent upon a change in the platelets at this time. They were not able to demonstrate the nature of this change although the role of platelets as modulators of the immune response is well established (Metcalf & Metcalf, 1972) and it is generally considered that (as yet to be fully defined) changes in the maternal response occur in early pregnancy.

Some pharmacological studies support a role of platelets in the establishment of pregnancy. Two pharmacological approaches have been used to inhibit PAF in early pregnancy (Spinks & O'Neill, 1988). Iloprost 5-(E)-(1S,5S,6R,7R)-7-hydroxy-6-(E)-(3S,4RS)-3-hydroxy-4-methyl-oct-1-en-6-yn-yl-bicylo3.3.0-octano-3-yliden-pentanoic acid is a stable analogue of prostacyclin which stimulates adenylcyclase activity leading to increased cellular cAMP and reduced cytoplasmic calcium. These effects inhibit the action of PAF in most cells. SRI 63-441 (*cis*-(±)-1-[2-hydroxy[tetrahydro-5-[(octadecylaminocarbonyl) oxy]methyl]-furan-2-yl]methoxy-phosphinyloxy]ethyl]-quinolinium hydroxide) is a specific PAF-receptor antagonist with potent pharmacological actions.

Both of these agents when administered to pregnant mice (on day 1–4 of pregnancy) significantly reduced the number of implantation sites. They did not act by having gross toxic effects on the embryo *in vitro* or *in vivo* (Spinks & O'Neill, 1988). A similar effect has been shown in the rat (Acker *et al.* 1988). They appear to act by prevention of implantation rather than its subsequent disruption. The earliest sign of implantation is a local increase in the vascular permeability surrounding the site of implantation. This can be visualized by high molecular weight dyes. Platelet activating factor inhibitors caused significantly fewer dye bands in the uterus on day 4 of pregnancy. There was no evidence of an effect of the antagonists on the early luteal endocrine profile (Spinks & O'Neill, 1988). To determine whether the PAF antagonist acted primarily at the maternal or embryonic level, an experiment was performed using reciprocal embryo transfers, in which blastocysts from mice treated with PAF-antagonist (SRI 63-441) or saline (controls), from days 1 to 4 of pregnancy, were transferred to day 4 pseudopregnant recipients which were also treated with SRI 63-441 or saline on days 1 to 4 of pregnancy. The antagonist (40 μg) was administered at 16:00 hours on day 1 and at 19:00 hours on days 2 to 4 of pregnancy. The percentage of the transferred embryos which implanted was determined on day 8 of pregnancy. Treatment of the donor female had a dramatic effect on the implantation rate, resulting in a reduction by 64% (from 40% to 14.3%, $P<0.04$), while treatment of the recipient female had no significant effect. These results suggest that PAF antagonists affected implantation at the embryonic level. Platelet activating factor antagonist also inhibited trophoblast outgrowth *in vitro* in a dose-dependent manner (Spinks *et al.* 1990), at doses that did not affect development from the one-cell to blastocyst stage (Acker *et al.* 1988). The inhibition of this process *in vitro* by PAF antagonists suggests that embryo-derived PAF may be an autocrine trigger for blastocyst activation and the resulting differentiation of the trophectoderm into invasive trophoblast.

This is not to say, however, that the activation of platelets does not act in a secondary role to promote pregnancy. Gasic and Gasic (1970) showed, in mice, that depletion of blood platelets, following intravenous injection of antiplatelet serum on days 4 and 7 of pregnancy, resulted in a 50% reduction in the number of successful pregnancies. Such treatment does not result in platelet activation and the accompanying release of important biologically active molecules but does lead to their destruction by the reticulo-endothelial system.

Possible roles for platelet activation and the consequent release of a variety of factors might include:

1 supporting embryo implantation into the endometrium; and
2 stimulating the maintenance of the corpus luteum.

There is preliminary evidence for both of these.

Role of platelets in embryo implantation

Implantation of the embryo into the uterus is a major hurdle to be overcome in order for pregnancy to ensue. The processes which initiate and control this event are far from clear. It involves modifications of the vasculature, maternal immune responses and promotion of cellular and tissue differentiation. The central role that platelets play in all of these processes and the evidence for activation of platelets in the pre- and peri-implantation period make them an attractive candidate for involvement in implantation.

An *in vitro* model for implantation exists, whereby blastocysts, in the presence of a complex culture environment, attach to the substratum of the culture vessel, undergo trophoblast outgrowth and transformation and display primary differentiation of the inner cell mass. This study, using the *in vitro* model, examines the role of platelet factors on the control of embryo implantation.

A study was performed to examine whether platelet-derived factors were necessary for the initiation and support of trophoblast outgrowth, by performing the classical test for platelet-derived trophic factors (O'Neill, 1986). Mouse blood was collected in trisodium citrate and underwent differential centrifugation to produce platelet-rich or platelet-poor plasma. The plasma was recalcified to cause a clot and activate platelets, where present. The resulting serum was used as a supplement to medium. Media supplemented with platelet-rich sera from either non-pregnant or pregnant mice supported blastocyst outgrowth to the same extent that fetal calf serum did. Serum from platelet-depleted plasma was totally incapable of supporting blastocyst outgrowth. Such serum produced from pregnant mice was capable of producing a small amount of blastocyst outgrowth, which is consistent with elevated levels of platelet-derived factors present in the serum of early-pregnant females due to the platelet activation caused by embryo-derived PAF. The active agents have yet to be identified but they were heat labile at 70 °C for 10 minutes but not at 56 °C for 30 minutes (O'Neill, 1986).

A range of secreted molecules from the platelet could conceivably have a role in supporting implantation. Cationic platelet derived growth factor (PDGF) is a potent mitogen for a wide range of cell types. Its effect on embryos is yet to be determined. Putative cell attachment factors, such as fibronectin, are also secreted by the platelet. Fibronectin coating of culture dishes was sufficient to support blastocyst outgrowth in defined culture media (Armant *et al.* 1986) and the kinetics of attachment and outgrowth were not different to complex media containing serum. It is thought that such attachment factors bind to surface proteoglycans, particularly heparin/heparan sulphate, on the embryonic surface. Of interest, a heparin-binding protein secreted by platelets upon activation, platelet factor 4 (PF4) also supports some outgrowth *in vitro* (Farach *et al.* 1987).

Thus, localized platelet activation by embryo-derived PAF may produce a range of molecules which support the attachment of the embryo to the uterine surface and thus promote the invasive growth associated with active implantation.

Role of platelet activation in the function of the corpus luteum

Platelets from a number of species produces the biogenic amine, serotonin (5-hydroxytryptamine). This has an extensive range of bio-activities, including the stimulation of the production of progesterone by the cells of the corpus luteum (Battista *et al.* 1989). Continued production of progesterone is essential for the maintenance of pregnancy. In females who do not achieve pregnancy the corpus luteum has a preprogrammed life-span. In pregnancy a number of mechanisms are in place to maintain and extend the function of the corpus luteum and these mechanisms are dependent on the presence of the early embryo. Data from a number of species, including the bovine, have shown that the progesterone concentration is higher in pregnant compared with non-pregnant animals even prior to implantation. Battista *et al.* (1989) have proposed that the activation of platelets by embryo-derived PAF may cause this. They have shown that relatively high concentrations of serotonin are present in the corpus luteum tissue and bovine platelets had a concentration of serotonin of 538.8 ng/litre $\times 10^8$ platelets. Co-incubation of luteal cells *in vitro* with washed platelets resulted in a significant enhancement of progesterone production. This occurred whether PAF was present or not. However, it is worth noting that under both circumstances platelets would have become activated: in the presence of PAF, by the PAF itself, in its absence, by the presence of Ca^{2+} in the culture media coupled with surface activation by the culture vessel. This enhancement of progesterone secretion was blocked by pre-incubation with the serotonin receptor antagonist, mianserin, but not by indomethocin.

These results suggest, in the bovine at least, that embryo-induced platelet activation may have a functional luteotrophic action by the secretion of active agents, probably serotonin, but possibly acting in concert with other platelet-derived mediators.

Conclusions

Thus, platelet activation may act physiologically to help support the initiation and maintenance of pregnancy by provision of embryotrophic attachment and luteotrophic factors. As well as this action of embryo-derived PAF via platelets, it has a more direct action. Platelet activating factor acts as a direct autocrine growth factor for the pre-implantation embryo (human and mouse); this action is essential for the initiation of pregnancy (O'Neill *et al.* 1989; Ryan *et al.* 1989, 1990a,b), furthermore PAF acts to suppress the oxytocin induced secretion of the luteolysin $PGF_{2\alpha}$ from the ovine uterus (Battye *et al.* 1989). It remains to be determined whether this action is a direct action of PAF or is mediated by the activation of secondary cells such as platelets.

The production of embryo-derived PAF with its broad range of consequent actions including activation of blood platelets, provides a new paradigm for the understanding of the physiology of the establishment of pregnancy and presents possible new targets for therapeutic intervention.

The involvement of platelets in pathologies of pregnancy

Thrombocytopenia in pregnancy

Hypertension in pregnancy

For the practising obstetrician this is probably the most common presentation of thrombocytopenia. It is seen in about 15% of pre-eclamptics and 30% of eclamptics (Ritchard *et al.* 1976; Kleckner *et al.* 1977). In early pre-eclampsia the platelet count drops slightly (Redman *et al.* 1978), probably secondary to consumption and a shorter platelet life-span (Rakoczi *et al.* 1979; Boner *et al.* 1980). Even without any change in the number of platelets the platelets tend to be younger and larger in pre-eclamptic women (Stubbs *et al.* 1986). Platelet activation is changed. Platelet-activation tests such as measuring platelet-specific protein, β-thromboglobulins, platelet 5-hydroxytryptamine levels and platelet aggregation tests all confirm these changes in pre-eclampsia (Redman *et al.* 1977; Whigham *et al.* 1978; Douglas *et al.* 1982).

The causes of the platelet changes in pre-eclampsia are not well understood. It is tempting to postulate that it is caused by a change in prostanoid metabolism altering the balance between prostacyclin and thromboxane affects on platelet aggregation and vascular tone. This would explain many other features of the micro-angiopathic affects of pre-eclampsia. However, only 15–29% of women with pre-eclampsia show a reduction in their platelet count (Kleckner *et al.* 1977) and it is hard, therefore, to contemplate this as a universal cause.

In severe pre-eclampsia, disseminated intravascular coagulation (DIC) can occur. This is much more likely if hepatic involvement also occurs (Killam *et al.*

1975). As the consumption of coagulation factors proceeds and the activation of the fibrinolytic system exacerbates the coagulopathy the platelet count will begin to decrease as well.

The third presentation of thrombocytopenia and pre-eclampsia is the HELLP (haemolysis, elevated liver transaminases and low platelet count) syndrome (Weinstein, 1982). These patients present with haemolytic anaemia, elevated liver transaminases and low platelet counts. They often have relatively benign hypertension and often feel well. The fall in platelet count can be dramatic and can often start or go on for a few days after delivery. Monitoring of the platelet count post partum is therefore very important. Occasionally these patients present with fulminating hepatorenal failure, DIC, and very high blood pressure.

The management of these hypertension-associated thrombocytopenias is based on gestation, severity of hypertension, other biochemical changes, and the laboratory and clinical evidence of coagulopathies. Systemic lupus erythematosus, auto-immune thrombocytopenia and drug-induced thrombocytopenia should be excluded. The mild changes in platelet counts in mild to moderate pre-eclampsia do not alter the management of the patient and no treatment is needed. In severe pre-eclampsia and eclampsia there is often multisystem failure with the coagulation system being just one of many systems failing. A dramatic fall in the platelet count is generally an indication for delivery. If Caesarian section is indicated then a platelet transfusion will be necessary if the platelet count is below $50\,000 \times 10^9$/litre. If vaginal delivery is contemplated then the usual haemostatic measures of syntocinon, ergometrine, rapid delivery of the placenta and meticulous haemostasis of the episiotomy site will often be enough to maintain haemostasis after delivery. This is because the principal haemostasic action after delivery is uterine contraction.

Most anaesthetists would consider an epidural anaesethic contraindicated if the platelet count is less than $100\,000 \times 10^9$/litre. Intramuscular injections should be avoided and the patient should be delivered in a hospital with ready access to blood products. There is no evidence that heparin, steroids or gammaglobulin infusions are of value. Long-term treatment of pre-eclampsia with low-dose aspirin appears to be efficacious in early trials (Trudinger *et al.* 1988). Aspirin given in this way does not affect platelet counts but does affect platelet function in a minimal and predictable way.

Disseminated intravascular coagulation

Modern obstetric management and the option of early delivery because of improved neonatal care has meant that obstetric DIC is now relatively uncommon. Acute causes of DIC in pregnancy include placental abruption, infection, termination of pregnancy, amniotic fluid embolism, uterine rupture and incompatible blood transfusion. More chronic causes include fetal death-*in-utero* and pre-eclampsia (Colvin, 1985).

Thrombocytopenia in DIC is secondary to consumption of platelets because of the multiple thrombotic lesions that form during the process. Other possibilities for thrombocytopenia in DIC are adhesion to damaged endothelial surfaces, aggregation of platelets by thrombin, immune complexes and endotoxins (Romero & Duffy, 1980).

Thrombocytopenia is only one aspect of DIC and it must be managed with an emphasis on a number of priorities. The first is to treat the cause. In placental abruption the uterus should be emptied as quickly as possible. Infection must be treated very aggressively and may need definitive surgical management. Trauma to the genital tract must be repaired.

General resuscitation must be undertaken to maintain homeostasis. Blood pressure, arterial oxygenation, urine output and biochemical balance have to be maintained. Replacement of blood products needs to be tailored to the specific deficiencies and to the clinical situation. If the patient is exanguinating then fresh-screened whole blood is best. If volume is being maintained then concentrates of platelets, blood factors, fresh frozen plasma and packed cells are best used. The theoretical problem of 'feeding the fire' with coagulation products does not occur in clinical practice (Colvin, 1985).

If the DIC is secondary to a retained death-*in-utero* and for whatever reason the foetus cannot be delivered then low-dose heparin therapy can be used. If this is used then the platelet count should be kept above $50\,000 \times 10^9$/litre (Laros, 1986) using platelet infusions.

Auto-immune thrombocytopenia purpura

Because auto-immune thrombocytopenia purpura (AITP) occurs most commonly in young women it is relatively common in pregnant women. The antibody to the platelets is usually IgG (Van Leeuwen *et al.* 1981) which can cross the placenta and affect the fetal platelets. Even if the woman has had a splenectomy to increase the platelet count the fetal reticulo-endothelial system will still clear the antibody-linked platelets and cause fetal and neonatal thrombocytopenia with its inherent birth risks.

The maternal platelet count generally correlates very poorly with the fetal platelet count (Kelton *et al.* 1982). Measurement of maternal serum platelet antibody correlates reasonably well with the neonatal platelet count although there appear to be individual exceptions (Scott *et al.* 1984). Measurement of platelet-associated IgG is a less accurate predictor (Cines *et al.* 1982; Kelton *et al.* 1982).

Initial management is aimed at raising the maternal platelet count. Corticosteroids are the main method and the platelet count is aimed to be kept above $50\,000 \times 10^9$/litre. Of all patients 70–90% will have some response. Splenectomy is relatively contraindicated in pregnancy because of the 10% maternal mortality, high premature labour rate and high rate of fetal loss (Tancer, 1960). These figures are now 30 years old but there appear to be no more recent figures. Maternal immunosuppression therapy is also contraindicated in pregnancy.

Recently intravenous IgG infusions have been used with good success. This is thought to work partly through retico-endothelial blockade but also through other unknown actions (Bussell & Hilgartner, 1984). The platelet count starts rising about 4 days after the start of treatment, peaks 5 days later and stays elevated for approximately 3 weeks. About 80% of women respond. The disadvantages of this therapy are the occasional non-responder or partial responder and the possibility of blood-borne infections being transmitted (Lever *et al.* 1984) (although some manufactured products appear to be free of this complication).

The mode of delivery is difficult to assess. Most clinical practitioners will perform a Caesarian section if the maternal platelet count is below $50\,000 \times 10^9$/litre. If the maternal platelet count is above $50\,000 \times 10^9$/litre then fetal scalp vein sampling has been advocated by Scott *et al.* (1980). However, the cervix needs to be at least 2–3 cm dilated before this can be done. Our clinical practise is to do this on all labouring women with a diagnosis of AITP.

Allo-immune thrombocytopenia

The platelet antigen PL^{A1} is possessed by 98% of women. If they are negative for the antigen, and the fetus carries the antigen then antiPL^{A1} antibodies can be formed and cross the placenta. This can cause severe neonatal and fetal thrombocytopenia. Only 1–2% of pregnancies are affected, but perinatal mortality is 25–35%. First pregnancies are often affected (Surainder *et al.* 1981).

The risk of serious *in-utero* haemorrhage is high. The diagnosis of allo-immune thrombocytopenia is made either after an affected pregnancy or by detection of maternal platelet antibodies (not a routine antenatal investigation). It has not always been possible to detect PL^{A1} so other antibodies may be involved.

If the diagnosis is made during pregnancy then intra-uterine platelet estimations and transfusions via cordocentesis appears to be the treatment of choice. The transfusions use PL^{A1} negative platelets. Once delivered the neonate can be transfused with washed maternal platelets if no PL^{A1} negative platelets are available. Steroids and gammaglobulin infusions are also used (Colvin, 1985).

Systemic lupus erythematosus

About a third of patients with systemic lupus erythematosus (SLE) have thrombocytopenia although it is very rarely less than $30\,000 \times 10^9$/litre (Hughes, 1979). The thrombocytopenia often occurs long before any clinical manifestations of SLE. As long as the platelet count remains above $50\,000 \times 10^9$/litre, little needs to be done about it. If the count falls below $50\,000 \times 10^9$/litre then steroid therapy is indicated. These patients often have platelet-associated IgG (McMillan, 1983). The main clinical problem with these patients is the possible presence of lupus anticoagulant and anticardiolipin antibodies. Paradoxically this causes thrombosis rather than haemorrhage. These can be deep venous thromboses, pulmonary embolus, cerebrovascular occlusion and renal vessel occlusion (Colvin, 1985). There is also a higher rate of spontaneous abortion, death-*in-utero* and perinatal mortality.

Thrombotic thrombocytopenia purpura and haemolytic ureamic syndrome

Thrombotic thrombocytopenia purpura (TTP) is a very rare syndrome consisting of thrombocytopenia, microangiopathic anaemia, renal impairment, neurological dysfunction and fever (Colvin, 1985). Haemolytic uraemic syndrome (HUS) is similar, except that it occurs more often in children, often in epidemic form, often after gastrointestinal (GIT) upsets and renal failure is more common. Both of these syndromes possibly occur more commonly in pregnancy but their rarity precludes an absolute answer.

Thrombotic thrombocytopenia purpura is not diagnosed by a single investigation. The platelet count is usually low, fibrinogen degradation products are low and clotting studies are normal (distinguishing this disease from DIC). Haemolytic anaemia is diagnosed from the blood film. Gingival biopsy may demonstrate hyaline thrombi in small arterioles in about 50% of cases (Myers *et al.* 1980). It appears that large numbers of Factor VIII: vWF multimers are present when these patients are in remission which may be of some potential help in management (Moake *et al.* 1982).

Treatment is difficult especially when pregnant but prednisone, oral antiplatelet aggregation drugs (aspirin and dipyridamole) and plasma exchange are usually first line. Fresh frozen plasma will occasionally give quite remarkable results (Colvin, 1985). Prostacyclin infusions can be considered but results have been poor (Machin, 1984). As discussed before, splenectomy and immunosuppression should be avoided in pregnancy.

Drug-induced thrombocytopenia

There are many drugs which are associated with thrombocytopenia. Some of the most common ones are shown in Table 9.1 in a list compiled by Romero and Duffy (1980).

The actions of drug-induced thrombocytopenias are often not known but possible mechanisms are depression of bone marrow production or release, immune-related platelet destruction or direct toxic effects (Romero & Duffy, 1980). There is no evidence of increased drug-induced thrombocytopenia in pregnancy.

Heparin-induced thrombocytopenia is of particular interest. The reported incidence is extremely variable. It is thought to be immune-related. The platelet count starts declining 3–8 days after therapy begins and reaches its lowest point 2–3 days later. If heparin is stopped the count returns to normal generally within 5 days. It is paradoxically associated with increased thrombo-embolism.

Table 9.1 Drugs associated with thrombocytopenia

Analgesics	*Anticoagulants*
Acetaminophen	Heparin
Acetylsalicylic acid	*Anticonvulsants*
Oxyphenbutazone	Barbiturates
Antibacterial drugs	Diphenylhydantoin
Ampicillin	*Antihypertensive drugs*
Cephalothin	Alpha-methyldopa
Isoniazid	Diazoxide
Para-amino salicyclate (PAS)	Hydralazine
Rifampicin	Hydralazine
Ristocetin	*Cardiac drugs*
Sulphonamides	Digitoxin
Diuretics	Quinidine
Acetazolamide	*Miscellaneous*
Furosemide	Oestrogens
Thiazides	Alcohol

Treatment of drug-associated thrombocytopenia is to cease all medications. Steroids and platelet infusions are of only short-term benefit if at all. If close to delivery the possibility of a low fetal platelet count should be considered and possibly checked.

Infection

Thrombocytopenia can occur in almost all types of infections. If the patient becomes septic it is much more common. The incidence in septicaemia has been reported to be as high as 77% (Riedler *et al.* 1971). The cause of thrombocytopenia in these infections is often a combination of bone marrow depression and platelet destruction. For example, decreased fetal and neonatal bone marrow production of platelets occurs in CMV and rubella infection. Platelet destruction can also occur either by direct endothelial damage or accelerated clearance by the reticulo-endothelial system. For example clostridial infection of retained products of conception will often result in thrombocytopenia secondary to toxin-mediated destruction.

Haemorrhage-related thrombocytopenia

Despite modern preventative measures the occasional pregnant woman will still have either a massive antepartum or postpartum haemorrhage. These are usually related to problems of placentation. Even if DIC does not ensue these patients will often have a low platelet count because of the sheer extent of blood loss.

Post-transfusion purpura

This is a rare syndrome occurring about 1–2 weeks after transfusion (Morrison & Mollison, 1966). It occurs in women who are platelet-specific antigen Pl^{A1} negative. This is only 2% of the population. The syndrome will present 1–2 weeks after transfusion with haemorrhagic manifestations. The platelet count is low, bone marrow megakaryocyte numbers are normal and platelet antibodies are positive (Abramson *et al.* 1974; Romero & Duffy, 1980).

The thrombocytopenia resolves in about 2 weeks but can go on for longer. If severe, plasmaphoresis or exchange transfusion can be contemplated.

Medical diseases in pregnancy

Many medical diseases will have thrombocytopenia as part of their syndrome. For example, severe hepatitis or cirrhosis of the liver often exhibit associated thrombocytopenia. Leukaemias, especially if treated with cytotoxic therapy, and pancytopenias will often have decreased platelet counts. Sometimes treatment of these patients will be compromised by the fact that they are pregnant and the patient may come to delivery still with a low platelet count. The management of the delivery is based on the level of the count and its short-term treatment possibilities.

Functional platelet diseases

A prolonged bleeding time in the face of a normal platelet count and normal coagulation studies characterize qualitative platelet disorders. These are rare but can be primary or secondary. An example of a primary disorder is the Bernard–Soulier syndrome (BSS). This is a disease of the defective platelet membrane 1B (Laros, 1986). Another example is Glanzmann's thromboasthenia, where the platelets have a defect in glycoproteins IIb and IIIa (Laros, 1986).

If at least two classes of platelet-specific subcellular granules are deficient then platelet function is also affected.

Secondary forms of functional platelet diseases include drug ingestation. Aspirin is easily the most important and most common. Aspirin irreversibly inhibits the cyclooxygenase enzyme necessary for the synthesis of thromboxane (Romero & Duffy, 1980). The effect can last for a week and as little as a single 300-mg dose will be effective. There is early evidence that this can be put to therapeutic use in some diseases of pregnancy which have a microvascular component, for example, pre-eclampsia (Trudinger *et al.* 1988).

Diseases such as uraemia, myeloproliferative disorders and protein disorders can also result in functional platelet deficiencies.

Thrombocytosis

Essential or primary thrombocythemia is a myeloproliferative disease. It occurs usually in patients between 30 and 60 years old (Gurs, 1960). It is a rare disease and even rarer in pregnant women. Not only is the platelet count extremely high but platelet function is deranged. The Polycythemia Vera Study Group now accepts $600\,000 \times 10^9$/litre as the lower limit for diagnosis. The platelets show decreased aggregation (Jones *et al.* 1988). The disease can present clinically with either thrombotic and/or haemorrhagic symptoms but may also be completely asymptomatic. It is thought to be more benign in younger patients (Houghland & Silverstein, 1978), but this is controversial (Mercer *et al.* 1988).

There are only a small number of cases reported with pregnant patients. There does appear to be an increase in early and later pregnancy failures, placental problems and fetal growth (Jones *et al.* 1983; Falconer *et al.* 1987; Mercer *et al.* 1988). However, some authors question whether the small number of anecdotal cases is enough to support this (Linares *et al.* 1988).

Most authors seem to use platelet anti-aggregating therapy (aspirin and/or dipyridamol). Some authors use heparin in addition, and some use phoresis (Mercer *et al.* 1988). They claim anecdotal improvements in pregnancy outcome compared with their patients' previous histories. Some authors query the use of platelet anti-aggregating drugs because of the lack of scientific evidence and the lack of knowledge about whether the obstetric complications are secondary to haemorrhagic or thrombotic affects.

References

Abramson, N., Eisenberg, P.D. & Aster, R.H. (1974) Post transfusion purpura. Immunologic aspects and therapy. *New En J Med* **291**, 1163.

Acker, G., Hecquet, F., Etienne, A., Braquet, P. & Mencia-Huerta, J.M. (1988) Role of platelet activating factor (PAF) in the ovoimplantation in the rat: Effect of the specific PAF-acether antagonist, BN 52021. *Prostaglandins* **35**, 233–241.

Armant, D.R., Kaplan H.A. & Lennarz, W.J. (1986) Fibronectin and laminin promote *in vitro* attachment and outgrowth of mouse blastocysts. *Develop Biol* **116**, 519–523.

Aster, R.H. (1966) Pooling of platelets in the spleen: Role in the pathogenesis of 'hypersplenic' thrombocytopenia. *J Clin Invest* **45**, 645–656.

Battista, P.J., Alila, H.W., Rexroad, C.E. & Hansel, W. (1989) The effects of platelet-activating factor and platelet-derived compounds on bovine luteal cell progesterone production. *Biol Reprod* **40**, 769–775.

Battye, K.M., Evans. G. & O'Neill, C. (1989) A role for platelet activating factor in maintenance of the ovine corpus luteum. *Proc Aust Soc Reprod Biol* **21**, 32.

Bonen, B., Fournie, A., Sie P., Grandjean, H., Bierme, R. & Pontannier, G. (1980) Platelet production time, uricaemia and some hemostasis tests in pre-eclampsia. *Eur J Obstet Gynaecol Reprod Biol* **11**, 85–94.

Brodsky, I., Dennis, L.H., Kahn, S.B. & Brady, L.W. (1966) Normal mouse erythropoieses. The role of the spleen in mouse erythropoiesis. *Cancer Res* **26**, 198–201.

Bussell, J.M. & Hilgartner, M.V. (1984) The use and mechanism of action of intravenous immunoglobulin in the treatment of immune haematological disease. *Br J Haematol* **56**, 1–7.

Camussi, G., Tetta, C. & Bussolino, F. (1983) Inhibitory effect of prostacyclin (PGI_2) on neutropenia induced by intravenous injection of platelet-activating factor (PAF) in the rabbit. *Prostaglandins* **25**, 343–351.

Cines, D.B., Dusak, B., Tomaski, A., Mennuti, M. & Schreiber, A.D. (1982) Immune thrombocytopenic purpura and pregnancy. *New Engl J Med* **306**, 826–831.

Collier, M., O'Neill, C., Ammit, A.J. & Saunders, D.M. (1988) Biochemical and pharmacological characterisation of human embryo-derived platelet activating factor. *Human Reprod.* **3**, 993–998.

Colvin, B.T. (1985) Thrombocytopenia. In Letsky, E.A. (ed.), *Haematological Disorders in Pregnancy. Clinics in Haematology 14*, pp. 661–681. W.B. Saunders, London.

Douglas, J.T., Shah, M., Lowe, G.D.O., Belch, J.J.F., Forbes, C.D. & Prentice, C.R.M. (1982) Fibrinopeptide A and beta-thromboglobulin in pre-eclampsia and pregnancy hypertension. *Thromb Haematol* **47**, 54–55.

Falconer, J., Pineo, G., Blahey, W., Bowen, T., Docksteader, B. & Jadusingh, I. (1987) Essential thrombocythemia associated with recurrent abortions and fetal growth retardation. *Am J Hematol* **25**, 345–347.

Farach, M.C., Tang, J.P., Decker, G.L. & Carson, D.D. (1987) Heparin/Heparan sulfate is involved in attachment and spreading of mouse embryos *in vitro*. *Develop Biol* **123**, 401–410.

Frojmovic, M.M. & Milton, J.G. (1982) Human platelet size, shape, and related functions in health and disease. *Physiol Rev* **62**, 185–261.

Gasic, G.J. & Gasic, T.B. (1970) Total suppression of pregnancy in mice by post-coital administration of neuraminidase. *Proc Natl Acad Sci USA* (1970), **67**, 793–798.

Grayson, J. & Mendel, D. (1965) *Physiology of the Splanchnic Circulation*. Edward Arnold Ltd, London.

Gunz, F.W. (1960) Hemorrhagic thrombocythemia: A critical review. *Blood* **15**, 706.

Guyton, A.C. (1971) *Textbook of Medical Physiology*, 5th edn. W.B. Saunders Co., Philadelphia.

Horger, E.O. & Keane, M.W.D. (1979) Platelet disorders in pregnancy. *Clin Obstet Gynecol* **4**, 843–857.

Hougland, H.C. & Silverstein, M.N. (1978) Primary thrombocythemia in the young patient. *Mayo Clin Proc* **53**, 578.

Hughes, G.R.V. (1979) Systemic lupus erthematosus. In Hughes, G.R.V. (ed.), *Connective Tissue Diseases*. Blackwell Scientific Publications, Oxford.

Jones, E.C., Mosesson, M.W., Thomason, J.L. & Jackson, T.C. (1988) Essential thrombocythemia in pregnancy. *Obstet Gynaecol* **71**, 501–503.

Kelton, J.C., Inwood, M.J., Barr, R.M. *et al.* (1982) The prenatal prediction of thrombocytopenia in infants of mothers with clinically diagnosed immune thrombocytopenia. *Am J Obstet Gynecol* **144**, 449–54.

Killam, A., Dillard, S., Patton, R. & Pederson, P. (1975) Pregnancy induced hypertension complicated by acute liver disease and disseminated intravascular coagulation. *Am J Obstet Gynecol* **123**, 823–828.

Kleckner, H.B., Giles, H.R. & Corrigan, J.J. (1977) The association of maternal and neonatal thrombocytopenia in high-risk pregnancies. *Am J Obstet Gynecol* **128**, 235–238.

Laros, R.K. (1986) Acquired coagulation disorders. In Laros, R.K. (ed.) *Blood Disorders in Pregnancy*, 1st edn. Lea and Febiger, Philadelphia.

Layendecker, S.J. & McDonald, T.P. (1982) The relative roles of the spleen and bone marrow in platelet production in mice. *Exp Hematol.* **10**, 334–342.

Lever, A.M.L., Webster, A.D.B., Brown, D. & Thomas, H.C. (1984) Non A, Non-B-Hepatitis occurring agammaglobulinaemic patients after intravenous immunoglobulin. *Lancet* **ii**, 1062–1064.

Linares, M., Pastor, E., Jarque, I., Sanz, G. & Sanz, M. (1988) Essential thrombocythemia and pregnancy. *Am J Hematol* **28**, 66 (letter).

Machin, S.J. (1984) Thrombcytopenic purpura. *Br J Haematol* **56**, 191–197.

McMillan, R. (1983) Immune thrombocytopenia. *Clin Haematol* **12**, 64–88.

Mercer, B., Drouin, J., Jolley, E. & d'Anjou, G. (1988) Primary thrombocythemia in pregnancy: A report of two cases. *Am J Obstet Gynecol* **159**, 127–128.

Metcalf, W.K. & Metcalf, N.F. (1972) Platelets, pregnancy and phytohemagglutinin. *Am J Obstet Gynecol* **114**, 602–606.

Moake, J.L., Rudy, C.K., Troll, J.H. *et al.* (1982) Usually large plasma factor VIII: Von Willebrand factor multimers in chronic relapsing thrombotic thrombocytopenic purpura. *New Engl J Med* **307**, 1432.

Morrison, F.S. & Mollison, P.L. (1966) Post transfusion purpura. *New Engl J. Med* **275**, 243.

Myers, T.H., Waken, C.T., Ball, E.D. & Tremont, S.J. (1980) Thrombotic thrombocytopenic purpura: Combined treatment with plasmapherosis and antiplatelet agents. *Ann Intern Med* **92**, 149.

O'Dell, T.T. & Murphy, J.R. (1974) Effects of degree of thrombocytopenia of thrombopoietic response. *Blood* **44**, 147–156.

O'Neill, C. (1985a) Thrombocytopenia is a initial maternal response to fertilisation in mice. *J Reprod Fert* **73**, 567–577.

O'Neill, C. (1985b) Examination of the causes of early pregnancy associated thrombocytopenia in mice. *J Reprod Fert* **73**, 578–585.

O'Neill, C. (1985c) Partial characterisation of the embryo-derived platelet activating factor in mice. *J Reprod Fert* **75**, 375–380.

O'Neill, C. (1986) The role of blood platelets in the establishment of pregnancy. In Han, J. (ed.) *Pregnancy Proteins In Animals*, pp. 225–234. Walter de Gruyter, Berlin.

O'Neill, C., Amos, E., Mote, P. & Gidley-Baird, A. (1986) Histological and Ultrastructural evidence for platelet activation in the Reproductive Tract. *Proc Aust Soc Reprod Biol* **18**, 11.

O'Neill, C., Collier, M. & Saunders, D.M. (1988) Embryo-derived PAF: Its diagnostic and therapeutic future. *Ann NY Acad Sci* **541**, 398–406.

O'Neill, C., Gidley-Baird, A.A., Pike, I.L., Porter, R.N., Sinosich, M.J. & Saunders, D.M. (1985a) Maternal blood platelet physiology and luteal phase endocrinology as a means of monitoring pre and post implantation embryo viability following *in vitro* fertilisation. *J in vitro Fertiliz Embryo Trans* **2**, 59–65.

O'Neill, C., Pike, I.L., Porter, R.N., Gidley-Baird,

A.A., Sinosich, M.J. & Saunders, D.M. (1985b) Maternal recognition of pregnancy prior to implantation — methods of monitoring embryonic viability *in vitro* and *in vivo*. *Ann NY Acad Sci* **442**, 429–439.

O'Neill, C., Ryan, J.P., Collier, M., Saunders, D.M., Ammit, A.J. & Pike, I.L. (1989) Supplementation of IVF culture media with platelet activating factor (PAF) increased the pregnancy rate following embryo transfer. *Lancet* **ii**, 769–772.

Pennington, D.G., Lee, N.L.Y., Roxborough, A.E. & McCready J.R. (1976) Platelet density and size: The interpretation of heterogeneity. *Br J Haematol* **37**, 365–370.

Pritchard, J.A., Cunningham, F.G. & Mason, R.A. (1976) Coagulation changes in eclampsia: Their frequency and pathogenesis. *Am J Obstet Gynecol* **124**, 855–864.

Rakoczi, I., Tallian, F., Bagdany, S. & Gati, I. (1979) Platelet life-span in normal pregnancy and pre-eclampsia as determined by a non-radiosotope technique. *Thromb Res* **15**, 553–556.

Redman, C.W.G., Allington, M.J., Bolton, F.G. & Stirrat, G.M. (1977) Plasma β-thromboglobulin in pre-eclampsia. *Lancet* **ii**, 248.

Redman, C.W.G., Bonnar, J. & Beilin, L.J. (1978) Early platelet consumption in pre-eclampsia. *Br Med J* **1**, 467–469.

Riedler, G.F., Straub, P.W. & Frick, P.G. (1971) Thrombocytopenia in speticemia. *Hel Med Acta* **36**, 23.

Romero, R. & Duffy, T.P. (1980) Platelet disorders in pregnancy. *Clin. Perinatol* **7**, 327–348.

Ryan, J.P., O'Neill, C. & Wales, R.G. (1990a) Oxidate metabolism of energy substrates by preimplantation mouse embryos in the presence of platelet activating factor. *J Reprod Fert* (in press).

Ryan, J.P., Spinks, N.R., O'Neill, C., Ammit, A.J. & Wales, R.G. (1989) Platelet activating factor (PAF) production by mouse embryos *in vitro* and its effects on embryonic metabolism. *J Cell Biochem* **40**, 387–395.

Ryan, J.P., Spinks, N.R., O'Neill, C. & Wales, R.G. (1990b) Implantation potential and fetal viability of mouse embryos cultured in media supplemented with platelet activating factor. *J Reprod Fert* (in press).

Sasaki, K. & Ito, T. (1981) Effects of estrogen and progesterone on the spleen of the mouse: A light and electron microscopic study. *Arch Histol Jap* **44**, 203–213.

Sasaki, K., Matsumura, G. & Ito, T. (1981) Effects of pregnancy on erythropoiesis and splenic red pulp of the mouse: A quantitative electron microscopic study. *Arch Histol Jap* **44**, 429–438.

Scott, J.R. Cruikshank, D.P., Kochenour, N.K., Pitkin, R.M. & Warenski, J.C. (1980) Fetal platelet counts in obstetric management of immunologic thrombocytopenic purpura. *Am J Obstet Gynecol* **136**, 495–499.

Scott, J.R., Rote, N.S. & Cruikshank, D.P. (1983) Antiplatelet antibodies and platelet counts in pregnancies complicated by autoimmune thrombocytopenic purpura. *Am J Obstet Gynecol* **145**, 932–939.

Sejeny, S.A., Eastham, R.D. & Baker, S.R. (1975) Platelet counts during normal pregnancy. *J Clin Pathol* **28**, 812–813.

Spinks, N.R. & O'Neill, C. (1988) Antagonists of embryo-derived platelet activating factor prevent implantation of mouse embryos. *J Reprod Fert (1988)*, **84**, 89–98.

Spinks, N.R., Ryan, J.P. & O'Neill, C. (1990) Antagonists of embryo-derived platelet activating factor act by inhibiting the mouse embryos capacity for implantation. *J Reprod Fert* (in press).

Stubbs, T.M., Lazarchik, J., Van Dorsten, J.P., Cox, J. & Loadholt, C.B. (1986) Evidence of accelerated platelet production and consumption in non thrombocytopenic pre-eclampsia. *Am J Obstet Gynecol* **155**, 263–265.

Surainder, S.Y., Bellar, B., Choudry, A., Chilis, T.J. & Rao, S. (1981) Isoimmune thrombocytopenia: Coordinated management of mother and infant. *Obstet Gynecol* **57**, 124–128.

Tancer, M.L. (1960) Idiopathic thrombocytopenic purpura and pregnancy. *Am J Obstet Gynecol* **79**, 148.

Trudinger, B.J., Cook, C.M., Thompson, R.S., Giles, W.B. & Connelly, A. (1988) Low dose aspirin therapy improves fetal weight in umbilical placental insufficiency. *Am J Obstet Gynecol* **159**, 681–685.

Van Leeuwen, E.F., Helmerhorst, F.M., Engelfriet, C.P. & Von Dem Borne, A.E.G. (1981) Maternal autoimmune thrombocytopenia and the newborn. *Br Med J* **283**, 104.

Weinstein, L. (1982) Syndrome of hemolysis elevated liver enzymes and low platelet count. A severe consequence of hypertension in pregnancy. *Am J Obstet Gynecol* **142**, 159–167.

Whigham, K.A.E., Howie, P.W., Drummond, A.H. & Prentice, C.R.M. (1978) Abnormal platelet function in pre-eclampsia. *Br J Obstet. Gynaecol* **85**, 28–32.

10: The Contribution of Platelets to Pulmonary Embolism

John E. Kaplan and Asrar B. Malik

Introduction

Platelets are frequently an important component of emboli found within the pulmonary circulation. In addition to contributing to obstruction of pulmonary vessels, platelets release a myriad of bioactive molecules. The functional consequences of platelet embolization, particularly with respect to pulmonary vessels and airways, has been a fertile field of investigation.

Pulmonary embolism can be considered to embrace two significantly different pathologies. The first results as a complication of venous thrombosis. This syndrome occurs upon dislodgement of thrombi which usually originate in the deep veins of the leg. Platelets can be observed in thrombi as relatively homogeneous zones of degranulated and partially degranulated platelets separated by erythrocytes enmeshed in fibrin. Leukocytes are generally present along the margins of these platelet masses. Fibrin strands attached directly to the platelet masses are most dense in these regions. Thrombi can have quite variable platelet content. The platelet content depends, mainly, on maintained blood flow which continues to deliver platelets to the site of the thrombus. This produces a white 'head' on the thrombus facing the upstream direction. These venous thrombi contain variable, often low, platelet content. Platelets may also become involved in the response to such pulmonary embolism as a result of platelet attachment to the thrombi after detachment from the vein and as a result of secondary thrombosis after occlusive embolization in the pulmonary vasculature.

Pulmonary embolism also includes microemboli that may develop in response to injury, sepsis and with pathologies associated with the initiation of disseminated thrombosis. Circulating platelet aggregates with the potential to embolize in the lungs have been demonstrated (Wu & Hoak, 1974). Microemboli containing platelets, fibrin and leukocytes are frequently associated with pulmonary dysfunction. The findings of pulmonary platelet sequestration and thrombocytopenia associated with the adult respiratory distress syndrome (ARDS) have implicated a role for the platelet in the development of pulmonary insufficiency and oedema.

The goal of this chapter is to review the role of platelets in pulmonary embolism. Emphasis will be placed on disseminated microembolization rather than large pulmonary emboli because of our more complete understanding of the contribution of platelets in the former process. The functional consequences of platelet embolization, particularly those which lead to pulmonary dysfunction, will be stressed. In addition, we will describe current studies of the interaction of platelets with pulmonary endothelium.

A large body of data has contributed to the concept that platelet emboli are involved in the pathophysiology of pulmonary oedema and the resultant ARDS. These studies have indicated that platelet aggregation and release influence the pulmonary pressor response, not only by mechanical obstruction but primarily as the result of release of vasoactive materials (Vaage & Hauge, 1977; Vaage, 1977, 1982). Evidence indicates an important role for platelet release products in the induction of increased airway resistance (Vaage & Hauge, 1977; Vaage, 1982). Increases in pulmonary capillary hydrostatic pressure can contribute to haemodynamically related alterations in pulmonary fluid balance (i.e. pulmonary oedema), whereas both vascular and airway responses may impair gas exchange as a result of ventilation–perfusion mismatching.

Less information exists concerning the possibility that platelet emboli contribute to the enhanced pulmonary vascular permeability and oedema formation. Data have clearly suggested that platelet products have the capacity to induce vascular permeability changes (Mustard *et al.* 1965; Nachman *et al.* 1972; Niewiarowski, 1977; Nachman, 1978); augmented permeability occurs in association with the development of thrombocytopenia and pulmonary sequestration of platelet aggregates (Vaage & Hauge 1977; Vaage, 1982). No clear evidence however, has linked platelets to the aetiology of increased pulmonary vascular permeability. Similarly, no evidence has been found to rule out such a possibility. These questions are further complicated by the concept that platelets may contribute to the maintenance of the integrity of vascular endothelium and its ability to act as a permeability barrier (Gimbrone *et al.* 1969; Johnson, 1971).

The probable basis for the unresolved role of the platelet derives from several facts. The platelet is a highly complex, and extremely reactive, cell fragment which interacts with most of the plasma and cellular participants of the inflammatory responses. Thus, platelets may not only contribute directly to the pulmonary vascular and airway response as effector cells but also can affect other cellular and plasma components, thereby leading to the generation of secondary signals. Moreover, studies addressing the role of the platelet in pulmonary dysfunction have been performed in numerous species utilizing highly variable experimental models and approaches. It is clear that platelets from different species are not equally reactive.

Platelet role and response in models of experimentally induced pulmonary dysfunction

The suggestion that platelet microembolization participates in the development of ARDS derives from the findings that acute lung injury in patients and experimental models is generally associated with the development of thrombocytopenia (Hill *et al.* 1975). Platelet sequestration and the histological determination of microemboli containing platelets, as well as fibrin and leukocytes, also indicate the involvement of platelets (Orell, 1971). These findings have been reinforced by the observation that agents which induce platelet aggregation, either as a primary effect or as part of a more complex response, induce ARDS-like syndromes which include increases in transcapillary fluid filtration and pulmonary oedema. A wide variety of experimental animal models of acute pulmonary dysfunction including those induced by trauma (Berman *et al.* 1971; Beal *et al.* 1987), haemorrhage (Bo & Hognestad, 1972), endotoxin (Stein & Thomas, 1967; Bredenberg *et al.* 1980; Almqvist *et al.* 1983), bacteria (Ljungquist & Schwartz, 1975), adenosine diphosphate (ADP) (Jorgensen *et al.* 1970; Vaage *et al.* 1974; Vaage, 1982), collagen (Bo & Hognestad, 1972; Vaage *et al.* 1974, 1976, 1978; Vaage & Gjesdal, 1976; Vaage & Hauge, 1977; Vaage 1980, 1982), thrombin (Mustard *et al.* 1965; Busch *et al.* 1974; Tahamont & Malik, 1983), antiplatelet serum (Vaage *et al.* 1974), glass beads (Mlczoch *et al.* 1978; Binder *et al.* 1980; Vaage, 1982), barium sulphate (Bo *et al.* 1974), protamine sulphate (Radegran & McAslan, 1972), fibrinogen degradation product D (Luterman *et al.* 1977; Manwaring *et al.* 1978; Manwaring & Curreri, 1980a), blood clots (Mayer *et al.* 1981), and transfusion of blood (Mayer *et al.* 1981) and blood components (Berman *et al.* 1976) have been associated with thrombocytopenia and/or pulmonary platelet sequestration. The pulmonary alterations (i.e. pulmonary hypertension, pulmonary vasoconstriction, and airway constriction), are in part ameliorated by prior induction of thrombocytopenia. There is a high incidence of thrombocytopenia in patients with acute respiratory failure of a variety of aetiologies (Hill *et al.* 1975; Schneider *et al.* 1980). Pulmonary platelet sequestration, as a corollary, has been demonstrated by external scintigraphy after injection of radiolabelled platelets and histologically in lung biopsy and autopsy specimens (Orell 1971; Schneider *et al.* 1980). Platelet survival time is decreased in these patients and platelet turnover is increased (Schneider *et al.* 1980). Both these changes are consistent with platelet consumption without depression of thrombopoiesis.

Several groups utilizing standardized animal models of shock, tissue injury, and sepsis have implicated a role for platelet embolization in pulmonary dysfunction. Hardaway and Johnson (1963) and McKay and Csavossy (1965) reported that endotoxin produces rapid thrombocytopenia and intravascular platelet aggregation in the pulmonary circulation. Stein and Thomas (1967) found that animals rendered thrombocytopenic by prior injection of endotoxin or after treatment with a serotonin antagonist did not respond to endotoxin injection with increased airway resistance and decreased lung compliance. Bo and Hognestad (1972) similarly determined that haemorrhagic hypotension resulted in a pulmonary pressor response and that thrombocytopenia obviated this effect. Bergentz *et al.* (1971) noted that labelled platelets were trapped in the lung during shock and trauma (Peer & Schwartz, 1973; Thorne *et al.* 1979). Subsequent studies confirmed these findings after tissue injury (Peer & Schwartz, 1973; Thorne *et al.* 1979), and during sepsis and haemorrhage (Ljungquist & Schwartz, 1975). Thrombocytopenia has been shown to ameliorate the early pulmonary hypertension occurring with endotoxin in dogs (Bredenberg *et al.* 1980) but is without effect in sheep (Snapper *et al.* 1984). McDonald *et al.* (1983) also found that thrombocytopenia produced no alteration in the pulmonary haemodynamic response to infusion of activated complement in sheep. However, the lack of a role of platelets in complement-induced pulmonary pressor response may derive from the lack of C3b receptors on sheep platelets (Henson & Ginsberg, 1981). These studies suggest that platelets mediate vascular and airway constriction, although they are not the exclusive mediators of these changes. Platelet-derived humoral mediators, such as serotonin, have been implicated as mediators of the vascular and airway response (Vaage, 1982).

Platelets and pulmonary dysfunction during experimentally induced pulmonary embolism

Various studies have utilized models to simulate pulmonary embolism including the infusion of platelet aggregating agents. In a series of studies Vaage and co-workers (Aursnes & Vaage, 1973; Vaage *et al.* 1974, 1976, 1978; Vaage & Gjesdal 1976; Vaage & Hauge 1977; Vaage, 1982) reported on the effects of experimentally induced platelet aggregation on pulmonary function. They primarily utilized soluble collagen infusion and to a lesser extent platelet aggregation induced by adenosine diphosphate, antiplatelet serum, and barium sulphate. These studies showed that the airway and vascular constriction depended on the presence of platelets and a stimulus which would induce platelet release as well as aggregation (Vaage *et al.* 1974; Vaage & Gjesdal, 1976). The increased pulmonary vascular resistance could be prevented by infusion of a vasodilator with the aggregating agent (Bo & Hognestad, 1972). In further studies a role for vagal reflex bronchoconstriction and for arachidonic acid metabolites in the response of airway and pulmonary vascular smooth muscle was implicated (Vaage, 1976; Vaage *et al.* 1978).

In addition, platelets have been implicated in other models of pulmonary embolism. Radegran and McAslan (1972) reported that the pulmonary response to injection of protamine sulphate in heparin-treated dogs, or to injection of thrombin, could be inhibited by acetylsalicylic acid. Mlczoch *et al.* (1978) reported that thrombocytopenic and antiplatelet drugs ameliorated the pulmonary hypertension and hypoxia seen with glass bead embolization. Binder *et al.* (1980) reported a similar effect in sheep after glass bead embolization. Manwaring *et al.* (1978) and Manwaring and Curreri (1980a,b) reported that platelets were an important component of the pulmonary dysfunction induced by infusion of fibrinogen degradation product D. Both the thrombocytopenia and the respiratory failure were inhibited by the antihistamine, diphenhydramine. Minnear *et al.* (1982) demonstrated that thrombocytopenia protected against the hypoxic response mediated by ADP-induced platelet aggregation. Brigham and Owen (1975a,b) and

Thompson *et al.* (1986) have demonstrated pulmonary vascular hypertension and hypoxemia following injection of 5-HT, a major platelet dense granular component. Thompson *et al.* (1986) also reported that 5-HT receptor blockade with ketanserin inhibited the increase in pulmonary vascular resistance and prevented hypoxemia and thrombocytopenia following infusion of an autologous clot. Ogletree (1982) and co-workers (Ogletree & Brigham, 1980) made similar observations after infusion of sodium arachidonate or a thromboxane mimic; therefore, arachidonate products released after platelet aggregation may be responsible for the pulmonary effects of platelet aggregation. Lelcuk *et al.* (1987) have similarly reported that inhibition of thromboxane synthesis moderates the increase in physiological shunt before intravenous infusion of clotted blood rich in platelets.

Platelets, vascular permeability, and pulmonary oedema

There is considerably more controversy regarding the role played by platelets in increased pulmonary vascular permeability and the development of pulmonary oedema. Transfusion of stored blood containing platelets leads to the development of endothelial damage and pulmonary oedema in dogs (Mayer *et al.* 1981). This effect is prevented by particulate filtration and has been attributed to platelet-rich microthrombi (Mayer *et al.* 1981). Berman *et al.* (1976) attributed the increase in pulmonary vascular permeability after transfusion of fresh blood to platelets.

Several studies support the capacity of platelets to induce endothelial damage and increased vascular permeability. Mustard *et al.* (1965) reported that stimulated platelets release permeability factors as judged by albumin accumulation in rabbit skin. Nachman (1978) and co-workers (Nachman *et al.* 1972) reported a permeability-enhancing activity in rabbit skin as a result of extracted cationic proteins obtained from platelet granules. The enhanced permeability was biphasic with an acute response dependent on histamine. The latter response was characterized by tissue leukocytosis secondary to complement activation and generation of C5a. Bignold (1980) reported that platelets injected into rat joints induced increased vascular permeability in synovial vessels. Erythrocytes, leukocytes, and plasma did not produce this effect. Braunstein *et al.* (1980) demonstrated that subcutaneous injection of platelet pellets (but not brain, heart, or kidney) induced an inflammatory response which included intense oedema. They suggested that the response may have been the result of the effects of the infiltrated leukocytes.

Jacob *et al.* (1982) have reported that platelets enhance the ability of complement-activated neutrophils to adhere to, and damage, cultured endothelial cells. This effect was mimicked by 5-HT and inhibited by 5-HT antagonists. These data indicate that platelets are capable of increasing vascular permeability. They also suggest that granulocytes are direct effectors, while platelets may regulate this action. This platelet–granulocyte interaction may be an important factor contributing to lung vascular injury. Previous data, however, do not directly address the response of the pulmonary vasculature. Further support for a platelet–granulocyte interaction comes from the studies of Redl *et al.* (1983) who found that granulocyte aggregation induced by *N*-formyl-met-leu-phe or zymosan-treated serum was augmented by platelets.

Several studies have evaluated the ability of platelets to modulate oxidant-induced lung injury and granulocyte secretion of superoxide anion. Granulocytes have been implicated as important effectors of lung injury during microembolization (Tahamont & Malik, 1983). This appears to be mediated, in part, by granulocyte secretion of superoxide anion and other reactive oxygen intermediates. McGarrity *et al.* (1988) showed that platelets inhibit neutrophil superoxide generation induced by *N*-formyl-met-leu-phe. This activity was present in platelet lysates and was attributed to adenosine nucleotides. Moon *et al.* (1989) found that platelets inhibit basal levels of neutrophil superoxide secretion under stirring conditions. This effect was attributed to adenosine as it could be destroyed by adenosine deaminase. Cronstein *et al.* (1986) have reported that neutrophil superoxide generation is inhibited by adenosine. Ward *et al.* (1988) found that platelets and platelet release products increase neutrophil superoxide anion production elicited in response to immune complexes. They again identified the active moiety as released adenine nucleotides. Moon *et al.* (1989) found that platelets enhanced neutrophil superoxide anion generation elicited by either thrombin or platelet activating factor (PAF). This activity was not present in the supernatant of platelets or platelet lysates but could be detected in the membrane pellet of platelet lysates. Activity was not prevented by PAF receptor antagonists or inhibition of cyclooxygenase or lipoxygenase. Platelets also possess antioxidant enzyme systems including catalase (Del Principe *et al.* 1985) and the glutathione redox cycle (Bryant *et al.* 1982). Heffner *et al.* (1988) have reported that platelets protect isolated lungs against oxidant injury induced by hydrogen peroxide. Thus, platelets may modify neutrophil superoxide production in either direction depending on the activation state of the platelet and may also directly protect against oxidant-induced lung injury as may occur in pulmonary embolism.

The evidence for the role of the platelet in the development of increased pulmonary vascular permeability in association with pulmonary microembolization is equivocal. Jorgensen *et al.* (1970) reported that there was transient formation of gaps in the endothelial lining upon infusion of ADP. Significant endothelial damage with loss of cells underneath mural platelet aggregates developed 2–24 hours post injection. These observations were made in several microcirculatory beds including the lung. Minnear *et al.* (1982), over a shorter time course and with a lower dose, found that ADP infusion in sheep was associated with increased pulmonary lymph flow and lymph protein clearance, but little if any change in permeability. However, Manwaring *et al.* (1978) found that fibrinogen degradation product D infusion in rabbits increased the pulmonary vascular leak of albumin and fluid accumulation, and that this did not occur in thrombocytopenic animals.

Vaage *et al.* (1976) reported that collagen increased the hydraulic conductivity of pulmonary exchange vessels in perfused rabbit lungs and that platelets were necessary for this response.

Two studies (Binder *et al.* 1980; Tahamont & Malik, 1983) have reported the influence of thrombocytopenia upon the pulmonary response to microembolization by glass beads and thrombin, respectively. Both groups have reported that thrombocytopenia ameliorated the pulmonary pressor response but neither found that protection was induced against the increase in permeability. However, in both cases the doses were chosen based upon the quantity of thrombin or beads necessary to produce the same increase in pulmonary vascular resistance (Tahamont & Malik, 1983) or pulmonary arterial pressure (Binder *et al.* 1980) as in the control animals. These studies utilized approximately twice the level of embolizing agents as did the control groups. These data can probably be interpreted as suggesting that platelets are not solely responsible for increasing pulmonary vascular permeability. Since the same permeability response required twice the agent in the platelet-depleted state, one might speculate that platelets were involved, perhaps as an adjunct to the granulocyte response. Of interest is the finding that when granulocytes were depleted prior to thrombin infusion, the thrombocytopenic response to thrombin was significantly attenuated, suggesting a granulocyte–platelet interaction. Snapper *et al.* (1984), however, reported that thrombocytopenia produced no changes in the increased lung fluid and soluble exchange observed in endotoxemic sheep.

Brigham and Owen (1975a,b) and Ogletree and Brigham (1980) have evaluated pulmonary fluid dynamics after infusion of several platelet mediators. They found that while sodium arachidonate, thromboxane mimic (U 46619), 5-HT and histamine all elicited increased transvascular fluid flux, only histamine appeared to increase lung vascular permeability.

Several reports suggest that PAF or acetyl glyceryl ether phosphorylcholine functions as an important mediator of pulmonary vascular airway changes. Platelet activating factor is produced by platelets as well as mast cells, endothelial cells, granulocytes, macrophages and monocytes. It has effects on many cell types including the capability to induce platelet aggregation and release. It is an important effector of granulocyte activation and constriction of both vascular and bronchiolar smooth muscle. This combination of sources and activities suggests that PAF is a potential mediator of pulmonary dysfunction during embolization. Initial studies by Mojarad *et al.* (1983) and Heffner *et al.* (1983) demonstrated that PAF produced pulmonary oedema, but differed on the ascribed mechanisms. Mojarad *et al.* (1983), studying dogs, found an increase in protein-rich pulmonary lymph in the absence of haemodynamic changes and suggested a direct effect of PAF on vascular permeability. Heffner *et al.* (1983), studying isolated rabbit lungs, found oedema induced by perfusion with platelets stimulated by PAF. This was accompanied by pulmonary hypertension suggesting oedema secondary to increased pulmonary capillary pressure.

Studies by Burhop *et al.* (1986a,b) indicated an involvement of PAF in both the pulmonary hypertensive response and the increased vascular permeability. Christman *et al.* (1988) documented changes in pulmonary mechanics in response to PAF. These findings have by and large been supported by other investigators (Hamasaki *et al.* 1984; Toyofuku *et al.* 1988). It is not entirely clear whether the oedematogenic qualities of PAF relate to a change in pulmonary vascular permeability or to increases in pulmonary microvascular pressure. Most investigators addressing this question (Hamasaki *et al.* 1984; Burhop *et al.* 1986a,b; Christman *et al.* 1988) have presented data consistent with increased permeability. Several reports (Bjork *et al.* 1983; Handley *et al.* 1984; Humphrey *et al.* 1984) have demonstrated the capacity of PAF to increase permeability in non-pulmonary vascular beds. Direct effects on endothelial cell permeability were found in human umbilical vein culture (Bussolino *et al.* 1987), but not in bovine pulmonary artery (Burhop *et al.* 1986b). Heffner *et al.* (1983) and Bolin *et al.* (1987), however, both using isolated rabbit lungs, report oedema due solely to increased intravascular pressure. It appears that in most experimental systems, pulmonary oedema in association with PAF is the result of both an increase in vascular permeability and increased intravascular hydrostatic pressure. Moreover, the pulmonary vascular hypertension in response to PAF appears to be mediated in part by cyclooxygenase products, probably thromboxane A_2 (Burhop *et al.* 1986b; Christman *et al.* 1988) while later components of the response are independent of thromboxane and possibly exerted directly (Toyofuku *et al.* 1988).

Platelet activating factor has been implicated as an effector of the pulmonary pathophysiological response to models of embolism induced by infusion of other mediators. The plasma and lung tissue levels of PAF increase following endotoxin infusion (Chang *et al.* 1987). Pulmonary haemodynamic and permeability changes induced by endotoxin were ameliorated by PAF receptor antagonists. Receptor antagonists have also been utilized to invoke a role for PAF in the pulmonary haemodynamic alteration on infusion of thrombin (van der Zee *et al.* 1988) and tissue necrosis factor (Horvath *et al.* 1989).

The extent to which the effects attributed to PAF are platelet dependent remains an open question. It has been clearly demonstrated that intravascular PAF results in pulmonary vascular accumulation of platelets and granulocytes (Humphrey *et al.* 1984). Christman *et al.* (1988) found that platelet depletion attenuated pulmonary hypertension, reduced thromboxane levels, and permitted more rapid recovery of changes in lung mechanics after PAF injection. They found, however, that PAF had profound effects despite platelet depletion. Vargaftig *et al.* (1980) and Halonen *et al.* (1981) showed that the platelet depletion eliminated or reduced the change in lung mechanics induced by PAF. The maximal PAF-induced changes in pulmonary arterial pressure in perfused lungs required platelets (Heffner *et al.* 1983). None the less, several investigators (Hamasaki *et al.* 1984; Christman *et al.* 1988) have found notable pulmonary haemodynamic and vascular permeability responses to PAF in the absence of platelets. These data collectively suggest that both platelet-dependent and platelet-independent effects are required for the mediation of the responses.

Platelet adhesion to endothelial cells

Adhesion of platelets to the vascular walls is an initial event in the development of intravascular thrombosis associated with vascular injury, and may be important in pulmonary microembolism. Although most studies envisage this process as being initiated by platelet adherence to exposed subendothelium, platelets are capable of adhering directly to endothelium (Curwen *et al.* 1980; Hoak *et al.* 1980; Radomski *et al.* 1987; Sneddon & Vane, 1988; Venturini *et al.* 1988; Kaplan *et al.* 1989a).

It is becoming increasingly clear that endothelial cells are active and important regulators of vascular processes including haemostasis and thrombosis. Because of the ability of endothelial cells to become adhesive to other circulating cells as well as their documented ability to regulate thrombotic processes, it has been hypothesized that exposure of endothelial monolayers to thrombin would promote platelet adhesiveness via an interaction with the endothelium. Experiments have been performed to evaluate whether exposure of sheep pulmonary artery endothelial cells to thrombin augmented the adherence of platelets to the endothelial monolayer (Kaplan *et al.* 1989a). Addition of thrombin to co-incubated platelets and endothelial cells or pre-incubation of endothelium with thrombin, which was removed prior to the addition of platelets, both resulted in augmentation of platelet adherence to the endothelium. This process was dose-dependent over a range of 0.002 units/ml thrombin up to 20 units/ml of thrombin. Adherence was dependent upon the presence of divalent cations. Gamma-thrombin, a proteolytically active thrombin with a modified cell receptor recognition site, is not active in this response nor are active site-inhibited thrombins. Gamma-thrombin at high concentrations (10^{-7} M) augments platelet adherence in co-incubation experiments. Several pieces of data suggest that augmented platelet adhesiveness results from the retention of active thrombin on the endothelial cells. If endothelial cells were pretreated with thrombin, and either hirudin or the specific thrombin inhibitory tripeptide phenylalanyl-prolyl-arginine chloromethylketone was added after pre-incubation with thrombin, the endothelial cells no longer stimulated platelet adhesiveness. In addition, the augmented platelet adhesiveness was prevented in thrombin pre-incubated endothelial cells by adding a 1000-fold excess of thrombin in which the active site was inhibited by diisopropylfluorophosphate. This latter observation suggests that specific saturable receptors are responsible for this action. These observations have been repeated with sheep vascular segments and isolated perfused rat lungs.

Since evidence indicates that increased leukocyte adhesion to endothelial cells in response to thrombin is, in part, dependent on PAF, the potential role of PAF in this response was investigated. Preincubation of endothelial cells with PAF did not increase platelet adhesion of endothelial cells. The addition of L-652, 731 or WEB 2086, specific PAF receptor inhibitors, was not effective in reducing the augmented platelet adherence which followed thrombin exposure (Kaplan *et al.*, unpublished observations).

Additional evidence suggests that platelet adherence is associated with platelet activation. Scanning electron microscopy studies (Kaplan *et al.* 1989a) indicate that the addition of thrombin to co-incubated endothelial cells and platelets results in the deposition of dense compact aggregates of platelets which have clearly undergone shape change. When endothelial cells are pre-incubated with thrombin, there are looser aggregates but still clear evidence that the adherent platelets are activated in terms of shape change and extension of pseudopodia. In both co-treated and pretreated systems, the aggregates are adherent over the endothelial surface and not limited to interendothelial junctions. The electron micrographs suggest that the subendothelial matrix is not being exposed. Further evidence of platelet activation is provided by data on serotonin release. Endothelial cells pre-incubated with thrombin are capable of causing platelets to release their serotonin stores. Unlike adhesion, this response is independent of the presence of divalent cations; and, unlike the case with cultured monolayers, adherence to thrombin-treated rat lungs interestingly showed single platelets (Venturini *et al.* 1988). These were activated as indicated by extension of pseudopodia, shape change and degranulation. Platelets were found in pulmonary capillaries and none were observed in large vessels.

Promotion of platelet adherence to endothelial cells is not a general property of platelet aggregators in that the response is not reproduced by PAF, ADP, arachidonic acid, or calcium ionophore A23187 in either pre-incubation or co-incubation. Johnson and Helgeson (1988) have demonstrated attachment of collagen-stimulated platelets to endothelial cells. Co-incubation with phorbol esters which activate protein kinase C also results in augmented platelet adherence (Kaplan *et al.* 1989b). Phorbol esters which are not activators of protein kinase C are inactive in this response. Based on these studies we evaluated the influence of the protein kinase C inhibitor, H7, on this response. Pretreatment of platelets with H7 eliminated the increase in platelet adherence seen with thrombin stimulation and reduced the effect of the phorbol esters, suggesting a protein kinase C mediated effect. The effect of exogenously activated phospholipase C, which should produce the endogenous diacylglycerols resulting in protein kinase C activation, were also assessed. Phospholipase C resulted in dose-dependent increases in platelet adherence to endothelium and this effect could be similarly inhibited by H7.

Further studies have begun to evaluate the ability of the endothelial cells to modify these responses. Evidence suggests that thrombin treatment of endothelial cells is associated with decrease in endothelial cell levels of 13-hydroxyoctadecadienoic acid (13-HODE) (Buchanan *et al.* 1985) and that addition of exogenous 13-HODE can reduce thrombin-stimulated platelet adhesion to endothelial cells (Tloti *et al.* 1989). Additional studies have demonstrated that platelet adhesion in the presence of thrombin is augmented by the addition of haemoglobin to the system and decreased by the addition of superoxide dismutase to the system (Venturini *et al.* 1989), suggesting a possible modulation of this effect by endothelial derived relaxing factor.

Platelets and the maintenance of endothelial integrity

A potentially important aspect of platelet function during pulmonary embolism may derive from the ability of platelets to 'support' endothelial function. Considerable evidence has indicated that platelets are important in supporting the integrity of the vascular barrier. Danielli (1940) first implicated platelets as factors regulating vascular barrier function. He found that the addition of platelets to a perfusate reduced oedema formation in the perfused hind limb. Some of the first clinical observations that platelets are involved in maintaining vascular integrity came from Kraner (1961) and Gaydos *et al.* (1962) when they reported that thrombocytopenia is often associated with purpuric haemorrhage due to 'low capillary resistance' (i.e. fragile capillaries). Johnson *et al.* (1964), after conducting ultrastructure studies on the effect of thrombocytopenia on human skin, found that 'vascular integrity is dramatically improved immediately following platelet transfusions'. They referred to this as the 'endothelial supporting function of platelets'. Gimbrone *et al.* (1969) concurred with Johnson *et al.* (1964), after performing functional and anatomical studies on isolated thyroids using platelet-rich and platelet-poor plasma perfusate. The conclusion was drawn that 'platelets "nurture" the microcirculation in some way'. Dodds *et al.* (1973) reported similar studies and conclusions with isolated perfused rat kidneys. Roy and Djerassi (1972) and Aursnes (1974) reported that thrombocytopenic animals demonstrated elevations in erythrocyte content of lymph and in the vascular disappearance rate of [^{125}I]albumin, respectively, and that these changes could be reversed by platelet administration. These findings were reinforced by Kitchens and Weiss (1975) who reported structural changes in the endothelium of capillaries and post-capillary venules within 6 hours of rendering an animal thrombocytopenic, although Miles and Hurley (1983) did not observe such changes in similar studies. Recent studies by McDonagh (1986) have shown that platelet depletion increases coronary microvascular permeability to fluorescein isothiocyanate-labelled albumin in the perfused rat heart 'and that these changes are ameliorated by perfusion with platelet-rich plasma. It has been demonstrated that platelets reduce the susceptibility of the vascular barrier to injury. Scratch injury to the endothelial cell monolayers was more readily repaired in the presence of platelets, and DNA synthesis was increased (Maca *et al.* 1977). These observations provide evidence for a supportive role for platelets with regard to vascular integrity, possibly mediated by a direct effect upon endothelial cells. Fantone *et al.* (1984) reported that platelet-depleted rats were more sensitive to lung injury induced by α-napthyl thiourea using morphometric criteria as well as lung water accumulation.

Studies by Lo *et al.* (1988) provided the first direct evidence of a permeability defect in the pulmonary vasculature of intact thrombocytopenic animals. Sheep which had been chronically depleted of platelets with polyclonal rabbit antisheep platelet antibodies developed the characteristic petechia that are seen in thrombocytopenic patients. Under normal pulmonary vascular pressures, lymphatic flow and protein content were within normal range. However, with elevated left atrial pressures, lymph flow was greatly elevated and there was no decrease in lymph protein content. Animals developed severe pulmonary oedema at left atrial pressures (20–25 mmHg) which are normally well tolerated. These effects were rapidly prevented by transfusion of platelet-rich plasma. These observations led to a direct evaluation of the influence of platelets upon the albumin permeability of cultured pulmonary artery endothelial cells grown to confluence on polycarbonate filters (Shepard *et al.* 1989b). In this system there was a dose-dependent decrease in albumin permeability.

Three hypotheses have been offered to explain the postulated support of endothelial barrier function by platelets. The first, originally stated by Danielli (1940) and reasserted by Tranzer and Baumgartner (1967) suggested that platelets act by physically blocking 'pores' or 'gaps' that allow for the passage of protein out of the vessel. This could be interpreted as maintenance of vascular wall integrity by virtue of an ongoing expression of normal haemostatic function. Others have suggested that platelets support endothelial barrier function by a trophic function. Cronkite *et al.* (1961), Wojcik *et al.* (1969) and Johnson *et al.* (1964) concluded that platelets or platelet components were directly incorporated into endothelial cells. More recently Shepro and D'Amore (1984) have suggested that the permeability-decreasing effect of platelets is humorally mediated by the release of granular constituents from the platelet. Several investigators have demonstrated morphological, metabolic, and trophic influences of platelets upon endothelial cells in culture (Busch *et al.* 1976; D'Amore & Shepro, 1977; D'Amore, 1978). Saba and Mason (1975) and Maca *et al.* (1977) reported that co-culture with platelets or addition of platelet secretion products, ADP and 5-HT, augmented the growth rate of human umbilical vein endothelial cells. D'Amore (1978) and D'Amore and Shepro (1977) found that platelets and several platelet secretion products enhanced endothelial proliferation. They implicated augmented Ca^{2+} influx as a common pathway in this response. Maca *et al.* (1977) reported that human umbilical vein endothelial cells that were cultured with platelets dispersed more evenly with greater contiguity of the monolayer and with a more elongated morphology.

Recent data (Shepard *et al.* 1989b) support the contention that the permeability decreasing effect of platelets is humorally mediated. These effects cannot be explained by platelet plugging of endothelial gaps. The permeability-decreasing effect in the endothelial monolayer was found using both platelet-conditioned media and the supernatant of platelets lysed by sonication. The permeability-decreasing activity of platelets was eliminated by fixation of platelets with paraformaldehyde, and occurred with few platelets adherent to the monolayer. The activity was not altered by platelet activation with ADP, which augments granule release, or with thrombin, which augments both granule release and adherence to endothelial cells. Platelet inhibition with aspirin or prostaglandin E_1 similarly failed to alter the permeability-decreasing activity of platelets.

It has been demonstrated that certain amines which are found in, and released from, platelets can decrease endothelial cell permeability (Bottaro *et al.* 1986a). There appears, however, to be variability in terms of the source of endothelial cells used to assay the barrier function. 5-HT decreases permeability with bovine aortic intimal endothelial cells (Bottaro *et al.* 1986b) but not with endothelial cells derived from cerebral microvessels (Bottaro *et al.* 1986a) or pulmonary artery endothelium (Shepard *et al.* 1989b). Ketanserin, an antagonist for the 5-HT_2 receptor on endothelial cells, the serotonergic receptor on endothelial cells, did not prevent the decrease in albumin permeability by either platelets or platelet lysate supernatant. Moreover, the addition of increasing concentrations of serotonin to pulmonary endothelial monolayers did not influence endothelial permeability.

Shepard *et al.* (1989b) applied both platelets and lysate supernatant to the monolayers along with propranolol, a β-adrenergic receptor antagonist, since catecholamines may reduce endothelial permeability via activation of β-receptors (Bottaro *et al.* 1986a; Minnear *et al.* 1986). Propranolol did not prevent the effect of either the platelets or the lysate supernatant. Thus, the platelet effect on endothelial cell permeability does act solely through endothelial β-adrenergic receptors. The data of Minnear *et al.* (1986) have demonstrated that isoproterenol decreases albumin flux with the pulmonary artery endothelial cells. However, the possibility that these amines contribute to the decrease in permeability in concert with other platelet-derived substances remains to be determined.

Recent studies have pursued the isolation of platelet-derived substances which decrease pulmonary endothelial permeability to macromolecules. These studies suggest two active factors, a low molecular weight compound, possibly adenosine (Shepard *et al.* 1989a), and a larger substance, possibly a peptide (Paty *et al.* 1989).

Concluding remarks

The contribution of platelets to the pulmonary airway and vascular responses to embolization is complex and not yet fully defined. It has been clearly demonstrated that platelets are components of both macro- and microemboli of the pulmonary vascular bed. Platelets and platelet-derived mediators contribute to the vascular and airway components of the pulmonary pressor responses and airway constriction.

It has been demonstrated that platelets may, in a fashion that remains ill-defined, mediate changes which lead to increased vascular permeability. However, a cause and effect relationship between platelets and increased pulmonary vascular permeability has been neither definitively demonstrated nor ruled out. Platelets have been shown to regulate the capability of other cells included in pulmonary emboli, in particular, granulocytes, to produce lung vascular injury. The data here are controversial since some studies indicate that platelets and platelet-derived products reduce neutrophil activation, whereas other data indicate the opposite effect of platelets. Recent studies have demonstrated the direct interaction of platelets with pulmonary endothelium in terms of both adherence and the regulation of pulmonary vascular barrier function. These data taken together support the likelihood that platelets contribute in a significant way to the pulmonary vascular and airway dysfunction associated with pulmonary embolism.

Acknowledgements

This work was supported by Program Project Grant HL-32418 from the Heart, Lung and Blood Institute of National Institutes of Health.

References

Almqvist, P., Duenzig, M. & Schwartz, S.I. (1983) Effect of naloxone on endotoxin-induced pulmonary platelet sequestration. *Acta Chir Scand* **149**, 23–26.

Aursnes, I. (1974) Increased permeability of capillaries to protein during thrombocytopenia: An experimental study in the rabbit. *Microvasc Res* **7**, 283–295.

Aursnes, I. & Vaage, J. (1973) Changes in peripheral lymph during intravascular aggregation of blood platelets. *Acta Physiol Scand Suppl* **369**, 61.

Beal, S.L., Reed II, R.L., Heimbach, D., Chi, E. & Reynold, L. (1987) Pulmonary microembolism: A cause of lung injury. *J Surg Res* **43**, 303–310.

Bergentz, S.-E., Lewis, D.H. & Ljungquist, U. (1971) Trapping of platelets in the lung after experimental injury. In Ditzel, J. & Lewis, D.M. (eds) *Symposium on the Lung in Shock*. S. Karger, Basel.

Berman, I.R., Smulson, M.E., Pattengale, P. & Schoenbach, S.F. (1971) Pulmonary microembolism after soft tissue injury in primates. *Surgery* **70**, 246–253.

Berman, I.R., Iliescu, H., Ransom, J.H.C. & Eng, K. (1976) Pulmonary capillary permeability — a transfusion lesion. *J Trauma* **16**, 471–480.

Bignold, L.P. (1980) Importance of platelets in increased vascular permeability evoked by experimental haemarthrosis in synovium of the rat. *Pathology* **12**, 169–179.

Binder, A.S., Kageler, W., Perel, A., Flick, M.R. & Staub, N.C. (1980) Effect of platelet depletion on lung vascular permeability after microemboli in sheep. *J Appl Physiol* **48**, 414–420.

Bjork, J., Lindbom, L., Gerdin, B., Smedegard, G., Arfors, K.-E. & Benveniste, J. (1983) Paf-acether (platelet-activating factor) increases microvascular permeability and affects endothelium–granulocyte interaction in microvascular beds. *Acta Physiol Scand* **119**, 305–308.

Bo, G. & Hognestad, J. (1972) Effects on the pulmonary circulation of suddenly induced intravascular aggregation of blood platelets. *Acta Physiol Scand* **85**, 523–531.

Bo, G., Hognestad, J. & Vaage, J. (1974) The role of blood platelets in pulmonary responses to microembolization with barium sulfate. *Acta Physiol Scand* **90**, 244–251.

Bolin, R.W., Martin, T.R. & Albert, R.K. (1987) Lung endothelial and epithelial permeability after platelet-activating factor. *J Appl Physiol* **63**, 1770–1775.

Bottaro, D., Shepro, D., Peterson, S. & Hechtman, H.B. (1986a) Serotonin, norepinephrine, and histamine mediation of endothelial cell barrier function *in vitro*. *J Cell Physiol* **128**, 189.

Bottaro, D., Shepro, D. & Hechtman, H.B. (1986b) Heterogeneity of intimal and microvessel endothelial cell barriers *in vitro*. *Microvasc Res* **32**, 389–398.

Braunstein, Jr., P.W., Ceunod, H.F., Joris, I. & Majno, G. (1980) Platelets, fibroblasts and inflammation. Tissue reaction to platelets injected subcutaneously. *Am J Pathol* **99**, 53–66.

Bredenberg, C.E., Taylor, G.A. & Webb, W.R. (1980) The effect of thrombocytopenia on the pulmonary and systemic hemodynamics of canine endotoxin shock. *Surgery* **87**, 59–68.

Brigham, K.L. & Owen, P.J. (1975a) Mechanism of the serotonin effect on lung transvascular fluid and protein movement in awake sheep. *Circ Res* **36**, 761–770.

Brigham, K.L. & Owen, P.J. (1975b) Increased sheep lung vascular permeability caused by histamine. *Circ Res* **37**, 647–657.

Bryant, R.W., Simon, T.C. & Bailey, J.M. (1982) Role of glutathione peroxidase and hexose monophosphate shunt in the platelet lipoxygenase pathways. *J Biol Chem* **257**, 14937–14943.

Buchanan, M.R., Haas, T.A., Lagarde, M. & Guichardant, M. (1985) 13-Hydroxyocta-decadienoic acid is the vessel wall chemorepellant factor, LOX. *J Biol Chem* **260**, 16056–16059.

Burhop, K.E., van der Zee, H., Bizios, R., Kaplan, J.E. & Malik, A.B. (1986a) Platelet activating factor: Pulmonary vascular response in awake sheep and role of cyclooxygenase metabolites. *Am Rev Respir Dis* **134**, 548–554.

Burhop, K.E., Garcia, J.G.N., Selig, W.M., Lo, S.K., van der Zee, H., Kaplan, J.E. & Malik, A.B. (1986b) Platelet activating factor increases lung vascular permeability to protein. *J Appl Physiol* **61**, 2210–2217.

Busch, C., Lindquist, O. & Saldeen, T. (1974) Respiratory insufficiency in the dog induced by pulmonary microembolism and inhibition of fibrinolysis. *Acta Chir Scand* **140**, 255–266.

Busch, C., Heldin, C.-H., Wasteson, A. & Westermark, B. (1976) Stimulation of endothelial cell proliferation by a factor released from human platelets. *Bibl Anat* **16**, 219–222.

Bussolino, F., Camussi, G., Aglietta, M., Braquet, P., Bosia, A., Pescarmona, G., Sanavio, F., D'Urso, N. & Marchisio, P.C. (1987) Human endothelial cells are target for platelet-activating factor. *J Immunol* **139**, 2439–2446.

Chang, S.-W., Fedderson, C.O., Henson, P.M. & Voelkel, F. (1987) Platelet-activating factor mediates hemodynamic changes and lung injury in endotoxin-treated rats. *J Clin Invest* **79**, 1498–1509.

Christman, B.W., Lefferts, P.L., King, G.A. & Snapper, J.R. (1988) Role of circulating platelets and granulocytes in PAF-induced pulmonary dysfunction in awake sheep. *J Appl Physiol* **64**, 2033–2041.

Cronkite, E.P., Bond, V.P., Fliedner, T.M., Paglia, D.A. & Adamik, E.R. (1961) Studies on the origin, production and destruction of platelets. In Johnson, S.A., Monto, R.V., Rebuck, J.W. & Horn Jr R.C. (eds) *Blood Platelets*, Int. Henry Ford Hospital Symp. X, Detroit. Little, Brown. & Co. Boston.

Cronstein, B.N., Levin, R.I., Belanoff, J., Weissman, G. & Hirschhorn, R. (1986) Adenosine: an endogenous inhibitor of neutrophil-mediated injury to endothelial cells. *J Clin Invest* **78**, 760–770.

Curwen, K.D., Gimbrone, M.A. & Handlin, R.I. (1980) *In vitro* studies of thrombo-resistance: The role of prostacyclin (PGI_2) in platelet adhesion to cultured normal and virally transformed human vascular endothelial cells. *Lab Invest* **42**, 366–374.

D'Amore, P.A. (1978) Platelet-endothelial interaction and the maintenance of the microvasculature. *Microvasc Res* **15**, 137–145.

D'Amore, P.A. & Shepro, D. (1977) Stimulation of growth and calcium influx in cultured, bovine, aortic endothelial cells by platelets and vasoactive substances. *J Cell Physiol* **92**, 177–183.

Danielli, J.F. (1940) Capillary permeability and oedema in the perfused frog. *J Physiol* **98**, 109–129.

Del Principe, D., Menichelli, A., De Matteis, W., Di Corpo, M.L., Di Guilio, S. & Finazzi-Agro, A. (1985) Hydrogen peroxide has a role in the aggregation of human platelets. *FEBS Lett* **185**, 142–146.

Dodds, W.J., Raymond, L.R.S.L. & Pert, J.H. (1973) Isolated kidney perfusion: A model for testing platelet function. *Proc Soc Exp Biol Med* **144**, 189–194.

Fantone, J.C., Kunkel, R.G. & Kinnes, D.A. (1984) Potentiation of α-napthyl thiourea-induced lung injury by prostaglandin E_1 and platelet depletion. *Lab Invest* **50**, 703–710.

Gaydos, L.A., Freireich, E.J. & Mantel, N. (1962) The quantitative relationship between platelet count and hemorrhage in patients with acute leukemia. *New Engl J Med* **266**, 905–909.

Gimbrone, M.A., Aster, R.H., Cotran, R.S., Corkery, J., Jandl, J.H. & Folkman, J. (1969) Preservation of vascular integrity in organs perfused *in vitro* with a platelet-rich medium. *Nature* **222**, 33–36.

Halonen, M., Palmer, J.D., Lohman, I.C., McManus, L.M. & Pinckard, R.N. (1981) Differential effects of platelet depletion on the physiologic alterations of IgE anaphylaxis and acetyl glyceryl ether phosporylcholine. *Am Rev Respir Dis* **124**, 416–421.

Hamasaki, Y., Mojarad, M., Saga, T., Tai, H.-H. & Said, S.I. (1984) Platelet-activating factor raises airway and vascular pressures and induces edema in lungs perfused with platelet-free solution. *Am Rev Respir Dis* **129**, 742–746.

Handley, D.A., Arbeeny, C.M., Lee, M.L., Van Vaten, R.G. & Saunders, R.N. (1984) Effect of platelet activating factor on endothelial permeability to plasma macromolecules. *Immunopharmacology* **8**, 137–142.

Hardaway, R.M. & Johnson, D. (1963) Clotting mechanism in endotoxin shock. *Arch Int Med* **112**, 775–782.

Heffner, J.E., Shoemaker, S.A., Canham, E.M., Patel, M., McMurty, I.F., Morris, H.G. & Repine, J.E. (1983) Acetyl glyceryl ether phosphorylcholine-stimulated human platelets cause pulmonary hypertension and edema in isolated rabbit lungs. Role of thromboxane A_2. *J Clin Invest* **71**, 351–357.

Heffner, J.E., Katz, S.A., Halushka, P.V. & Cook, J.A. (1988) Human platelets attenuate oxidant injury in isolated rabbit lungs. *J Appl Physiol* **65**, 1258–1266.

Henson, P.M. & Ginsberg, M.H. (1981) Immunological reactions of platelets. In Gordon J.L. (ed.) *Platelets in Biology and Pathology*, Vol. 5, pp. 265–308. Elsevier/North Holland Biomedical Press, New York.

Hill, R.N., Shibel, E.M., Spragg, R.G. & Moser, K.M. (1975) Adult respiratory distress syndrome: early predictors of mortality. *Trans Am Soc Artif Intern Organs* **21**, 199–204.

Hoak, J.C., Czervionke, R.L., Fry, G.L. & Smith, J.B. (1980) Interaction of thrombin and platelets with the vascular endothelium. *Fed Proc* **39**, 2606–2609.

Horvath, C.J., Kaplan, J.E., Moon, D.G. & Malik, A.B. (1989) Role of platelet activating factor (PAF) in the tumor necrosis factor (TNFa)-induced increase in lung vascular permeability. *FASEB J* **3**, A2723.

Humphrey, D.M., McManus, L.M., Hanahan, D.J. &

Pinckard, R.N. (1984) Morphologic basis of increased vascular permeability induced by acetyl glyceryl ether phosphorylcholine. *Lab Invest* **50**, 16–25.

Jacob, H.S., Moldow, C.F., Flynn, P.J., Weisdorf, D.J., Vercellotti, G.M. & Hammerschmidt, D.E. (1982) Therapeutic ramifications of the interaction of complement, granulocytes, and platelets in the production of acute lung injury. *Ann NY Acad Sci* **384**, 489–495.

Johnson, C.M. & Helgeson, S.C. (1988) Platelet adherence to cardiac and non-cardiac endothelial cells in culture: lack of a prostacyclin effect. *J Lab Clin Med* **112**, 372–379.

Johnson, S.A. (1971) Platelets and thrombosis: Interaction with components of the vessel wall. In (eds) Brinkhouse, K.M., Shermer, R.W. & Mostofi F.K. *The Platelet*, pp. 198–214. Williams & Wilkins, Baltimore.

Johnson, S.A., Balboa, R.S. & Dessel, B.H. (1964) The mechanism of the endothelial supporting function of intact platelets. *Exp Mol Pathol* **3**, 115–127.

Jorgensen, L., Hovig, T., Rowsell, H.C. & Mustard, J.F. (1970) Adenosine diphosphate-induced platelet aggregation and vascular injury in swine and rabbits. *Am J Pathol* **61**, 161–176.

Kaplan, J.E., Moon, D.G., Weston, L.K., Minnear, F.L., Del Vecchio, P.J., Shepard, J.M. & Fenton, J.W. (1989a) Platelets adhere to thrombin treated endothelial cells *in vitro*. *Am J Physiol* **257**, H423–H433.

Kaplan, J.E., Weston, L.K., Venturini, C.M., Del Vecchio, P.J. & Fenton II, J.W. (1989b) Platelet adherence to endothelial cells is promoted by activators of platelet protein kinase C. *FASEB J* **3**, A458.

Kitchens, C.S. & Weiss, L. (1975) Ultrastructural changes of endothelium associated with thrombocytopenia. *Blood* **46**, 567–578.

Kraner, J. (1961) Capillary resistance and its relation to bleeding. In Johnson, S.A., Monto, R.W., Rebuck, J.W. & Horn Jr, R.C. (eds), *Blood Platelets*. Int. Henry Ford Hospital Symp. X, Detroit Little, Brown. & Co., Boston.

Lelcuk, S., Klausner, J.M., Merhav, A. & Rozin, R.R. (1987) Effect of OKY 046, a thromboxane synthetase inhibitor, on lung vascular permeability after pulmonary embolism in sheep. *Thorax* **42**, 676–680.

Ljungquist, U.E. & Schwartz, S.I. (1975) Pulmonary platelet trapping during shock and pulmonary embolism. *J Surg Res* **18**, 559–565.

Lo, S.K., Burhop, K.E., Kaplan, J.E. & Malik, A.B. (1988) Role of platelets in maintenance of pulmonary vascular permeability to protein. *Am J Physiol* **254**, H763–H771.

Luterman, A., Manwaring, D. & Curreri, P.W. (1977) The role of fibrinogen degradation products in the pathogenesis of the respiratory distress syndrome. *Surgery* **82**, 703–709.

McDonagh, P.F. (1986) Platelets reduce coronary microvascular permeability to macromolecules. *Am J Physiol* **251**, H581–H587.

McDonald, J.W.D., Ali, E., Morgan, E., Townsend, E.R. & Cooper, J.D. (1983) Thromboxane synthesis by causes other than platelets in association with complement-induced pulmonary leukostasis and pulmonary hypertension in sheep. *Circ Res* **52**, 1–6.

McGarrity, S.T., Stephenson, A.H., Hyers, T.M. & Webster, R.O. (1988) Inhibition of neutrophil superoxide anion generation by platelet products: role of adenine nucleotides. *J Leuk Biol* **44**, 411–421.

McKay, D.G. & Csavossy, I. (1965) Ultrastructural study of the intravascular effects of bacterial endotoxin. *Fed Proc* **24**, 456.

Maca, R.D., Fry, G.L., Hoak, J.C. & Loh, P.T. (1977) The effects of intact platelets on cultured human endothelial cells. *Thromb Res* **11**, 715–727.

Manwaring, D. & Curreri, P.W. (1980a) The role of platelet aggregation and release in fragment D-induced pulmonary dysfunction. *Ann Surg* **192**, 103–107.

Manwaring, D. & Curreri, P.W. (1980b) Platelet mediation of fragment D-induced respiratory distress syndrome. *Surg Forum* **31**, 242–243.

Manwaring, D., Throning, D. & Curreri, P.W. (1978) Mechanism of acute pulmonary dysfunction induced by fibrinogen degradation product D. *Surgery* **84**, 45–54.

Mayer Jr, J.E., Kersten, T.E. & Humphrey, E.W. (1981) Effects of transfusion of emboli and aged plasma on pulmonary capillary permeability. *J Thorac Cardiovasc Surg* **82**, 358–364.

Miles, R.G. & Hurley, J.V. (1983) The effect of thrombocytopenia on the ultrastructure and reaction to injury of vascular endothelium. *Microvasc Res* **26**, 273–290.

Minnear, F.L., Moon, D.G. & Hill, L.A. (1986) Thrombin-induced increase in pulmonary endothelial permeability *in vitro*: protective effect of isoproterenol. *Ann NY Acad Sci* **485**, 432–435.

Minnear, F.L., Moon, D.G., Kaplan, J.E. & Malik, A.B. (1982) Effect of ADP-induced platelet aggregation on lung fluid balance in sheep. *Am J Physiol* **242**, H645–H651.

Mlczoch, J., Tucker, A., Weir, E.K., Reeves, J.T. & Grover, R.F. (1978) Platelet-mediated pulmonary hypertension and hypoxia during pulmonary microembolism. Reduction by platelet inhibition. *Chest* **14**, 648–653.

Mojarad, M., Hamasaki, Y. & Said, S.I. (1983) Platelet-activating factor increases pulmonary microvascular permeability and induces pulmonary edema: a preliminary report. *Clin Respir Physiol* **19**, 253–256.

Moon, D.G., van der Zee, H., Krasodomski, J., Morton, K., Fenton II, J.W. & Kaplan, J.E. (1989) Platelet modulation of neutrophil production of superoxide anion. *FASEB J* **3**, A235.

Mustard, J.F., Movat, H.Z., Macmorine, D.R.L. & Senyi, A. (1965) Release of permeability factors from the blood platelet. *Proc Soc Exp Biol Med* **119**, 988–991.

Nachman, R.L. (1978) The platelet as an inflammatory cell. In de Gaetano, G. & Garattini, S. (eds) *Platelets:*

A Multidisciplinary Approach, pp. 199–203. Raven Press, New York.

Nachman, R.L., Weksler, B. & Ferris, B. (1972) Characterization of human platelet vascular permeability-enhancing ability. *J Clin Invest* **51**, 549–556.

Niewiarowski, S. (1977) Proteins secreted by the platelet. *Thromb Haemost* **38**, 925–938.

Ogletree, M.L. (1982) Pharmacology of prostaglandins in the pulmonary microcirculation. *Ann NY Acad Sci* **384**, 191–206.

Ogletree, M.L. & Brigham, K.L. (1980) Arachidonate raises vascular resistance but not permeability in lungs of awake sheep. *J Appl Physiol* **48**, 581–586.

Orell, S.R. (1971) Lung pathology in respiratory distress following shock in the adult. *Acta Pathol Microbiol Scand* **79**, 65–76.

Paty, P.S.K., Sherman, P.F., Shepard, J.M., Weston, L.K., Moon, D.G. & Kaplan, J.E. (1989) Preliminary characterization of a platelet derived endothelial permeability decreasing factor. *FASEB J* **3**, A6286.

Peer, R.M. & Schwartz, S.I. (1973) Prevention of pulmonary platelet trapping following trauma. *Surg Forum* **24**, 5–7.

Radegran, K. & McAslan, C. (1972) Circulatory and ventilatory effects of induced platelet aggregation and their inhibition by acetylsalicylic acid. *Acta Anaesth Scand* **16**, 76–84.

Radomski, M.W., Palmer, R.M.J. & Moncada, S. (1987) The role of nitric oxide and cGMP in platelet adhesion to vascular endothelium. *Biochem Biophys Res Commun* **148**, 1482–1489.

Redl, H., Hammerschmidt, D.E. & Schlag, G. (1983) Augmentation by platelets of granulocyte aggregation in response to chemotaxins: studies utilizing an improved cell preparation technique. *Blood* **61**, 125–131.

Roy, A.J. & Djerassi, I. (1972) Effects of platelet transfusions: plug formation and maintenance of vascular integrity. *Proc Soc Exp Biol Med* **139**, 137–142.

Saba, S.R. & Mason, R.G. (1975) Effects of platelets and certain platelet components on growth of cultured human endothelial cells. *Thromb Res* **7**, 807–812.

Schneider, R.C., Zapol, W.M. & Carvalho, A.C. (1980) Platelet consumption and sequestration in severe acute respiratory failure. *Am Rev Respir Dis* **122**, 445–451.

Shepard, J.M., Paty, P.S.K., Sherman, P.F., Weston, L.K. & Kaplan, J.E. (1989a) Role of adenosine in platelet mediated enhancement of endothelial barrier function. *FASEB J* **3**, A6290.

Shepard, J.M., Moon, D.G., Weston, L.K., Del Vecchio, P.J., Minnear, F.L., Malik, A.B. & Kaplan, J.E. (1989b) Platelets decrease albumin permeability of endothelial cell monolayers. *Microvasc Res* **37**, 256–266.

Shepro, D. & D'Amore, P.A. (1984) Physiology and biochemistry of the vascular wall endothelium. In Renkin, E.R. & Michel, C.C. (eds) *Handbook of Physiology: A Critical Comprehensive Presentation of Physiological Knowledge and Concepts*, Vol. IV, Section 2, Ch. 4, American Physiological Society.

Snapper, J.R., Hinson, J.M., Hutchison, A.A., Lefferts, P.L., Ogletree, M.L. & Brigham, K.L. (1984) Effects of platelet depletion on the unanesthetized sheep's pulmonary response to endotoxemia. *J Clin Invest* **74**, 1782–1791.

Sneddon, J.M. & Vane, J.R. (1988) Endothelium-derived relaxing factor reduces platelet adhesion to bovine endothelial cells. *Proc Natl Acad Sci USA* **85**, 2800–2804.

Stein, M. & Thomas, D.P. (1967) Role of platelets in the acute pulmonary response to endotoxin. *J Appl Physiol* **23**, 47–52.

Tahamont, M.V. & Malik, A.B. (1983) Granulocytes mediate the increase in pulmonary vascular permeability after thrombin embolism. *J Appl Physiol* **54**, 1489–1495.

Thompson, J.A., Millen, J.E., Glauser, F.L. & Hess, M.L. (1986) The role of 5-HT_2 receptor inhibition in pulmonary embolization. *Circ Shock* **20**, 299–309.

Thorne, L.J., Kuenzig, M. & Schwartz, S.I. (1979) Effects of acetylsalicylic acid and prostaglandin on post-traumatic pulmonary platelet sequestration. *Surg Forum* **30**, 1745–177.

Tloti, M.A., Moon, D.G. & Kaplan, J.E. (1989) Thrombin inhibits 13-hydroxyoctadecadionic acid (13-HODE) production by cultured sheep pulmonary artery endothelial cells. *FASEB J* **3**, A457.

Toyofuku, T., Kobayashi, T., Koyama, S. & Kusama, S. (1988) Pulmonary vascular response to platelet-activating factor in conscious sheep. *Am J Physiol* **255**, H434–H440.

Tranzer, J.P. & Baumgartner, H.R. (1967) Filling gaps in the vascular endothelium with blood platelets. *Nature* **216**, 1126–1128.

Vaage, J. (1976) Vagal reflexes in the bronchoconstriction occurring after induced intravascular platelet aggregation. *Acta Physiol Scand* **97**, 94–103.

Vaage, J. (1977) Intravascular platelet aggregation and acute respiratory insufficiency. *Circ Shock* **4**, 279–290.

Vaage, J. (1980) The role of platelets in post-traumatic pulmonary insufficiency. *Acta Chir Scand* **499**, 141–159.

Vaage, J. (1982) Intravascular platelet aggregation and pulmonary injury. *Ann NY Acad Sci* **384**, 301–318.

Vaage, J. & Gjesdal, K. (1976) Lung responses and platelet release reaction following induced intravascular platelet aggregation in the cat. *Scand J Clin Lab Invest* **36**, 641–648.

Vaage, J. & Hauge, A. (1977) Small airway constriction and closure after induced intravascular platelet aggregation. *Acta Physiol Scand* **100**, 221–230.

Vaage, J., Bo, G. & Hognestad, J. (1974) Pulmonary responses to intravascular platelet aggregation in the cat. *Acta Physiol Scand* **92**, 546–556.

Vaage, J., Nicolaysen, G. & Waaler, B.A. (1976) Aggregation of blood platelets and increased hydraulic conductivity of pulmonary exchange vessels. *Acta Physiol Scand* **98**, 175–184.

Vaage, J., Wiberg, T. & Scott, E. (1978) Release of prostaglandin-like substances and lung reactions to induced intravascular platelet aggregation in cats. *Scand J Clin Lab Invest* **38**, 337–347.

van der Zee, H., Moon, D.G., Morton, K., Fenton, II, J.W., Gudewicz, P.W. & Kaplan, J.E. (1988) The PAF antagonist WEB 2086 attenuates thrombin-induced leukopenia and thrombocytopenia in sheep. *FASEB J* **2**, A1576.

Vargaftig, B.B., Lefort, J., Chignard, M. & Benveniste, J. (1980) Platelet-activating factor induces a platelet-dependent bronchoconstriction unrelated to the formation of prostaglandin derivatives. *Eur J Pharmacol* **65**, 185–192.

Venturini, C.M., Krebs, S.W. & Kaplan, J.E. (1988) Platelets adhere to thrombin treated endothelium under flow conditions. *FASEB J* **2**, A1163.

Venturini, C.M., Del Vecchio, P.J. & Kaplan, J.E. (1989) Thrombin induced platelet adhesion is modified by endothelial derived relaxing factor (EDRF). *Biochem Biophys Res Commun* **157**, 349–354.

Ward, P.A., Cunningham, T.W., McCulloch, K.K., Phan, S.H., Powell, J. & Johnson, K.J. (1988) Platelet enhancement of O_2^- responses in stimulated human neutrophils: Identification of platelet factor as adenine nucleotide. *Lab Invest* **58**, 37–47.

Wojcik, J.D., Van Horn, D.L., Webber, A.J. & Johnson, S.A. (1969) Mechanism whereby platelets support the endothelium. *Transfusion* **9**, 324–335.

Wu, K.K. & Hoak, J.C. (1974) A new method for the quantitative detection of platelet aggregates in patients with arterial insufficiency. *Lancet* **ii**, 924–926.

11: Platelets and Renal Disease

J. Stewart Cameron

Introduction

Inflammation and coagulation; the endothelial cell

The study of mediators of injury in glomerular disease is still in progress, as we understand better the ways various cellular and humoral inflammatory cascades may interact. To study any individual component, it is usually necessary to isolate it to some extent in an experimental system, which immediately distorts the complex interactions taking place *in vivo*. It is clear that all the inflammatory systems listed in Table 11.1 interact with each other, sometimes at many points; so that whichever is triggered first, all the others are likely to be recruited sooner or later.

Thus platelet function cannot be considered in isolation from other systems, and when we consider coagulation, it is especially important to keep both fluid phase systems, cells (principally monocytes), platelets and endothelium in mind together; the endothelium takes an active rather than a passive part in both maintaining the free flow of blood in health, and in promoting thrombosis, vascular contraction and inflammation during injury. During injury of course, these act as protective mechanisms. Also, short of actual damage, glomerular function may be profoundly affected by a variety of humoral agents released from platelets, including angiotensin, platelet derived growth factor (PDGF) (Deuel & Huang, 1984), platelet activating factor (PAF); and acetyl glyceryl ether phosphorylcholine (AGEPC) (Schlondorff & Neuwirk, 1986) for all of which there are receptors in one glomerular cell or another. Arachidonate-derived products are of especial importance, including eicosanoids such as prostaglandins I_2 and E_2, and thromboxane A_2 (TXA_2) (Lianos, 1984) epoxyeicosatrienoic acids (EETs; Ballou *et al.* 1987), and leukotrienes. These effects are most prominent on the mesangial cells, which being contractile affect both glomerular blood flow and also the area for glomerular filtration. In addition TXA_2 promotes local collagen synthesis, and EETs division of mesangial cells (Harris *et al.* 1989).

The glomerulus itself is a mass of small hemiarterioles, that is, capillaries with smooth muscle cells investing one half of their circumference, on the mesangial side. These are covered with endothelium, and thus the crucial events in glomerular

Table 11.1 Mediator systems in inflammation

Cells	Humoral systems	Cell products
Polymorphonuclear leukocytes	Complement	Free oxygen radicals
Eosinophils	C3b, anaphylatoxins (C3a, C5a), C5–9	Eicosanoids:
T lymphocytes	Coagulation cascade-fibrinopeptides	prostaglandins
Monocytes	Kinins	leukotrienes
Platelets		Platelet activating factor
		Procoagulant activity

injury involve the endothelial cell (Neild & Gordge, 1988). The same is true of the peritubular capillaries, especially involved in allograft rejection but also in glomerulonephritis and lupus. It has long been known that if subendothelial collagen is exposed by loss of endothelial cell cover — by whatever mechanism — then platelets will gather and be powerfully stimulated to release and aggregate. Moreover it has been shown recently that injury of whatever origin may cause expression of procoagulant activity by endothelial cells (Bevilacqua *et al.* 1985), and that endothelial cells produce substances capable of relaxing endothelium derived relaxing factor (EDRF) and contracting (endothelin) local arteriolar myocytes (Vanhoutte, 1988; Yanigasawa *et al.* 1988). Immediately it is clear that experiments performed *in vitro* in the absence of endothelial cells, and even worse on washed platelets in the absence of plasma, are seen to be highly artificial, even if they are convenient.

The role of fibrin and other fluid phase reactants in glomerulonephritis and transplantation has been summarized elsewhere on a number of occasions (Kincaid-Smith, 1984; Hancock & Atkins, 1985) including our own recent review (Neild & Cameron, 1989), emphasizing the role of both monocytes (Holdsworth & Tipping, 1985) and endothelial cells (Bevilacqua *et al.* 1985) in expressing procoagulant activity. Reviews of the literature of platelets and nephritis which can be consulted elsewhere (George *et al.* 1975; Cameron, 1977; Parbtani & Cameron, 1980; Cameron 1984a,b; Neild & Cameron, 1989) have been published, and the topic has also been reviewed in a broader context (Remuzzi & Rossi, 1989). Platelet–endothelial interactions in renal injury have been reviewed in detail by Neild and Gordge (1988).

Platelets as inflammatory cells

Platelets share many functions with both monocytes and polymorphonuclear leukocytes (Nachman & Weksler, 1980) (see Chapter 5). Also, platelets can undertake a form of 'phagocytosis', although this resembles endocytosis into the platelet canalicular system, and true phagosomes are not formed, In passing we should not forget that the *dense granules* of most laboratory animals' platelets contain up to 10 or even 20 times the amount of amines that human and primate platelets do; this is only one of several differences which make extrapolation from animal to human models even more hazardous than usual. *Alpha* (α) *granule* contents are very important, in particular platelet factor 4 (PF4), β-thromboglobulin (β-TG), and the powerful mitogen, platelet derived growth factor (PDGF) (Deuel & Huang, 1984). Both PF4 and PDGF are powerful chemotactic agents for both monocytes and polymorphonuclear leukocytes (PMNs), and in addition PDGF can stimulate cultured glomerular endothelial and mesangial cells to proliferate (Tranqui *et al.* 1985). Platelets are also versatile and potent producers of eicosanoids (see Chapter 7) as are glomerular endothelial and mesangial cells (Lianos, 1984).

The role of platelets in glomerulonephritis

What is the evidence that platelets participate in glomerulonephritis? We can study the effects of mediators in various ways (Table 11.2) and can examine what the evidence may be for each of the headings 1–5 in the table.

Platelet *turnover studies* have been performed in patients with nephritis by a number of authors (George *et al.* 1974), including ourselves. This involves labelling the platelet with either ^{51}Cr or more recently, ^{111}In-oxine. In general platelet turnover was most accelerated in patients with focal segmental glomerulosclerosis (FSGS) and in mesangiocapillary glomerulonephritis (MCGN). In both groups of patients there was some correlation between the severity of vascular injury and the acceleration of platelet turnovers. There is, however, no good evidence that labelled platelets are taken up in excess in the kidneys; they may well be activated in the kidney and taken up in the spleen. In man, the proximity of the liver and spleen makes attempts to assess radioactivity in the kidney difficult (Rigby *et al.* 1980), and no experiments have been done in animals of counting the isolated kidney.

Findings in the kidney

It is impossible, using optical microscopy, to resolve individual platelets in vascular or tissue sections, and although on electron microscopy free platelets with obvious granules may be seen within capillaries, platelets which have discharged their granular contents, i.e. activated platelets, are almost impossible to identify from other cytoplasmic areas, although this can be done (Richman & Kasnic, 1982).

Table 11.2 Methods of study of mediator systems

1	Is turnover of mediator accelerated?
2	Is mediator present at site of injury?
3	Are products of activation present in circulation?
4	Does depletion of mediator abrogate injury?
5	Does use of antagonists of mediator abrogate or ameliorate injury?

Thus, in general one must rely on immune staining of platelet antigens to identify them in tissue. *Platelet-related antigens* have been demonstrated at sites of glomerular injury, using immunofluorescent techniques (Miller *et al.* 1981; Duffus *et al.* 1982). This material usually appears as finely granular focal and segmental aggregates. We have also shown that PF4 is present at the same sites as the platelet membrane antigens in human glomerulonephritis (Duffus *et al.* 1982), a point of particular importance in view of its biological activity. This protein is cationic at physiologic pH (pI 7.6) and therefore binds avidly to the negatively charged proteoglycan of the glomerular capillary (Barnes & Venkatachalam, 1985). This binding to, and masking of, negative charges might itself contribute to injury through induction of proteinuria, as happens with the infusion of other polycations. The presence of PDGF also at sites of glomerular injury in crescentic nephritis is suggested by the finding of increased expression of PDGF receptors in the glomeruli of this type of nephritis (Rubin *et al.* 1988). Unlike lupus nephritis, however (see below), we were unable to demonstrate PDGF itself at sites of injury in primary glomerulonephritis.

Platelet and plasma concentrations of platelet-released factors

Evidence of *systemic platelet activation* is strong in human glomerulonephritis. Circulating platelets are depleted of both dense granule contents (5-hydroxytryptamine (5-HT), (adenosine disphosphate (ADP) (Parbtani *et al.* 1979, 1980a) and α-granule products (β-TG, PF4) (Parbtani *et al.* 1979), whilst in the plasma, increased amounts of most of these products can be demonstrated. Caution must be excercised in interpreting some results from plasma, especially those for 5-HT and β-TG, since these accumulate with decreased renal function, unlike PF4. Crude indices of platelet aggregates, including the ratio of platelet counts in EDTA (which will disaggregate platelets) and in paraformaldehyde, suggest increased amounts of platelet aggregates in both MCGN and IgA nephropathy (Woo *et al.* 1980). The presence or absence of a nephrotic syndrome did not appear to affect the release of 5-HT or β-TG from platelets, although in nephrotic plasma platelets will aggregate spontaneously (see below).

Platelet agglutinating immune complexes

We found evidence of material with the characteristics of *immune complexes* in the plasma of patients with glomerulonephritis, which was capable of agglutinating platelets *in vitro* (Kasai *et al.* 1981). Subsequent studies of lupus and Henoch–Schonlein purpura nephritis have shown good correlations with disease activity (Kasai *et al.* unpublished work) and the amount of this material, although others have identified similar material in the blood of patients with the Kawasaki syndrome, a childhood vasculitis in which the kidney is *not* involved. Older work, and studies in whole animals, suggested that platelet release was most provoked by complexes in strong antibody excess, but a recent paper suggests that complexes of wider composition than this may also be capable of activating washed platelets at least (Battersby *et al.* 1985). Whether platelet activation may occur within the glomeruli by locally bound platelet-activating immune complexes is possible, but remains speculative.

Platelet depeletion experiments in animals

Thus there is ample evidence that platelets are activated in glomerulonephritis, and present within the glomeruli. But what role, if any, do they play in injury? The classical experiment is to study the effect, in an animal model of nephritis, of *platelet depletion*. Apart from the problem of profound species differences in platelet immunology and pharmacology mentioned above, the simple difficulty is that an animal depleted of platelets to a level where platelet action is insufficient usually bleeds to death, whilst if 5–10% of platelets continue to circulate, the general failure to demonstrate inhibition of injury (e.g. Sindrey *et al.* 1979) is no test of the hypothesis. However recently Johnson *et. al.* (1988), who studied a model of *in situ* endothelial antigen–antibody complex formation, employing sequential injection of concanavalin A (con-A) and anti-con-A antibody, succeeded in demonstrating a clear requirement for platelets in both injury and proteinuria, at least in this model.

Effects of antiplatelet drugs in animals and man

What of the effect of *antiplatelet drugs*? One problem is that platelets have at least three intracellular pathways by which activation is sustained, and a second is that the relevance of *in vitro* performance in standard aggregation tests to events *in vivo* is unknown. In human glomerulonephritis there have been anecdotal stories of the effect of antiplatelet agents since Kincaid-Smith's first descriptions (Kincaid-Smith *et al.* 1970), but in almost all studies (Futrakul *et al.* 1978) including our own (Cameron, 1976), the antiplatelet agents have been used as part of multiple drug regimes of varying complexity. However, the careful long-term study from the Mayo clinic (Donadio *et al.* 1984) on patients with MCGN provided convincing evidence of an action of aspirin and dipyridamole together, and is backed up by uncontrolled data using warfarin in addition in the same disease (Zimmerman *et al.* 1983). In animals, a number of earlier studies have shown varying effects of antiserotonin, antihistamine and antiplatelet drugs in models of serum sickness, and both dipyridamole (Koyama *et al.* 1985; Izumino *et al.* 1986) and ticlopidine (Izumino *et al.* 1986, 1987) have been reported recently to inhibit proteinuria (and also glomerular immune complex deposition) in rabbits with either serum sickness (Koyama *et al.* 1985; Izumino *et al.* 1986) or anti-glomerular basement membrane (GBM) nephritis (Izumino *et al.* 1986). In humans also, there appears to be an antiproteinuric effect of dipyridamole (Tojo *et al.* 1978; Ueda *et al.* 1986), but whether this is the result of an effect on glomerular haemodynamics is not clear yet.

Antiprostaglandin agents appear to be an attractive method of disease modification. Most cyclooxygenase inhibitors (such as indomethacin) inhibit proteinuria, but this appears to be a reversible effect depending upon a fall in renal blood flow and glomerular filtration rate (GFR). However, some have argued that improvements in histological appearances also occur in humans with glomerulonephritis under this treatment. Inhibition of TXA_2 production would inhibit monocyte as well as platelet activity, and one group found an improvement in rabbit serum sickness nephritis using imidazole, a TXA_2 inhibitor (Saito *et al.* 1984). However, in contrast we found that OKY-046 (an imidazole derivative) made both clinical and histological aspects of anti-GBM nephritis worse, (Shinkai & Cameron, 1987a) as did Remuzzi and co-workers using aspirin (Bertani *et al.* 1986), although they found that the other cyclooxygenase inhibitor, sulindac, appeared to improve the histological appearances. Niwa *et al.* (1988) showed that OKY-046 reduced proteinuria in patients with nephrotic syndromes of various aetiologies. It is worth remembering that *in vitro*, thromboxane inhibitors do not inhibit platelet aggregation — although they do so powerfully in association with small doses of aspirin (Bertelé *et al.* 1983).

On the basis that PDGF might be involved in the induction of injury, we used the *anti-PDGF* agent trapidil (Shinkai & Cameron, 1987b), which is effective in inhibiting cell proliferation both on 3T3 cells in culture and in arterial denuduation experiments *in vivo*. The model we chose was a model of severe 'accelerated' antiglomerular basement membrane antibody crescentic glomerulonephritis. Unfortunately, in this severe nephritis no amelioration of histological injury, uraemia or proteinuria was observed.

Conclusions

It is clear that platelets are involved in glomerular diseases, but whether they play an important role in the induction of injury is still unknown. It seems almost certain that they **do** play at the least a secondary role in perpetuating or amplifying injury; indeed they could scarcely fail to do so, when almost every form of injury to the glomerulus involves either or both of endothelial damage or exposure of subendothelial structures.

Platelets in lupus nephritis

The circulating platelet, release products and immune complexes

Thrombocytopenia is of course a common finding in systemic lupus (Miller *et al.* 1983), with or without nephritis. In general, this is the direct result of circulating antibody directed against platelet surface glycoproteins (Karpatkin *et al.* 1971).

However, thrombocytopenia correlates with the presence and severity of nephritis in lupus, and platelet turnover is accelerated in lupus with nephritis, the more so in the severe proliferative form of the disease (Clark *et al.* 1975). We showed also that intraplatelet 5-HT was lower in lupus than in any other form of nephritis we studied, and these data again correlated with proteinuria and other indices of the severity of nephritis (Parbtani *et al.* 1980b). Yet again, as in primary glomerulonephritis, plasma concentrations of platelet release proteins such as β-TG and PF4 were markedly elevated (Parbtani *et al.* 1979)

We found that these amine and α-granule depleted platelets were paradoxically hyperaggregable *in vitro* (Marchesi *et al.* 1981), even in the absence of a nephrotic syndrome, and thus should not be described as 'exhausted'. Obviously here is a possible amplification loop for further injury. One possible cause for this hyperaggregability seems to be that the platelets were bearing immune complexes, bound by the Fc receptors to the cell. Platelet-associated IgG is of course raised in lupus (Bonacossa *et al.* 1985; Howe & Lynch, 1987), and we confirmed this not only for lupus nephritis (Bennett *et al.* 1986) but also in primary glomerulonephritis; however, the nature of this IgG is not known — in lupus some is presumably specific antiplatelet antibody. We were able to show also that the serum of patients with lupus nephritis, as in glomerulonephritis, contained large quantities of platelet-agglutinating material, some of which was IgG and was of high molecular weight (Kasai *et al.* 1981); that is, it had the properties of platelet-agglutinating complexes.

However, a more precise demonstration of the presence of immune complexes on the platelet surface in lupus was the finding that both double-stranded DNA and its specific antibody were present on platelets, and moreover that DNAase removed both (Frampton *et al.* 1986); suggesting they were present in immune complex form (Taylor *et al.* 1985) rather than, for example, associated with the platelet DNA receptor. Thus circulating, amine-depleted platelets in lupus have immune complexes containing DNA and its specific antibody associated with their surface.

Findings in the kidney

In the kidney affected by lupus nephritis, we showed the presence of platelet-related antigen and PF4 using immunofluorescent techniques (Duffus *et al.* 1982), but unlike primary glomerulonephritis we were also able to identify PDGF in the glomeruli in lupus (Frampton *et al.* 1988) employing on this occasion an immunoperoxidase method. Like PF4, PDGF is a cationic protein (pI 10.2) which could bind readily to the polyanionic coat of the glomerular capillary wall. Camussi and co-workers (1986) likewise report the presence of platelet cationic proteins in the glomeruli of biopsies from patients with lupus nephritis, and have shown that the association is charge-dependent.

Other histological studies by Kant *et al.* (1981) point to the importance of glomerular capillary thrombi, which we have shown to contain platelets, PF4 and PDGF, in the progression of lupus nephritis. They found a correlation between the number of glomerular capillary thrombi in renal biopsies, and the subsequent finding of glomerulosclerosis, and of a decline in renal function. These findings have not been confirmed by other workers, however (Leaker *et al.* 1987). On occasion, in lupus the glomerular capillary thrombi are so severe that acute renal failure is caused (Ponticelli *et al.* 1974), and in a few patients a thrombotic thrombocytopenic (TTP) purpura or haemolytic uraemic (HUS)-like syndrome can be observed (Gelfand *et al.* 1985); this is difficult to diagnose unless the red cell fragmentation is noticed, and is discussed below in the section on haemolytic-uraemic syndromes.

Antiphospholipid antibodies

In lupus and lupus-related disorders it is well known that antiphospholipid antibodies may be present (Harris *et al.* 1985), and that this antibody is associated with the *in vitro* 'lupus anticoagulant' phenomenon (Rosner *et al.* 1987). In this state, the presence of a prolongation of some *in vitro* phospholipid-dependent tests is associated *in vivo* with thrombosis, usually venous, and also recurrent abortions (Harris *et al.* 1985). We showed that some 40% of our patients with lupus nephritis (Frampton *et al.* 1987), even after immunosuppressive treatment, had detectable antiphospholipid antibody present, sometimes of all three isotypes: IgA, IgM and IgG. The presence of this antibody correlated with the finding of glomerular thrombi in renal biopsies taken at the same time, suggesting a role for the antiphospholipid antibody in the pathogenesis or progression of the nephritis.

The mechanisms by which the antiphospholipid antibodies lead to thrombosis *in vivo* are unknown. To study this we (Frampton & Cameron, 1988) prepared purified antiphospholipid antibodies from lupus sera and examined their specificity. As others have reported, they reacted preferentially with negatively charged phospholipids, but these native polyclonal antibodies did not react at all with DNA, which has been reported for mouse monoclonal antibodies. When normal platelets were exposed to the antibody, there was no aggregation since phospholipids such as phosphatidylserine are not exposed on the outer leaflet of the resting platelet plasma membrane. During activation, however, these are exposed, and we found that previous treatment with subthreshold doses of ADP, thrombin or collagen would render the treated platelets highly susceptible to aggregation and thromboxane release by the purified antiphospholipid antibody. Khamashta *et al.* (1988) have reported similar results, using disintegrated platelets.

This might explain why in lupus, either circulating immune complexes or antiphospholipid antibodies may each be associated with good health and an absence of thrombosis. It may require the coincidence of immune complex-activated platelets and the antiphospholipid antibody to precipitate intraglomerular, and peripheral venous thrombosis.

Implications for treatment

Given the strong evidence for the involvement of platelets in glomerular injury in lupus nephritis, it is logical to use antiplatelet agents as part of the therapy given to these individuals. Although this is quite a widespread practice, it is impossible to see an effect of these agents alone against the background of varying spontaneous disease activity and changes in immunosuppressive treatment. In general, formal anticoagulation has been used only in patients with peripheral thrombosis.

Platelet hyperaggregability in the nephrotic syndrome

Nephrotic individuals have a well-documented tendency to thrombosis (Cameron, 1984b; Livio, 1989). Despite major changes in many procoagulant and regulator proteins of the coagulation cascade in nephrotics, which have been emphasized and widely discussed, the net effect of these changes is, in the majority of nephrotic patients, often trivial in functional terms. It seems more likely to me that the thrombotic tendency of nephrotic patients depends to a major extent on platelet hyperaggregability (Cameron, 1984b; Cameron *et al.* 1988).

The *platelet count* in nephrotic patients has variously been reported as either normal or raised (see Cameron, 1984b; Livio, 1989, for a review) but the elevation, if present, is usually mild. However, there is agreement that platelets from nephrotic patients are hyperaggregable to ADP stimulation *in vitro* when in their own plasma, on occasion aggregating spontaneously; this hyperaggregability could be reversed by adding concentrated urine protein to the *in vitro* system (Bang *et al.* 1973). Thus it seemed that some factor, or factors, present in plasma modulate platelet function and are lost in the urine in nephrotics.

Silver and co-workers (Silver *et al.* 1973; Bills *et al.* 1976) showed that *albumin* modulates arachidonic-acid-induced aggregation, and addition of pure albumin either *in vitro* (Yoshida & Aoki, 1978; Remuzzi *et al.* 1979a; Stuart *et al.* 1980), or *in vivo* by infusion (Remuzzi *et al.* 1979a) to nephrotic platelets both restore hyperaggregability to normal. Those patients with a plasma albumin below 20 g/litre showed the greatest effect. The production of TXA_2 (or malonaldehyde, as a general indicator of prostaglandin production) by platelets *in vitro* is greater at lower ambient albumin concentrations (Yoshida & Aoki, 1978; Stuart *et al.* 1980; Jackson *et al.* 1982; Schiepatti *et al.* 1984). It seems possible, therefore, that binding sites for arachidonate on the albumin compete with the cyclooxygenase (which leads to TXA_2 production), for arachidonate released from membrane lipids by phospholipase A. Thus, the hyperaggregability of nephrotic platelets appeared to be explained.

While this is clearly an important mechanism in nephrotic platelet hyperaggregability, it is not, however, the whole story. First, hypoalbuminaemia itself reduces the production of endogenous arachidonate from the membrane lipid

(Stuart *et al.* 1980), which may explain the minor hyperaggregability of nephrotic platelet rich plasma to collagen (which leads to endogenous arachidonate release) when compared to the effect of exogenously added arachidonate (Jackson *et al.* 1982), in a non-physiological *in vitro* system. In addition, there is no increase in TXA_2 generation in the presence of demonstrated hyperaggregability to collagen (Jackson *et al.* 1982).

Hyperlipidaemia is also a prominent feature of the nephrotic syndrome, either hypercholesterolaemia alone, or together with hypertriglyceridaemia. Lipoproteins bind to platelets (Aviram & Brook, 1983), low density lipoproteins (LDL) enhancing and high density lipoproteins (HDL) inhibiting aggregation; these effects may be mediated through effects on adenylate cyclase (Colli *et al.* 1985), since intraplatelet cAMP levels are one of the main controls of aggregation and release. Hyperlipidaemia is associated, in nephrotics, with spontaneous aggregation (Jackson *et al.* 1982). Ambient lipids 'label' platelet membrane lipids — for example, if ω3-unsaturated fatty acids are fed, which is associated with a decrease in platelet aggregability and an increase in bleeding time (Galloway *et al.* 1985). There are also opposing effects of LDL and HDL on endothelial cell production of prostacyclin (PGI_2) (Nordoy *et al.* 1978), which is a powerful modulator of platelet activity. The effects of nephrotic hyperlipidaemia on *in vitro* hyperaggregability and *in vivo* thrombosis deserve more exploration.

We must also consider the question of the **charge** on platelets. Like all cells, platelets have a net negative charge on their surface, as can be demonstrated by electrophoresis. Using an indirect assessment of charge using the binding of the cationic dye Alcian blue, Levin and co-workers (1985) suggested that in children with the steroid-responsive nephrotic syndrome there was a reduced net negative charge on the platelets and red cells. This might more readily lead to platelet aggregation, and spontaneous red cell aggregation has been described in nephrotics (Ozanne *et al.* 1983) as well as spontaneous platelet aggregation (Jackson *et al.* 1982; Levin *et al.* 1985). Levin and co-workers suggested that this phenomenon might relate specifically to the pathogenesis of minimal-change nephrotic syndrome, but others either found the same effect in all nephrotics of whatever histology (Boulton Jones *et al.* 1986), or could not confirm the data at all, even using Alcian blue (Feehally *et al.* 1986). Recently, direct measurements of platelet charge in nephrotics using electrophoresis have shown no difference in charge from normal (Cohen, H.T. *et al.* 1988), so the significance of the data based on studies using Alcian blue binding is doubtful at the moment.

However, we (Bennett & Cameron, 1987) have found hyperaggregability to ristocetin — a cationic compound — in nephrotic adults irrespective of underlying histology. This hyperaggregability appeared to be independent of the depletion of albumin, or the availability of arachidonate, which of course is not needed for aggregation using ristocetin. The hyperaggregability to ristocetin described probably relates most to the elevated levels of von Willebrand factor found in almost all nephrotics (Bennett & Cameron, 1987; Cameron *et al.* 1988), to which ristocetin binds in a triple complex with the platelet. However, in addition the amount of IgG present on (and in) the platelets was reduced in proportion to the reduction in serum IgG found in all nephrotics. This reduction in surface protein would reduce the negative charge, and this could affect aggregability also.

It is clear that there may be a number of factors involved in platelet hyperaggregability in the nephrotic syndrome, and also that it may provide an important component of a 'vicious circle' of damage in glomerular disease leading to profuse proteinuria.

Platelet involvement in haemolytic-uraemic syndromes

The presence of thrombocytopenia, along with evidence of red cell fragmentation, is of course central to the definitions of both the haemolytic-uraemic syndrome (HUS) (Gasser *et al.* 1955; Kaplan & Remuzzi, 1989) and thrombotic thrombocytopenic purpura (TTP) (Amorosi & Ultmann, 1966; Rossi, 1989). In the latter condition, systemic effects, and in particular central nervous system (CNS) signs and symptoms are usually present, whereas in HUS the condition usually manifests itself only in the kidney and renal failure, often requiring dialysis, is common. The other major difference is that HUS is predominantly a disease of young children, either sporadically and in micro-epidemics (which may represent two different forms of the syndrome) whilst the rarer TTP affects mainly adults. In some patients, the histological changes associated with HUS are present apparently without changes in the peripheral blood film. This condition has been termed 'malignant nephrosclerosis' by some renal pathologists (Bohle *et al.* 1977).

Much evidence suggests that HUS is just what its name implies, a syndrome in which a variety of circumstances may lead to a final common pathway of endothelial damage and unrestrained intravascular platelet aggregation (Kaplan & Drummond, 1978; Drummond, 1985; Neild, 1987; Kaplan & Remuzzi, 1989). This, rather than primary generation of fibrin, appears to be the primary event in the syndrome. Most authors view TTP to be another end of the HUS spectrum, with a considerable number of overlap cases being seen (Remuzzi, 1987). Another route to an almost identical syndrome is via accelerated hypertension with micro-angiopathy and haemolytic anaemia.

Platelet involvement

Apart from the obvious and usually severe thrombocytopenia, platelet consumption and turnover — and by inference production — have all been shown to be greatly accelerated in both HUS and TTP by studies on reinjected radiolabelled platelets (Harker & Schlichter, 1972; Berberich *et al.* 1974; Riella *et al.* 1976) with a half-life of the circulating platelet population of less than 1 day in some cases. The circulating platelets are depleted of both dense granule and α-granule contents (Fong & Kaplan, 1982; Edelfonti *et al.* 1985; Walters *et al.* 1988), whilst plasma levels of platelet-released substances are elevated (Claris Appiani *et al.* 1982; Fong & Kaplan, 1982; Walters *et al.* 1988). Platelets and platelet antigens are present in the thrombi seen within the glomeruli and afferent arterioles in both HUS and TTP (Miller *et al.* 1981; Churg & Strauss, 1985). During the acute phase of the disease, the circulating amine-depleted platelet population is hypoaggregable (Fong & Kaplan, 1982; Walters *et al.* 1988) and although normal aggregation returns, the platelets remain hyporesponsive to PGI_2 (Bloom *et al.* 1985) and we have consistently observed hyperaggregability to collagen, ADP and arachidonate during the recovery phase whilst intraplatelet amines remain low (Trompeter *et al.*, unpublished observations).

Thus, platelets are clearly involved centrally in the pathogenesis of the HUS syndrome of all types. The problems lie in the direction of exactly what role platelet aggregation might play. Primary fibrin generation seems not to be present and fibrin turnovers are normal (Berberich *et al.* 1974), and fibrinopeptide concentrations are low in HUS. Current ideas suggest that the intense platelet activation, consumption and release characteristic of this syndrome are secondary results of events occurring either in the endothelium of blood vessels, or because of aggregatory substances in the circulation; rather than that a primary platelet abnormality is the major cause of injury. Naturally, however, having been activated, platelets will contribute to the generation and amplification of injury through release of vasoactive and mitogenic platelet contents. Levin *et al.* (1986) have adduced evidence of activation of PDGF in HUS.

Endothelial abnormalities in HUS

The nature and genesis of the primary endothelial injury is still the subject of speculation. As precipitating agents, the role of *Escherichia coli* capable of exerting toxicity on vero cells cultured *in vitro* (verotoxin) has received much support recently (Drummond, 1985; Karmali *et al.* 1985; Lancet editorial, 1987). Other bacteria, such as *Shigella*, *Yersinia* and *Campylobacter*, several viruses, and agents such as mitomycin C (Giroux *et al.* 1985) and cyclosporin A (Brown *et al.* 1986) which are directly toxic to endothelial cells have also been found to play a role in the induction of clinical HUS. Neuraminidase-mediated injury may also occur in HUS associated with pneumococcal sepsis (Rose *et al.* 1985), and a variety of other circumstances such as snakebite, oral contraceptives and pregnancy may precipitate HUS, perhaps in individuals who are genetically susceptible (see below). Anti-endothelial cell antibodies have been described in HUS (Leung *et al.* 1988), but these may arise secondary to endothelial injury rather than as a primary event.

Endothelium is now known to be capable, when activated by stimuli such as interferon gamma, of expressing HLA-DR (Bevilacqua *et al.* 1985) and procoagulant activity (Holdsworth *et al.* 1985). To complicate matters further, endothelial cells are now thought to be capable of expressing an antigen identical to platelet glycoprotein Ib as well (Asch *et al.* 1988; Sprandio *et al.* 1988).

Endothelial generation of PGI_2

Great interest has been shown in the ability of the endothelium to secrete the platelet anti-aggregatory substance prostacyclin (PGI_2) in the HUS (Remuzzi *et al.* 1978). The ability of sera from patients with HUS to support PGI_2 production from endothelial cells *in vitro* has been shown to be low in a proportion of patients with HUS (Remuzzi *et al.* 1978), especially those with a sporadic onset (Walters *et al.* 1988), rather than those occurring in epidemic clusters. In the sporadic cases a strong family history may be found (Remuzzi *et al.* 1979b), sometimes in association with the inability to generate PGI_2 in the affected family members, suggesting an inherited predisposition. One current problem is that the factor (or factors) which promote PGI_2 synthesis by endothelium have not been characterized fully (Deckmyn *et al.* 1985). In TTP, accelerated degradation of PGI_2 has been described also (Chen *et al.* 1981) suggesting the existence of PGI_2 stabilizing factors in plasma.

These discussions are of more than theoretical interest, since many observers have suggested (Remuzzi *et al.* 1978; Misiani *et al.* 1982) that plasma infusion or plasma exchange may benefit HUS and TTP, following the first observations in 1977 (Byrnes & Khurana, 1977). A recent careful prospective controlled trial in children with severe HUS, however, showed little benefit from this treatment over conservative and supportive measures including dialysis (Loirat *et al.* 1988), and in a variable and sometimes relapsing disease with a high remission rate, as in the case of HUS, the effects of treatment are particularly difficult to evaluate.

Platelet aggregating substances in HUS and TTP

The presence of platelet aggregating substances has been suggested by several observers, mostly in patients with TTP (Lian *et al.* 1983), but also in cases of epidemic HUS (Monnens *et al.* 1985), whose nature or natures are at present obscure; although a molecular weight of 37 000 has been suggested, together with a binding-inactivating protein present in normal plasma of molecular weight 150 000 in the best-studied example (Siddiqui & Lian, 1985). The relation of this factor to von Willebrand factor (vWF) concentrations and multimer pattern is not yet clear.

In HUS, levels of circulating vWF are greatly increased, as one expects after endothelial injury, during which vWF is released from endothelium (Brown *et al.* 1986). A large proportion of this circulating vWF consists of multimers of high molecular weight (Rose *et al.* 1985). When vWF is added to TTP plasma *in vitro*, its platelet aggregant activity was increased (Kelton *et al.* 1984). Siddiqui and Lian (1985) demonstrated, however, that neither IgG itself nor antibody directed against the platelet glycoprotein Ib (GpIb) receptor for vWF inhibited the aggregatory activity of TTP plasma, findings confirmed by Kelton (1987) who did, however, obtain inhibition with a monoclonal antibody against GPIIb–IIIa.

In contrast, Moake (1985) has identified an abnormal multimeric pattern of vWF in relapsing TTP **between** attacks, which disappeared, either when thrombocytopenia appeared, or between attacks when cryoprecipitate was infused, and Murphy *et al.* (1987) describe a clear interaction between platelet aggregating material and vWF in a similar pattern.

Finally, an interesting observation is that when normal plasma is incubated with *E. coli* verotoxin, platelet aggregating ability was generated (Rose *et al.* 1985). In addition to all these factors, red cell stroma and nucleotides released from fragmented red cells will obviously also promote platelet aggregation.

Clearly the presence of platelet aggregating material — of whatever type — free in the plasma, would again support a role for plasma **exchange**, which in this case should be superior to plasma **infusion**.

Treatment

Apart from plasma exchange, the proposed central role for a deficiency of PGI_2 production (Remuzzi *et al.* 1978) and the ample evidence of platelet activation summarized above, suggest a role for both PGI_2 infusions and for antiplatelet agents. It is disappointing to report that there is almost no evidence that either antiplatelet agents (Kaplan & Drummond, 1978; Goldstein *et al.* 1979; del Zoppo, 1987) or PGI_2 infusion (Defreyn *et al.* 1982) are effective in altering the course of established TTP or HUS (see Kaplan & Remuzzi, 1989, for review of treatment).

Platelet dysfunction in uraemia and platelet activation during haemodialysis

Introduction

The haemostatic defect found in uraemia has been known clinically since the time of Bright. It is complex, and has been reviewed in several recent articles (Deykin, 1983; Andrassy & Ritz, 1985; Jubelierer, 1985; Livio *et al.* 1985; Remuzzi, 1988; Gotti & Remuzzi, 1989), and especially from the platelet point of view by Remuzzi and Pusineri (1989). In uraemia, the striking findings are a very prolonged bleeding time (15–30 minutes or more compared with control values of 5–6 minutes) (Lewis *et al.* 1956) whilst conventional *in vitro* tests of coagulation such as prothrombin or kaolin–cephalin times are normal (Larsson, 1971), and the platelet count is normal or near-normal. Immediately, these data suggest a qualitative defect of platelet function, or of platelet interaction with vWF and/or the endothelium. Study of the problem is complicated by superimposed effects of haemodialysis, with exposure of blood to extracorporeal circuits containing bio-incompatible membranes (Addonizio & Colman, 1982) plus treatment with heparin; unfortunately, some authors have not distinguished adequately between studies in uraemic patients receiving, or not receiving, haemodialysis.

Platelets in uraemia

Platelet function in uraemia has been studied for more than 30 years. Numerous studies, reviewed in Remuzzi and Pusineri (1989) show that a modest *thrombocytopenia*, insufficient in itself to cause haemostatic problems, is quite common in uraemia, despite a normal number of megakaryocytes in the bone marrow. Uptake of [^{75}S-]selenomethionine into platelets is reduced, however (Gafter *et al.* 1987), suggesting some reduction in thrombopoiesis. Survival of injected labelled platelets is normal (Stewart, 1967). Thrombopoietin production from the kidney has not been measured in uraemia.

Defective *platelet adhesion* was one of the first aspects of platelet function to be reported abnormal in uraemia (Salzman & Neri, 1966; Stewart & Castaldi 1967). This may depend in part on the *anaemia of renal failure*, since platelet adhesion improves, by an unknown mechanism, with increasing haematocrit (Eknoyan *et al.* 1969; Turitto & Weiss, 1980). In parallel with these data, Livio *et al.* (1982), Cohen *et al.* (1988) and many others provide ample data to show that bleeding times can be shortened in uraemics by red cell transfusions, and a similar effect is noted following erythropoietin administration to uraemic subjects (Moia *et al.* 1987). The possible role of vWF is discussed below.

In vitro platelet aggregation in uraemia is a controversial topic (see Remuzzi and Pusineri, 1989, for detailed review). Both physiological stimuli such as ADP, adrenaline, thrombin, serotonin and arachidonic acid have been studied, and also aggregation dependent upon surface actions such as that induced by collagen, immune complexes and kaolin. Most of this work has been done *in vitro* on stirred platelet-rich plasma (which contains a variably lower concentration of platelets in uraemia than normal because of anaemia), or on washed platelets resuspended in saline; using different agents in differing concentrations, in patients with or without haemo- or peritoneal dialysis, and with differing degrees of uraemia; dose responses and thresholds have in general not been studied.

Thus, some differences of opinion are inevitable, and relevance to events *in vivo* speculative. Reduced aggregation to ADP (Castaldi *et al.* 1966; Evans *et al.* 1972) and thrombin (Salzman & Neri, 1966; Evans *et al.* 1972) have been most often described. However, other authors have failed to note decreased aggregation in uraemic patients, and whilst this perhaps arises because of effects from concomitant haemodialysis (see below) in some data, other careful studies (Gordge *et al.* 1988) have failed to show defective aggregation in patients not yet receiving dialysis. Phospholipid (*platelet factor III*) is also reported to be diminished in uraemia (Altschuter *et al.* 1960).

Platelet nucleotide content is reduced in uraemia (Eknoyan & Brown, 1981), both ADP and serotonin, and ATP content is low, with reduced ATP release in response to a variety of agents (di Minno *et al.* 1985). Thus, uraemic platelets may be considered to have an acquired storage pool defect. *Intraplatelet cyclic AMP* is increased in uraemic platelets (Vlakoyannis & Schoeppe, 1982), which might contribute to the failure of aggregation, since a fall in cAMP is a prerequisite for aggregation in response to most (but not all) aggregatory agents (see Chapter 3). In addition, *intraplatelet calcium concentration* is elevated (Gura *et al.* 1982), which reverses almost to normal on treatment with 1α-OH vitamin D. *Parathyroid hormone* (PTH) is elevated in almost all severe uraemic subjects (Arnaud, 1973), and regulates intracellular Ca^{2+}, stimulating adenyl cyclase and raising intracellular cAMP. *In vitro*, PTH was found by Remuzzi and co-workers (Remuzzi *et al.* 1981; Benigni *et al.* 1985) to inhibit platelet aggregation; however, this finding is controversial (Leithner *et al.* 1984).

Platelet production of *thromboxane* in response to a variety of agents has been reported as low in uraemic platelets (Smith & Dunn, 1982; Remuzzi *et al.* 1983). However, in both these studies the patients were on regular haemodialysis treatment (see below), and di Minno *et al.* (1985) could not confirm the findings. Winter *et al.* (1983a), studying non-dialysed patients, only found low platelet thromboxane B_2 (TXB_2) production in a subgroup of uraemic patients who also had low aggregation response and high aggregation thresholds to arachidonic acid. Kyrle *et al.* (1988) found no difference between controls and dialysed uraemics in TXB_2 in blood coming from a standard cut.

Remuzzi and co-workers (1983) suggested that the failure to produce thromboxane A_2 was the result of a cyclooxygenase defect in the uraemic platelet, since endoperoxide production and prostaglandin E_2 (PGE_2) synthesis were also reduced during clotting, and PGH synthetase activity was normal; the thromboxane receptor appeared normal as judged by response to the synthetic agonist U46619. However, in the light of the data of Winter *et al.* (1983a) and Bloom *et al.* (1986), and their own subsequent data (Gaspari *et al.* 1987) cyclooxygenase inhibition, even if present, now seems probably not to be a critical step.

Platelet–vessel-wall interaction

The role of von Willebrand factor

All authors are agreed that von Willebrand factor (vWF) antigen concentrations are raised in uraemia (Kazatchkine *et al.* 1976; Remuzzi *et al.* 1977; Warrell *et al.* 1979; Turney *et al.* 1981). The multimeric structure of this antigenic material was in general normal (Mannucci *et al.* 1983; Livio *et al.* 1986b) although using prolonged electrophoresis Winter *et al.* (1983b) showed an excess of small fragments, and Gralnick *et al.* (1989) a deficiency of large multimers, despite careful use of proteases to prevent proteolysis after sampling. Gralnick *et al.* also confirmed the finding of Turney *et al.* (1981), that ristocetin-induced aggregation was reduced in uraemia, and Winter *et al.* (1984) noted decreased release of vWF from human uraemic forearm veins in response to ischaemia. Recently, Andrassy and co-workers (1988) have demonstrated by peptidic digestion and two-dimensional electrophoresis that the GpIb and IIb–IIIa platelet receptors for vWF are abnormal in uraemia. Thus a convincing story can be built up around ineffective vWF (perhaps proteolysed), together with a defective platelet receptor.

However, in contrast, others (Herrmann *et al.* 1977; Remuzzi *et al.* 1977; Warrell *et al.* 1979) did **not** find reduced vWF activity (ristocetin co-factor) in uraemia, or reduced ristocetin-induced aggregation (Jorgensen & Ingeberg, 1979); and despite the observations of Winter *et al.* (1984), the bleeding time in uraemia is consistently reversed towards normal by the administration of fresh cryoprecipitate rich in multimers of vWF (Janson *et al.* 1978) or deamino-8-D-arginine vasopressin (DDAVP) (Mannucci *et al.* 1983), which releases fresh multimeric vWF from vascular endothelium. True, DDAVP is also capable of this in patients with some varieties of von Willebrand disease, so a defect in vWF release is not excluded. Both Cases *et al.* (1988) and Gralnick *et al.* (1989) reported that vWF binds normally to uraemic platelets, but Escolar *et al.* (1988) found abnormal binding to the GPIIb–IIIa fibrinogen receptor. In addition, Weinstein *et al.* (1985) report abnormalities of coagulant Factor VIII (haemophilic factor) itself in uraemia, again possibly the result of abnormal proteolysis. Thus the role of vWF factor in platelet interactions and the haemostatic defect of uraemia is not yet clear.

The role of vascular protaglandin production

The other aspect of platelet function in relation to vessel walls is the production and release of PGI_2, which strongly inhibits platelet release (see Chapter 3). Vessels from uraemic animals (Silberbauer *et al.* 1978) and uraemic patients (Remuzzi *et al.* 1979c) produce increased amounts of PGI_2 *in vitro*, while uraemic platelets remain normally susceptible to this prostaglandin (Pusineri *et al.* 1980). Kyrle *et al.* (1988) found increased PGI_2 in blood from a standard cut, and also decreased release of β-TG. The increased production of PGI_2 has been attributed to increased amounts of a plasma prostacyclin-stimulating factor (PSF) in uraemia (Defreyn *et al.* 1980) but this has not been characterized fully (Deckmyn *et al.* 1985) and other PGI_2 stimulating factors may be present in uraemic plasma. Also, conjugated oestrogens restore the bleeding time to normal in uraemics *without* altering vascular PGI_2 (Livio *et al.* 1986a) — although equally no other haemostatic function studied was improved, and the role of this treatment in uraemic bleeding remains obscure, suggesting that there are as yet unexplored facets of the prolonged bleeding time in uraemic patients.

Effects of dialysis on platelet function in uraemia

Here we have two aspects to consider: the benefit gained from the removal, by dialysis, of substances potentially toxic to platelets; and the effects of exposure of platelets to foreign material in the extracorporeal circuit during haemodialysis, which will not be present during peritoneal dialysis.

Removal by dialysis of compounds toxic to platelets and improvement in platelet function

Stewart and Castaldi (1967) were amongst the first to report that haemodialysis immediately — but temporarily — improved platelet function; both the adhesion response to ADP and the generation of platelet factor III activity. These observations have been amply confirmed since (Rabiner, 1972; Lindsay *et al.* 1975; Nenci *et al.* 1979). Smith and Dunn (1981) showed that in addition thromboxane production is decreased (but see below). This suggests that substances of low molecular weight, capable of passing, by diffusion, through the cellulose membranes still generally in use, are — at least in part — responsible for the defects in platelet function found in uraemia. These factor(s) have not been characterized, but guanidinosuccinic acid (Eknoyan *et al.* 1969; Horowitz *et al.* 1970), phenolic acids (Rabiner & Molinas, 1970) and even urea itself (Eknoyan *et al.* 1969) have all been suggested as culprits, along with higher molecular weight substances in the 'middle' molecular mass range (500–2000 Da) (Gallice *et al.* 1980; Bazilinski *et al.* 1985), or somewhat smaller (Mabuchi & Nakahashi, 1983). The nature of the substance or substances responsible for reduced platelet function in uraemia remain obscure. Peritoneal dialysis, both intermittent and continuous (CAPD, continuous ambulatory peritoneus dialysis) appears equally capable of restoring platelet function to normal (Stewart & Castaldi, 1967; Lindsay *et al.* 1976; Nenci *et al.* 1979; Arends *et al.* 1981).

Platelet aggregation and release in response to extracoporeal haemodialysis circuits and anticoagulation

Haemodialysis for chronic renal failure is usually performed twice or (more usually) thrice weekly for 4 to 6 hours, using circuits consisting of access lines made from polyvinyl chloride tubing, sometimes with a lining of polycarbonate, and cellulose dialysis membranes of 0.7–1.5 m^2 in area, over which the blood is spread in a thin film to facilitate diffusion. In conventional dialysis, removal of solutes by convection (ultrafiltration) is trivial. Heparin is normally used to prevent coagulation in the dialyser circuit. Thus, both the materials used and the anticoagulants employed to prevent clotting in the extracorporeal circuit may induce platelet aggregation. Bleeding (Vicks *et al.* 1983), atheromatous vascular disease and thrombosis (Lindsay *et al.* 1972a) are all associated with long-term dialysis treatment.

Anticoagulation is usually by heparin given into the arterial line of the circuit at rates of up to 600 units/hour by syringe pump (Donati & Pangrazzi, 1989). This may be reversed at the end of dialysis with protamine sulphate. Initially to establish each patient's heparin requirements, the heparinization may be evaluated by whole blood activated partial thromboplastin time. Heparin is, of course, known to be capable of causing platelet aggregation (Zucker, 1979; King & Kelton, 1984) and thus may increase the thrombogenic potential during dialysis. Longer acting, low molecular weight heparins are under evaluation (Ljungberg *et al.* 1987), PGI_2 (Turney *et al.* 1980) has been used in high-risk patients, and calcium chelating agents are also under study (Scharschmidt *et al.* 1977; Flanigan *et al.* 1987). Finally dialysis at high blood flow rates without any heparin or other anticoagulant at all has its advocates (Casati *et al.* 1984; Sanders *et al.* 1985; Schwab *et al.* 1987).

In addition, the effects of the materials and the dialyser design on platelet activation must be considered (Addonizio & Colman, 1982; Schmitt *et al.* 1987). It had been known for 20 years that dialysers containing cellulose membranes, usually prepared by the cuprammonium process, caused acute thrombocytopenia with release of platelet contents (Addonizio & Colman, 1982; Endo *et al.* 1982; Hakim & Schafer, 1985). Sometimes this thrombocytopenia is severe enough to induce bleeding (Vicks *et al.* 1983) but more attention has recently been paid to the release of intraplatelet substances such as PF4 β-TG and TXA_2 (Addonizio *et al.* 1979; Endo *et al.* 1982; Hakim & Schafer, 1985; Schmitt *et al.* 1987).

This platelet activation with release of TXA_2 and other platelet contents, arising from platelet contact with dialyser membrane, probably accounts for the apparently conflicting data on platelet aggregability, and on release of TXA_2 and other contents, from platelets studied *ex vivo* from haemodialysed uraemic patients. These functions have been noted to be reduced (Smith & Dunn, 1981; Remuzzi *et al.* 1983), or normal (Winter *et al.* 1983a), or supranormal (Endo *et al.* 1982; Rylance *et al.* 1985; Bloom *et al.* 1986; Viener *et al.* 1986), by different authors, in parallel with similarly discordant results on aggregation responses. The combination of reduced platelet function from uraemia, complicated by activation from very strong stimuli in the extracoporeal circuit, might be expected to produce discordant results from time to time.

This disagreement may also arise from the different stimulating agents used (collagen, ADP, adrenaline, thrombin and arachidonic acid), the different dosages used, and different timing of samples in relation to dialysis. Remuzzi *et al.* (1982, 1983) pointed to the important fact that at **low** arachidonate concentrations of 0.25 mmol, platelets from uraemic subjects on haemodialysis produced more TXA_2 or malonaldehyde than normal platelets; whereas at *higher* concentrations in excess of 1 mmol, uraemic platelets produced less TXA_2. Finally it must not be forgotten that the majority of the TXA_2 released in extracorporeal circuits from blood arises *not* from platelets, but from other sources, notably monocytes (Mahiout *et al.* 1987).

The type of membrane used is clearly critical, and recently there has been much interest in polyacrylonitrile, polysulphone and other high-flux membranes, which appear to activate contact systems and cells much less than cellulose membranes (Schmitt *et al.* 1987), and which cause less thrombocytopenia and platelet release. This type of membrane is generally used in the high-convection dialysers used for continous arteriovenous haemofiltration (CAVH), or for continuous pumpless arteriovenous haemodialysis (CAVHD), in critically ill patients in acute renal failure. This type of treatment requires continuous anticoagulation, sometimes for many days, but even using heparin bleeding is remarkably rare (Stevens *et al.* 1988).

Antiplatelet agents in haemodialysis

Because of reliance on external arteriovenous teflon–silastic shunts in the early history of haemodialysis, which frequently thrombosed, together with their recent use for acute renal failure for intermittent haemodialysis, CAVH and CAVHD, there has been interest in preventing thrombosis of this foreign body in the circulation; thrombosis occurs despite the haemostatic defects mentioned above. An additional incentive was the high incidence of chronic vascular and myocardial disease suffered by the dialysis population. Low-dose aspirin (Lindsay *et al.* 1972b; Harter *et al.* 1979) with or without concomitant dipyridamole or its analogues, were found to reduce platelet losses in the dialysers, and an even lower dose of aspirin prolonged further the bleeding time in uraemics (Livio *et al.* 1986b; Gaspari *et al.* 1987). Ticlopidine and sulphinpyrazone (Woods *et al.* 1979) have been used also to minimize dialyser platelet losses.

Platelets and transplantation

Platelets are involved both acutely and chronically in the reaction which follows when an allograft, or especially a xenograft, is placed into a recipient. This is not surprising in view of the fact that, although the principal reaction in allograft rejection is a complex cell-mediated infiltration of the stroma of the organ, a variety of antibodies reacting with endothelium are also present *ab initio*, or induced later in many graft recipients, and endothelial injury is present in almost all host versus graft reactions.

Allografts

When an allograft (an organ from a different member of the same species) is placed into an incompatible recipient, a reaction called *rejection* begins, the precise nature of which still eludes us although it has been studied for more than

40 years. One of the major components of severe, especially acute rejection is vascular occlusion, leading to the death of the organ. Thrombosis of the *microcirculation*, both peritubular and glomerular in the kidney, is a prominent feature of this reaction (Mandel *et al.* 1979). Early platelet adhesion forms an important mechanism (Kincaid-Smith *et al.* 1969; Kincaid-Smith 1970), and the more severe and acute the rejection, the greater the platelet deposition with the vasculature.

'Hyperacute' rejection

Thus in severe acute, so-called 'hyperacute' rejection of allografted kidneys, which occurs in patients previously sensitized against alloantigens by pregnancy, blood transfusion, or rejection of a previous allograft, *thrombocytopenia* is common (Kissmeyer Nielsen *et al.* 1966; Colman *et al.* 1969; Pillay *et al.* 1973). Platelet adhesion is one of the earliest events in both experimental models (Leithner *et al.* 1981) and clinical transplantation (Colman *et al.* 1969), and the glomerular and peritubular capillaries of the kidney are choked with aggregates of partially released or completely degranulated platelets (Kissmeyer Nielsen *et al.* 1966; Colman *et al.* 1969; Simpson *et al.* 1970; Sharma *et al.* 1972). This reaction probably arises from endothelial cell damage which results in turn from anti-endothelial cell antibodies already present in the recipient ('preformed' antibodies).

Stable allografts and rejection in modified recipients

All these reactions are blunted, but not suppressed, by immunosuppressive drugs given to the allograft recipient, such as azathioprine and corticosteroids. Thus one finds that in chronically immunosuppressed allograft kidney recipients *platelet turnovers* are accelerated (George *et al.* 1974), radiolabelled platelets are sequestrated within allografts (Leithner *et al.* 1982a; Chandler *et al.* 1983; Fenech *et al.* 1984; Martin Comin *et al.* 1983), and released back into the circulation after treatment of rejection (Mowbray & Parayinanda, 1971). This has been used as a test for the presence of rejection, and appears reliable even in patients treated with cyclosporin (Collier *et al.* 1988). *Platelet aggregates* are visible in fine needle aspirates of rejecting kidneys (von Willebrand *et al.* 1985) as well as within glomerular capillaries in renal biopsies (Porter *et al.* 1967; Lowenhaupt & Nathan, 1968; Busch *et al.* 1975), and platelet release occurs, with the circulating *platelets depleted of amines* and *α-granule contents* (Capitanio *et al.* 1982; Frampton *et al.* 1983), together with raised plasma levels of *PF4* and β-*TG*; even when the graft is well functioning and has stable function, years after grafting (Frampton *et al.* 1983).

Paradoxically, as in lupus, these partially depleted platelets may be hyperaggregable *in vitro*, as judged by spontaneous aggregation *in vitro* (Cohen, H. *et al.* 1988), lowered thresholds to aggregating agents and *in vitro* production of TXB_2 in response to arachidonate (Frampton *et al.* 1983), although other authors have reported *hypo*aggregability in response to ADP and other agents (Capitanio *et al.*

1982). *Platelet-related antigens* are present as well as morphologically visible platelets in biopsies of allografts, together with PF4 (Frampton *et al.* 1983). In addition, PDGF receptors are expressed in excess of normal in rejecting allografts (Fellstrom *et al.* 1989) suggesting a role for platelet-released mitogens in the vascular proliferative lesions of chronic rejection (Rowlands *et al.* 1976).

The plasma of allograft recipients also contains immune complexes (Palosuo *et al.* 1976; Johny *et al.* 1981) with the possibility of immune complex–platelet interaction and release of platelet contents (von Felten *et al.* 1981) or aggregation, as discussed earlier in this chapter.

Antiplatelet agents in transplantation

All this evidence of platelet activation in allografted recipients, and the role of platelets in rejection, led to trials of antiplatelet agents in kidney transplantation; however, the results have been disappointing. Dipyridamole (Anderson *et al.* 1974; Mathew *et al.* 1974) had no effect on renal function, although an effect on the severity of vascular histological changes was suggested by Mathew *et al.* (1974). A benefit in terms of reduced renal artery stenosis by dipyridamole was also described (Kauffman *et al.* 1980). Cyproheptadine did not appear to have any effect (Jessing *et al.* 1976), although suphinpyrazone gave a brief benefit (Sharma *et al.* 1972) and aspirin gave rise to frequent gastrointestinal bleeding in recipients receiving corticosteroids (Kauffman *et al.* 1980). Prostacyclin had obvious problems of delivery, but has been used in acute rejection by some investigators (Leithner *et al.* 1981, 1982a). More recently, interest has centred on the use of *thromboxane synthetase inhibitors* and *thromboxane receptor antagonists*, but it is too early to say what results may be obtained.

Xenografts

Most species have pre-existing antibodies, which are not of dietary origin and are present in cord blood at birth, which are directed against antigens of other species (Auchincloss, 1988). Thus the rejection of a xenograft (a graft from one species into another) is usually hyperacute, and always involves endothelial injury. Platelets are prominent in the early thrombosis of the microvasculature (Rosenberg *et al.* 1969; Kemp *et al.* 1980) and in rejection of organs besides the skin such as xenografted skin and cornea. Prostacyclin (Munday, 1980; Munday *et al.* 1980) kept xenograft and hyperacute allograft reactions at bay for as long as it was infused, suggesting that platelets may have a primary role to play in the xenograft reaction. On the other hand, xenografts are rejected just as rapidly in the absence of platelets (Jorgensen *et al.* 1986). No other treatment appears able to abrogate the xenograft reaction at the moment; these early experiments may become more important as attention returns to xenografts (e.g. from the pig) as possible sources for human grafting (Auchincloss, 1988).

Effect of cyclosporin A on endothelium and platelets

Currently cyclosporin A, a cyclic 11-amino acid peptide, is a major immunosuppressant used in transplantation (Perico & Remuzzi, 1989). It appears to be capable of damaging endothelium (Zoja *et al.* 1986), causing vWF release (Brown *et al.* 1988), and inhibiting PGI_2 production (Neild *et al.* 1983). The mechanism of the prostaglandin effects may be through cyclooxygenase inhibition (Brown *et al.* 1988). At the same time a proaggregatory effect on platelets has been described (Vanrenterghem *et al.* 1985; Grace *et al.* 1987; Cohen, H. *et al.* 1988). As well as *in vitro* hyperaggreability, Cohen, H. *et al.* (1988) noted also decreased *in vitro* sensitivity to PGI_2. Thus, in addition to the effects on platelets of transplantation *per se* noted above, it is not surprising that capillary thrombi have been described in the glomeruli and peritubular capillaries in renal allografts under cyclosporin treatment (Neild *et al.* 1985) amounting to a clinical haemolytic uraemic syndrome in some patients (van Buren *et al.* 1985; Berden *et al.* 1987) which has been noted also in bone marow transplant recipients (Shulman *et al.* 1981), and therefore relates to the drug and not to the rejection process in the kidney, plus the drug.

Recurrent HUS

As well as the appearance *de novo* of an HUS in cyclosporin-treated renal allograft recipients, recurrence of the HUS clinically and in the allograft has been reported, although rather rarely (Leithner *et al.* 1982b; Bonsib *et al.* 1985; Hebert *et al.* 1986; Griño *et al.* 1988; van den Berg Wolf *et al.* 1988), even in patients receiving azathioprine for immunosuppression, and not cyclosporin. Risk factors for recurrence have not been worked out clearly, but the time elapsed from renal failure and the acute episode may be important.

Conclusions

With the large area of endothelium which must be present in such a vascular organ, it is hardly surprising that during immune and other injury to the kidney platelets are involved in the subsequent events. To what extent platelets are prime movers, or — probably more usually — secondary amplifiers of injury remains to be determined. In addition, the global toxicity of uraemia must, of necessity, affect platelets as it does all cells, and the addition of extracoporeal circuits containing bio-incompatible materials in order to treat uraemia brings in its train inevitable platelet activation. Thus both haematologists and nephrologists must be aware of the platelet in relation to the kidney in their clinical practice, as well as having available for study a number of models of interesting pathophysiology in their patients.

References

Addonizio, V.P. & Colman, R.W. (1982) Platelets and extracorporeal circulation. *Biomaterials* **3**, 9–15.

Addonizio, V.P., Smith, J.B., Guiod, L.R., Strauss, J.F., Colman, R.W. & Edmunds, L.H. (1979) Thromboxane synthesis and platelet protein release during simulated extracorporeal circulation. *Blood* **54**, 371–376.

Altschuler, G., Marcus, A. & Ulmann, H. (1960) Platelets and platelet phosphatides in uremia. *Blood* **16**, 133–137.

Amorosi, E.L. & Ultmann, J.E. (1966) Thrombotic thrombocytopenic purpura: report of 16 cases and review of the literature. *Medicine* **45**, 139–159.

Anderson, M., Dewar, P., Fleming, L.B., Hacking, P.M., Morley, A.R., Murray, S., Swinney, J., Taylor, R.M.R., Uldall, P.R. & Wardle, E.N. (1974) A controlled trial of dipyridamole in human renal transplantation and an assessment of platelet function studies in rejection. *Clin Nephrol* **2**, 93–99.

Andrassy, K. & Ritz, E. (1985) Uremia as a cause of bleeding. *Am J Nephrol* **5**, 313–319.

Andrassy, K., Koderisch, J. & Lamminger, C. (1988) Defective platelet membrane receptors as a cause of uremic bleeding. *Blut* **57**, 243 (abstr).

Arends, J.P., Krediet, R.T., Boeschoten, E.W., van der Lelie, J., Veenhof, C.H.N. & von dem Borne, A.E.G. Kr. (1981) Improvement in bleeding time, platelet aggregation and platelet count during CAPD treatment. *Proc Eur Dialysis Transpl Ass* **18**, 280–285.

Arnaud, C.D. (1973) Hyperparathyroidism and renal failure. *Kidney Int* **4**, 89–95.

Asch, A.S., Adelman, B., Fujimoto, M. & Nachman, R.L. (1988) Identification and isolation of a platelet GP1b– like protein in human umbilical vein endothelial cells and bovine aortic smooth muscle cells. *J. Clin Invest* **81**, 1600–1607.

Auchincloss, H. (1988) Xenogeneic transplantation: a review. *Transplantation* **46**, 1–20.

Aviram, M. & Brook, J.G. (1983) Platelet interactions with high and low density lipoproteins. *Atherosclerosis* **43**, 259–68.

Ballou, L.R., Lam, B.K., Wong, P.Y.-K. & Cheung, W.Y. (1987) Formation of *cis*-14,15-oxido-5,8,11-icosatrienoic acid from phosphatidylinositol in human platelets. *Proc Natl Acad Sci USA* **84**, 6990–6994.

Bang, N.U., Trygstad, C.W., Schoeder, J.E., Heidenreich, R.O. & Csiscko, B.M. (1973) Enhanced platelet function in glomerular renal disease. *J. Lab Clin Med* **81**, 651–5.

Barnes, J.L. & Venkatachalam, M.A. (1985) The role of platelets and polycationic mediators in glomerular vascular injury. *Sem Nephrol* **5**, 57–68.

Battersby, B., Sherwood, T., Winocour, P. & Virella, G. (1985) Human platelets aggregate during antigen–antibody reactions at different antigen–antibody ratios. *J Lab Clin Immunol* **15**, 57–61.

Bazilinski, N., Shaykh, M., Dunea, G., Mamdani, B., Patel, A. & Czapek, E. (1985) Inhibition of platelet function by middle molecules. *Nephron* **40**, 423–428.

Benigni, A., Livio, M., Dodesini, P., Schiepatti, A., Panigata, M., Mecca, G., de Gaetano, G. & Remuzzi, G. (1985) Inhibition of human platelet aggregation by parathyroid hormone: is cyclic AMP implicated? *Am J Nephrol* **5**, 243–247.

Bennett, A. & Cameron, J.S. (1987) Hyperaggregability of platelets to ristocetin in the nephrotic syndrome not dependent upon thromboxane production or serum albumin concentration. *Clin Nephrol* **27**, 182–188.

Bennett, A., Frampton, G. & Cameron, J.S. (1986) Platelet- associated IgG in idiopathic glomerulonephritis and the nephritis of systemic lupus erythematosus. *Br J Haematol* **62**, 695–703.

Berberich, F.R., Cuene, S.A., Chard, R.L. & Hartmann, J.R. (1974) Thrombotic thrombocytopenic purpura. Three cases with platelet and fibrinogen survival studies. *J Pediat* **84**, 503–509.

Berden, J.M.H., Netten, P., van Leissum, P.A., Hoitsma, A.J., Assman, K.J.M., Monnens, L.A. & Koene, R.A.P. (1987) Hemolytic uremic syndrome during cyclosporine immunsosuppression in renal allograft recipients. *Clin Transpl* **1**, 246–252.

Bertani, T., Benigni, A., Cutillco, F., Rocchi, G., Morelli, C., Carminati, C., Verroust, P. & Remuzzi, G. (1986) Effect of aspirin and sulindac in rabbit nephrotoxic nephritis. *J Lab Clin Med* **107**, 261–268.

Bertelé, V., Falanga, A., Tomasiak, M., Dejana, E., Cerletti, C. & de Gaetano, G. (1983) Platelet thromboxane synthetase inhibitors with low dose aspirin: possible resolution of the 'aspirin dilemma'. *Science* **220**, 517–519.

Bevilacqua, M.P., Pober, J.S., Majeau, G.R., Cotran, R.S., Gimbrone Jr, M.A. (1985) Interleukin-1 (IL-1) induces biosynthesis and cell surface expression of procoagulant activity in human vascular endothelial cells. *J Exp Med* **160**, 618–623.

Bills, T.K., Smith, J.B. & Silver, M.J. (1976) Metabolism of (14C) arachidonic acid by human platelets *Biochim Biophys Acta* **424**, 303–314.

Bloom, A., Hannaford, P.A., Greaves, M., Preston, F.E. & Brown, C.B. (1985) Haemolytic-uraemic syndrome: demonstration of abnormalities of platelet reactivity and insensitivity to prostaglandin 12. *Clin Nephrol* **23**, 85–88.

Bloom, A., Greaves, M., Preston, F.E. & Brown, C.B. (1986) Evidence against a platelet cyclooxygenase defect in uraemic subjects on chronic haemodialysis. *Br J Haematol* **62**, 143–149.

Bohle, A., Helmchen, U., Grund, H.V., Gartner, H.-V., Meyer, D., Bock, K.D., Bulla, M., Bunger, P., Dieckmann, L., Frotscher, U., Hayduk, K., Kosters, W., Strauch, M., Scheler, F. & Christ, H. (1977) Malignant nephrosclerosis in patients with hemolytic uremic syndrome (primary malignant nephrosclerosis). *Curr Top Pathol* **65**, 81–113.

Bonacossa, I.A., Chalmers, I.M., Rayner, H.L. & Hunter, T. (1985) Platelet bound IgG levels in patients with systemic lupus erythematosus. *J Rheumatol* **12**, 78–80.

Bonsib, S.M., Ercolani, L., Ngheim, D. & Hamilton, H.E. (1985) Recurrent thrombotic microangiopathy in a renal allograft. Case report and review of the literature. *Am J Med* **79**, 520–527.

Boulton-Jones, J.M., McWilliams, G. & Chardrachud, L. (1986) Variation in charge on red cells of patients with different glomerulopathies. *Lancet* **ii**, 186–189.

Brown, C.B., Wilson, D., Turner, D.R., Cameron, J.S., Ogg, C.S., Chantler, C. & Gill, D. (1974) Combined immunosuppression and anticoagulation in rapidly progressive glomerulonephritis. *Lancet* **i**, 1166–1172.

Brown, Z., Neild, G.H., Willoughby, J.J., Somia, N.V. & Cameron, J.S. (1986) Increased factor VIII as an index of vascular injury in cyclosporin toxicity. *Transplantation* **42**, 150–153.

Brown, Z., Neild, G.H. & Lewis, G. (1988) Mechanism of cyclosporin inhibition of prostacyclin synthesis by cultured human umbilical vein endothelial cells. *Transpl Proc* **20**, 654–657.

Busch, G.J., Martins, A.C.P., Hollenberg, N.K., Wilson, R.E. & Colman, R.W. (1975) A primate model of hyperacute renal allograft rejection. *Am J Pathol* **79**, 31–51.

Byrnes, J.J. & Khurana, M. (1977) Treatment of thrombotic thrombocytopenic purpura with plasma. *N Engl J Med* **297**, 1386–1389.

Cameron, J.S. (1976) The treatment of glomerulonephritis with inhibitors of coagulation. In Kluthe, R., Vogt, A. & Batsford, S.R. (eds) *Glomerulonephritis*, pp. 154–164. Thieme, Stuttgart.

Cameron, J.S. (1977) Platelets and glomerulonephritis. *Nephron* **18**, 253–258.

Cameron, J.S. (1984a) Platelets in glomerular disease. *Ann Rev Med* **35**, 175–180.

Cameron, J.S. (1984b) Thrombosis and thromboembolic complications of the nephrotic syndrome. *Adv Nephrol* **13**, 75–114.

Cameron, J.S., Ogg, C.S. & Wass, V.J. (1988) Complications of the nephrotic syndrome. In Cameron, J.S. & Glassock, R.J. (eds) *The Nephrotic Syndrome*, pp. 849–920, Marcel Dekker, New York.

Camussi, G., Tetta, C., Mazzucco, G., Monga, G., Roffelino, C., Alberton, M., Dellabona, P., Malavasi, F. & Vercellone, A. (1986) Platelet cationic proteins are present in glomeruli of lupus nephritis patients. *Kidney Int* **30**, 555–565.

Capitanio, A., Mannucci, P.M., Ponticelli, C. & Pareti, F. (1982) Detection of circulating released platelets after renal transplantation. *Transplantation* **33**, 298–301.

Casati, S., Moia, M., Graziani, G., Cantaluppi, A., Citterio, A., Paniucci, P.M. & Ponticelli, C. (1984) Haemodialysis without anticoagulants: efficiency and hemostatic aspects. *Clin Nephrol* **21**, 102–115.

Cases, A., Monteagudo, J., Escolar, G., Lopez, J., Revert, L., Castillo, R., de Marco, L. & Ruggieri, Z.M. (1988) Normal binding of native and asialo- von Willebrand factor to uremic platelets (UP). *Nephrol Dialysis Transpl* **3**, 531 (abstr).

Castaldi, P.A., Rozenberg, M.C. & Stewart, J.H. (1966) The bleeding disorder of uraemia: a qualitative platelet defect. *Lancet* **ii**, 66–69.

Chandler, S.T., Buckels, J., Hawker, R.J., Smith, N., Barnes, A.D. & McCollum, C.N. (1983) Indium labeled platelet uptake in rejecting renal transplants. *Surg Gynaecol Obstet* **157**, 242–246.

Chen, Y.-C., McLeod, B., Hall, E.R. & Wu, K.K. (1981) Accelerated prostacyclin degradation in thrombotic thrombocytopenic purpura. *Lancet* **ii**, 267–269.

Churg, J. & Strauss, L. (1985) Renal involvement in thrombotic microangiopathies. *Sem Nephrol* **5**, 46–56.

Claris Appiani, A., Edelfonti, A., Betinelli, A., Cossu, M.M., Palachni, M.L. & Rossi, E. (1982) The relationship between the plasma levels of factor VIII and platelet release products (beta thromboglobulin and platelet factor 4) in children with hemolytic uremic syndrome *Clin Nephrol* **17**, 195–199.

Clark, W.F., Lewis, M.L., Cameron, J.S. & Parsons, V. (1975) Intra renal platelet consumption in the diffuse proliferative glomerulonephritis of systemic lupus erythematosus. *Clin Sci* **49**, 247–252.

Cohen, H., Neild, G.H., Patel, R., Mackie, I.J. & Machin, S.J. (1988) Evidence for chronic platelet hyperaggregability and *in vivo* activation in cyclosporin-treated renal allograft recipients. *Thromb Res* **49**, 91–101.

Cohen, H.T., Singh, A.K., Kasinath, B.S. & Lewis, E.J. (1988) Red-cell surface charge in patients with nephrotic syndrome. *Lancet* **i**, 1459 (letter).

Colli, S., Maderna, P., Tremoli, E., Baraldi, A., Rovati, C.E., Gianfrancheschini, G. & Nicosia, S. (1985) Prostacyclin–lipoprotein interactions. Studies on human platelet aggregation and adenylate cyclase. *Biochem Pharmacol* **34**, 2451–2457.

Collier, B.D., Adams, M.B., Kauffman, H.M., Trembath, L., Hoffman, R.G., Tisdale, P.L., Rao, S.A., Hellman, R.S. & Isitman, A.T. (1988) Accurate diagnosis of renal transplant rejection by Indium-111 platelet imaging despite postoperative cyclosporin therapy. *Clin Nucl Med* **13**: 606–609.

Colman, R.W., Braun, W.E., Busch, G.H., Dammin, G.H. & Merrill, J.P. (1969) Coagulation studies in hyperacute and other forms of renal allograft rejection. *New Engl J Med* **281**, 685–691.

Deckmyn, H., Zoja, C., Arnout, J., Todisco, A., Van den Bulcke, F., D'Hondt, L., Hendrickx, N., Gresele, P. & Vermylen, J. (1985) Partial isolation and function of the prostacyclin regulating plasma factor. *Clin Sci* **69**, 383–393.

Defreyn, G., Vergara Dauden, M., Machin, S.J. & Vermylen, J. (1980) A plasma factor in uraemia which stimulates prostacyclin release from cultured endothelial cells. *Thromb Res* **19**, 695–699.

Defreyn, G., Proesmans, W., Machin, S.J., Lemmens,

F. & Vermylen J., (1982) Abnormal prostacyclin metabolism in the haemolytic uraemic syndrome: equivocal effect of prostacyclin infusions. *Clin Nephrol* **18**, 43–49.

del Zoppo, G.J. (1987) Antiplatelet therapy in thrombotic thrombocytopenic purpura. *Sem Hematol* **24**, 130–139.

Deuel, T.F. & Huang, J.S. (1984) Platelet-derived growth factor. Structure, function and roles in normal and transformed cells. *J Clin Invest* **74**, 669–676.

Deykin, D. (1983) Uremic bleeding (nephrology forum). *Kidney Int* **24**, 698–705.

di Minno, G., Martinez, J., McKean, M.-L., de la Rosa, J., Burke, J.F. & Murphy, S. (1985) Platelet dysfunction in uremia. Multifaceted defect partly corrected by dialysis. *Am J Med* **79**, 552–559.

Donadio, J.V., Anderson, C.F., Mitchell III, J.C., Holley, K.E., Ilstrup, D.M., Fuster, V. & Cheesbro, J.H. (1984) Membranoproliferative glomerulonephritis. A prospective clinical trial of platelet-inhibitor therapy. *New Engl J Med* **310**, 1421–1426.

Donati, M.B. & Pangrazzi, J. (1989) The use of heparin during haemodialysis. In Remuzzi, G. & Rossi, E.C. (eds) *Haemostasis and the Kidney*, pp. 309–317, Butterworth, London.

Drummond, K.N. (1985) Hemolytic-uremic syndrome—then and now. *New Engl J Med* **312**, 116–118.

Duffus, P., Parbtani, A., Frampton, G. & Cameron, J.S. (1982) Intraglomerular localisation of platelet-related antigens, platelet factor 4 and beta- thromboglobulin in glomerulonephritis. *Clin Nephrol* **18**, 298–302.

Edelfonti, A., Bettinelli, A., Mondonico, P., Claris Appiani, A., Picca, M., Cossu, M.M., Tentori, F., Giani, M. & Rossi, E. (1985) Intraplatelet serotonin (5-HT) in children with the hemolytic uremic syndrome. *Clin Nephrol* **23**, 207–211.

Eknoyan, G. & Brown, C.H. (1981) Biochemical abnormalities of platelets in renal failure. Evidence for decreased platelet serotinin ADP and magnesium dependent ATPase. *Am J Nephrol* **1**, 17–23.

Eknoyan, G., Waksman, S.J., Glueck, H.I. & Will, J.J. (1969) Platelet function in renal failure. *New Engl J Med* **280**, 823–826.

Endo, Y., Mamiya, S., Satoh, M., Takahashi, K. & Harada T. (1982) Plasma beta thromboglobulin and platelet factor 4 in patients with chronic renal failure and effect of haemodialysis. *Tohoku J Exp Med* **135**, 349–358.

Escolar, G., Cases, A., Monteagudo, J., Bastida, E., Lopez, J., Revert, L., Oridnas, A. & Castillo, R. (1988) Defective interaction of von Willebrand factor with GPIIb/IIIa in uremic platelets (PT). *Nephrol Dialysis Transpl* **3**, 531 (abstr).

Evans, E.P., Branch, P.A. & Bloom, A.L. (1972) A clinical and experimental study of platelet function in chronic renal failure. *J Clin Pathol* **25**, 745–753.

Feehally, J., Samanta, A., Kinghorn, H., Burden, A.C. & Walls, J. (1986) Red-cell surface charge in glomerular disease. *Lancet* **ii**, 635 (letter).

Fellstrom, B., Dimeny, E., Larsson, E., Klareskog, L., Tufuesson, G. & Rubin, K. (1989) Importance of PDGF receptor expression in accelerated atherosclerosis-chronic rejection. *Transpl Proc* **21**, 3689–3691.

Fenech, A., Smith, F.W., Power, D.A., MacLeod, A.M., Nicholls, A.J., Edward, N., Catto, G.R.D. & Bennett, B. (1984) The value of autologous indium (11In)-labelled platelets in the diagnosis of renal transplant rejection. *Clin Nephrol* **21**, 220–222.

Flanigan, M.J., Von Brecht, J., Freeman, R.M. & Lim, V.S. (1987) Reducing the hemorrhagic complications of hemodialysis: a controlled comparison of low-dose heparin and citrate anticoagulation. *Am J Kidney Dis* **9**, 147–153.

Fong, J.S.C. & Kaplan, B.S. (1982) Impairment of platelet aggregation in hemolytic uremic syndrome: evidence for platelet 'exhaustion'. *Blood* **60**, 564–570.

Frampton, G. & Cameron, J.S. (1988) Purified antiphospholipid antibodies (APA) from lupus nephritis patients enhance thromboxane (TxB2) production by activated platelets. *Kidney Int* **33**: 328 (abstr).

Frampton, G., Parbtani, A., Marchesi, D., Duffus, P., Livio, M., Remuzzi, G. & Cameron, J.S. (1983) *In vivo* platelet activation with *in vitro* hyperaggreagbility to arachidonic acid in renal allograft recipients. *Kidney Int* **23**, 506–513.

Frampton, G., Perl, S., Bennett, A., Cameron, J.S. (1986) Platelet-associated DNA and anti-DNA antibody in systemic lupus erythematosus with nephritis. *Clin Exp Immunol* **63**, 621–628.

Frampton, G., Cameron, J.S. & Hartley, R.B. (1987) Glomerular thrombi in lupus nephritis: an association with the presence of IgG anti-cardiolipin antibody *Nephrol Dialysis Transpl* **2**, 424 (abstr).

Frampton, G., Hildreth, G., Hartley, B., Cameron, J.S., Heldin, C.-H. & Wasteson, A. (1988). Could platelet-derived growth factor have a role in the pathogenesis of lupus nephritis? *Lancet* **ii**: 343 (letter).

Futrakul, P., Poshyachinda, M. & Mitrakul, D. (1978) Focal sclerosing glomerulonephritis: a kinetic evaluation of haemostasis and the effect of anticoagulant therapy: a controlled study. *Clin Nephrol* **10**, 180–186.

Gafter, U., Bessler, H., Malachi, T., Zevin D., Djaldetti, M. & Levi, J. (1987) Platelet count and thrombopoietic activity in patients with chronic renal failure. *Nephron* **45**, 207–210.

Gallice, P., Fournier, N., Crevat, P., Saingra, S., Fraysinnet, R., Murisasco, A. & Sicardi, F. (1980) *In vitro* inhibition of platelet aggregation by uremic middle molecules. *Biomedecine* **33**, 185–188.

Galloway, J.H., Cartwright, I.J., Woodcock, B.E., Greaves, M., Russell, R.G.G. & Preston, F.E. (1985) Effects of dietary fish oil supplementation on the fatty acid composition of the human platelet membrane: demonstration of selectivity in the incorporation of eicosapentenoic acid into membrane phospholipid pools. *Clin Sci* **68**, 449–54.

Gaspari, F., Vigano G., Orisio S., Bonati, M., Livio, M. & Remuzzi, G. (1987) Aspirin prolongs bleeding time in uremia by a mechanism distinct from cyclo-oxygenase inhibition. *J Clin Invest* **79**, 1788–1797.

Gasser, C., Gauthier, E., Steck, A., Siebenmann, R.E. & Oechslin, R. (1955) Hämolytisch-urämische Syndrome: Bilaterale Nierenrindennekrosen bei akuten erworbenen hämolytischen Anämien. *Schweiz Med Wschr* **38**, 905–919.

Gelfand, J., Truong, L., Stern, L., Pirani, C.L. & Appel, G.B. (1985) Thrombotic thrombocytopenic purpura syndrome in systemic lupus erythematosus: treatment with plasma infusion. *Am J Kidney Dis* **6**, 154–160.

George, C.R.P., Slichter, S.J., Quadracci, L.J., Striker, G.E. & Harker, L.A. (1974) A kinetic evaluation of hemostasis in renal disease. *New Engl J Med* **293**, 1111–1115.

George, C.R.P., Clark, W.F. & Cameron, J.S. (1975) The role of platelets in glomerulonephritis. *Adv Nephrol* **5**, 19–65.

Giroux, L., Bettez, L. & Giroux, L. (1985) Mitomycin-C nephrotoxicity: a clinico- pathological study of 17 cases. *Am J Kidney Dis* **6**, 28–34.

Goldstein, M.H., Churg, J., Strauss, L. & Gribetz, D. (1979) Haemolytic uraemic syndrome. *Nephron* **23**, 263–272.

Gordge, M.P., Faint, R.W., Rylance, P.B. & Neild, G.H. (1988) Platelet function and the bleeding time in progressive renal failure. *Thromb Haemost* **60**, 83–87.

Gotti, E. & Remuzzi, G. (1989) Uraemic bleeding: clinical presentation and management. In Remuzzi, G. & Rossi, E.C. (eds) *Haemostasis and the Kidney*, pp. 131–141. Butterworth, London.

Grace, A.A., Barradas, M.A., Mikhailidis, D.P., Jeremy, J.Y., Moorhead, J.F., Sweny, P. & Dandona, P. (1987) Cyclosporine A enhances platelet aggregation. *Kidney Int* **32**, 889–895.

Gralnick, H.R., Mckeown, L.P., Williams, S.B., Shafer B.C. & Pierce, L. (1989) Plasma and platelet von Willebrand factor defects in uremia. *Am J Med* **85**, 806–810.

Griño, J.M., Caralps, A., Carreras, L., Nogues, R., Castelao, A.M., Romero, R., Carreras, K. & Alsina, J. (1988) Apparent recurrence of hemolytic uremic syndrome in azathioprine treated allograft recipients. *Nephron* **49**, 301–304.

Gura, V., Creter, D. & Levi, J. (1982) Elevated thrombocyte calcium in uremia and its correction by 1 α (OH) vitamin D treatment. *Nephron* **30**, 237–239.

Hakim, R.M. & Schafer, A.I. (1985) Hemodialysis associated platelet activation and thrombocytopenia. *Am J Med* **78**, 575–580.

Hancock, W. & Atkins, R. (1985) Activation of coagulation pathways and fibrin deposition in human glomerulonephritis. *Sem Nephrol* **5**, 69–77.

Harker, L.A. & Slichter, S.J. (1972) Platelet and fibrinogen consumption in man. *New Engl J Med* **287**, 999–1006.

Harris, E.N., Gharavi, A.E. & Hughes, G.R.V. (1985) Anti-phospholipid antibodies. *Clin Rheum Dis* **11**, 591–609.

Harris, R.C., Homma, T., Falck, J., Badr, K.F. & Capdevila, J. (1989) Epoxyeicosatrienoic acids (EETs) are mitogens for cultured rat mesangial cells (CRMC) *Kidney Int*, **35**, 174 (abstr).

Harter, H.R., Burch, J.W., Majerus, P.W., Stanford, N., Delmez, J.A. Anderson, C.B. & Weerts, C.A. (1979) Prevention of thrombosis in patients on haemodialysis by low-dose aspirin. *New Engl J Med* **301**, 577–579.

Hebert, D., Sibley, R.K. & Mauer, S.M. (1986) Recurrence of hemolytic uremic syndrome in renal transplant recipients. *Kidney Int* **30** (Suppl), S51–S58.

Herrmann, R.P., Marshall, L.R. & Hurst, P.E. (1977) Bleeding in renal failure: a possible cause. *Br Med J* **i**: 1601–1602.

Holdsworth, S.R. & Tipping, P.G. (1985) Macrophage-induced glomerular fibrin deposition in experimental glomerulonephritis in the rabbit. *J Clin Invest* **76**, 1367–1375.

Horowitz, H.I., Stein, I.M., Cohen, B.D. & White, J.G. (1970) Further studies on the platelet inhibitory effect of guanidinosuccinic acid and its role in uraemic bleeding. *Am J Med* **49**, 336–345.

Howe, S.R. & Lynch, D.M. (1987) Platelet antibody binding in systemic lupus erythematosus. *J Rheumatol* **14**, 482–486.

Izumino, K., Iida, H., Asaka, M. & Sasayama, S. (1986) Effect of the antiplatelet agents ticlopidine and dipyridamole on experimental immune complex glomerulonephritis in rats. *Nephron* **43**, 56–61.

Izumino, K., Iida, H., Asaka, M. & Sasayama, S. (1987) Effect of the antiplatelet agents ticlopidine and dipyridamole on nephrotoxic serum nephritis in rats. *Nephron* **45**, 306–310.

Jackson, C.A., Greaves, M., Patterson, A.D., Brown, C.B. & Preston, F.E. (1982) Relationship between platelet aggregation, thromboxane synthesis and albumin concentration in nephrotic syndrome. *Br J Haematol* **52**, 69–77.

Janson, P.A., Jubelierer, S.J., Weinstein, M.J. & Deykin, D. (1978) Treatment of the bleeding tendency in uremia with cryoprecipitate. *New Engl J Med* **303**, 1319–1322.

Jessing, P., Agger, B. & Pedersen, F.B. (1976) Periactin ® (cyproheptadine hydbochloride) as a supplement to the immunosuppressive treatment in human cadaver kidney transplantation. *Scand J Urol Nephrol* **10**, 147–149.

Johnson, R.J., Alpers, C.E., Prizl, P., Schulze, M., Baker P., Pruchno, C. & Couser, W.G. (1988) Platelets mediate neutrophil-dependent immune complex nephritis in the rat. *J Clin Invest* **82**, 1225–1235.

Johny, K.V., Dasgupta, M.K., Kovithavongs, T. & Dossetor, J.B. (1981) Serial study of circulating immune complexes before and after renal transplantation. *Kidney Int* **19**, 332–340.

Jorgensen, K.A. & Ingeberg, S. (1979) Platelets and platelet function in patients with chronic uremia on maintenance hemodialysis. *Nephron* **23**, 233–236.

Jorgensen, K.A., Kemp, E., Barfort, P., Starklint, H.,

Larsen, S. & Munk-Andersen, G. (1986) Platelet aggregation is not essential for xenograft rejection. *Thromb Res* **43**, 87–90.

Jubelirer, S.J. (1985) Hemostatic abnormalities in renal disease. *Am J Kidney Dis* **5**, 219–225.

Kant, K.K., Pollak, V.E., Weiss, M.A., Glueck, H.I., Miller, M.A. & Hess, E.V. (1981) Glomerular thrombosis in systemic lupus erythematosus: prevalance and significance. *Medicine* **60**, 71–86.

Kaplan, B.S. & Drummond, K.N. (1978) The haemolytic uraemic syndrome is a syndrome. *New Engl J Med* **298**, 964–966.

Kaplan, B.S. & Remuzzi, G. (1989) The haemolytic uraemic syndrome. In Remuzzi, G. & Rossi, E.C. (eds) *Haemostasis and the Kidney*, pp. 201–236. Butterworth, London.

Karmali, M.A., Steele, B.T., Petric, M. & Lim, C. (1985) Sporadic cases of haemolytic-uraemic syndrome associated with faecal cytotoxin and cytotoxin-producing Escherechia coli in stools. *Lancet* **i**, 619–620.

Karpatkin, S., Strick, N., Karpatkin, M.B. & Siskind, G.W. (1971) Cumulative experience in the detection of antiplatelet antibody in 234 patients with idiopathic thrombocytopenic purpura, systemic lupus erythematosus and other clinical disorders. *Am J Med* **52**, 776–785.

Kasai, N., Parbtani, A., Cameron, J.S., Yewdall, V., Shepherd, P. & Verroust, P. (1981) Platelet-aggregating immune complexes and intra platelet serotonin in idiopathic glomerulonephritis and systemic lupus. *Clin Exp Immunol* **43**, 64–72.

Kauffman, H.M., Adams, M.B., Hebert, L.A. & Wakczak, P.M. (1980) Platelet inhibitors in human renal homotransplantation: randomized comparison of aspirin versus dipyridamole. *Transpl Proc* **12**, 311–313.

Kazatchkine, M., Sultan, Y., Caen, J.P. & Bariety, J. (1976) Bleeding in renal failure: a possible cause. *Br Med J* **ii**, 612–615.

Kelton, J.G., Moore, J., Santos, A. & Sheridan, D. (1984) Detection of a platelet agglutinating factor in thrombotic thrombocytopenic purpura. *Ann Intern Med* **101**, 589–593.

Kelton, J.G., Moore, J.C. & Murphy, W.G. (1987) Studies investigating platelet aggregation and release initiated by sera from patients with thrombotic thrombocytopenic purpura. *Blood* **69**, 924–928.

Kemp, E., Kemp, G. & Larsen, S. (1980) Survival of discordant renal xenografts up to 3 days. Assessment of function, light microscopy and immunofluorescent microscopy. *Scand J Urol Nephrol Suppl 54*, 100–155.

Khamashta, M.A., Harris, E.N., Gharavi, A.E., Derue, G., Gil, A., Vasquez, J.J. & Hughes, G.R.V. (1988) Immune mediated mechanism for thrombosis: antiphospholipid antibody binding to plate membranes. *Ann Rheum Dis* **47** 849–854.

Kincaid Smith, P. (1970) The pathogenesis of the vascular and glomerular lesions of rejection in renal allografts and their modification by antithrombotic and anticoagulant drugs. *Austral Ann Med* **3**, 201–214.

Kincaid Smith, P. (1984) Anti-coagulants are of value in the treatment of renal disease. *Am J Kidney Dis* **3**, 299–307.

Kincaid Smith, P., McKenzie, I.F.C., Morris, P.J. & Marshall, V.C. (1969) Biopsy features of early acute rejection in cadaveric renal grafts. *Transplantation* **1**, 287–289.

Kincaid Smith, P., Laver, M.C. & Fairley, K.F. (1970) Dipyridamole and anticoagulants in renal disease due to glomerular and vascular lesions. *Med J Austral* **1**, 145–151.

King, D.J. & Kelton, J.G. (1984) Heparin-associated thrombocytopenia. *Ann Intern Med* **100**, 535–540.

Kissmeyer Nielsen, F., Olsen, S., Peterson, V.P. & Fieldborg, O. (1966) Hyperacute rejection of kidney allografts associated with pre existing humoral antibodies against donor cells. *Lancet* **ii**, 662–665.

Koyama, A., Inage, H., Sano, M., Narita, M., Tojo, S., Neild, G.H. & Cameron, J.S. (1985) Platelet involvement in the nephritis of acute serum sickness in rabbits: protection by dipyridamole and FUT-175. *Clin Exp Immunol* **61**, 388–396.

Kyrle, P.A., Stockenhuber, F., Brenner, B., Gossinger, H., Korninger, C., Pabinger, I., Sunder-Plassmann, G., Balcke, P. & Lechner, K. (1988) Evidence for an increased generation of prostacyclin in the microvasculature and an impairment of the platelet α-granule release in chronic renal failure. *Thromb Haemost* **60**, 205–208.

Lancet editorial (1987) Unravelling HUS. *Lancet* **ii**, 1437–1439.

Larsson, S.O. (1971) On coagulation and fibrinolysis in renal failure. *Scand J Haematol* **15**(Suppl) 1–59.

Leaker, B., Fairley, K.F., Dowling, J. & Kincaid-Smith, P. (1987) Lupus nephritis: clinical and pathological correlation. *Q J Med* **62**, 163–179.

Leithner, C.H., Sinzinger, H. & Schwartz, M. (1981) Treatment of chronic kidney transplant rejection with prostacyclin-reduction of platelet deposition in the transplant; prolongation of platelet survival and improvement of transplant function. *Prostaglandins* **22**, 783–788.

Leithner, C., Sinzinger, H., Schwartz, M. & Pohanka, E. (1982a) Radiolabelled platelets and prostacyclin in diagnosis and treatment of transplant rejection. *Proc Eur Dialysis Transpl Assoc* **19**, 529–535.

Leithner, C., Sinzinger, H., Pohanka, E., Schwartz, M., Kretschmer, G. & Syre, G. (1982b) Recurrence of hemolytic uremic syndrome triggered by cyclosporin A after renal transplantation. *Lancet* **ii**, 1470 (letter).

Leithner, C., Kovarik, J., Sinzinger, H. & Woloszczuk, W. (1984) Parathyroid hormone does not inhibit platelet aggregation. *Lancet* **i**, 367–368.

Leung, D.Y.M., Moake, J.L., Havens, P.L., Kim, M. & Pober, J.S. (1988) Lytic anti-endothelial cell antibodies in haemolytic-uraemic syndrome. *Lancet* **ii**, 183–186.

Levin, M., Smith, C., Walters, M.D.S., Gascoine, P. &

Barratt, T.M. (1985) Steroid-responsive nephrotic syndrome: a generalised disorder of membrane negative charge. *Lancet* **ii**, 239–242.

Levin, M., Stroobant, P., Walters, M.D.S., Cheng, D.J., Waterfield, M.D. & Barratt, T.M. (1986) Platelet-derived growth factors as possible mediators of vascular proliferation in the sporadic haemolytic-uraemic syndrome. *Lancet* **ii**, 830–833.

Lewis, J.H., Zucker, M.B. & Ferguson, J.H. (1956) Bleeding tendency in uraemia. *Blood* **11**, 1073–1076.

Lian, E.C.-Y., Mui, P.T.K., Siddiqui, F.A. & Chiu, L.L.S. (1983) Purification and some properties of a protein obtained from normal human plasma which inhibits the platelet aggregation induced by thrombotic thrombocyctopenic purpura plasma. *Thromb Res* **33**, 69–76.

Lianos, E.A. (1984) Biosynthesis and role of arachidonic acid metabolites in glomerulonephritis. *Nephron* **37**, 73–77.

Lindsay, R.M., Prentice, C.R.M., Ferguson, D., Barton, J.A. & McNichol, G.P. (1972a) Reduction of thrombus formation on dialyzer membranes by aspirin and RA 233. *Lancet* **ii**, 1287–1291.

Lindsay, R.M., Prentice, C.R.M., Davidson, J.F. Burton, J.A. & McNichol, G.P. (1972b) Haemostatic changes during dialysis associated with thrombus formation on dialysis membranes. *Br Med J* **iv**, 454–458.

Lindsay, R.M., Moorthy, A.V., Koens, F. & Linton, A.L. (1975) Platelet function in dialysed and non-dialysed patients with chronic renal failure. *Clin Nephrol* **4**, 52–57.

Lindsay, R.M., Friesen, M., Koens, F., Linton, A.L., Oreopoulos, D. & de Veber, G. (1976) Platelet function in patients on long term peritoneal dialysis. *Clin Nephrol* **6**, 335–339.

Livio M. (1989) "Hypercoagulability" in the nephrotic syndrome. In Remuzzi, G. & Rossi, E.C. (eds) *Haemostasis and the Kidney*, pp. 145–152. Butterworth, London.

Livio, M., Gotti, E., Marchesi, D., Mecca, G., Remuzzi, G. & de Gaetano, G. (1982) Uraemic bleeding: role of anaemia and beneficial effect of blood transfusion. *Lancet* **ii**, 1013–1015.

Livio, M., Benigni, A. & Remuzzi, G. (1985) Coagulation abnormalities in uremia. *Sem Nephrol* **5**, 82–90.

Livio, M., Mannucci, P.M., Vigano, G., Mingardi, G., Lombardi, R., Mecca, G. & Remuzzi, G. (1986a) Conjugated estrogens for the management of bleeding associated with renal failure. *New Engl J Med* **315**, 731–735.

Livio, M., Benigni, A., Vigano, G., Mecca, G. & Remuzzi G. (1986b) Moderate doses of aspirin and risk of bleeding in renal failure. *Lancet* **i**, 414–416.

Ljungberg, B., Blombacke, M., Johnsson, H. & Lins, L.E. (1987) A single dose of a low molecular heparin fragment for anticoagulation during haemodialysis. *Clin Nephrol* **27**, 31–35.

Loirat, C., Sonsino, E., Hinglais, N., Jais, J.P., Landais, P. & Fermanian, J. (1988) Treatment of the childhood haemolytic uraemic syndrome with plasma. *Pediat Nephrol* **2**, 279–285.

Lowenhaupt, R. & Nathan, P. (1968) Platelet accumulation observed by electron microscopy in the early phase of renal allotransplant rejection. *Nature* **220**, 822–825.

Mabuchi, H. & Nakahashi, H. (1983) Isolation and partial characterization of platelet aggregation inhibitors in the blood of dialyzed patients. *Nephron* **35**, 112–115.

Mahiout, A., Joerres, A., Hiss, R., Meinhold, H. & Kessel, M. (1987) Effects of blood-dialyzer interaction on prostaglandins in uraemic patients and healthy man. *Nephrol Dialysis Transpl* **2**, 546–550.

Mandel, S.P., Schermer, R., Clark, R., Staab, E.V. & Webster, W.P. (1979) Thrombosis: a study of coagulation parameters and mechanisms during allograft rejection. *Thromb Haemost* **41**, 553–566.

Mannucci, P.M., Remuzzi, G., Pusineri, F., Lombardi, R., Valsecchi, C., Mecca, G. & Zimmerman, T.S. (1983) Deamino-8-D-arginine vasopressin shortens the bleeding time in uremia. *New Engl J Med* **308**, 8–12.

Marchesi, D., Parbtani, A., Frampton, G., Livio, M., Remuzzi, G. & Cameron, J.S. (1981) Thrombotic tendency in systemic lupus erythematosus *Lancet* **i**, 719 (letter).

Martin Comin, J., Roca, M., Grino, J.M., Paradell, C. & Caralps, C. (1983) Indium-111 labeled oxime autologous labeled platelets in the diagnosis of kidney graft rejection. *Clin Nucl Med* **8**, 7–10.

Mathew, T.H., Kincaid-Smith, P., Clyne, D.H., Saker, B.M., Nanra, R.S., Morris, P.J. & Marshall, V.C. (1974) A controlled trial of oral anticoagulants and dipyridamole in cadaveric renal allografts. *Lancet* **i**, 1307–1310.

Miller, K., Dresner, I.G. & Michael, A.F. (1981) Localization of platelet antigens in human kidney disease. *Kidney Int* **18**, 472–479.

Miller, M.H., Urowitz, M.B. & Gladman, D.D. (1983) The significance of thrombocytopenia in systemic lupus erythematosus. *Arthritis Rheum* **26**, 1181–1186.

Misiani, R., Claris Appiani, A., Edelfonti, A., Gotti, E., Bettinelli, A., Giani, M., Rossi, E., Remuzzi, G. & Mecca, G. (1982) Haemolytic uraemic syndrome: therapeutic effect of plasma infusion. *Br Med J* **285**, 1304–1306.

Moake, J.L., Byrnes, J.J., Troll, J.H., Rudy, C.K., Hong, S.L., Weinstein, M.J. & Colanino, N.M. (1985) Effects of fresh frozen plasma and its cryosupernatant fraction on von Willebrand factor multimeric forms in chronic relapsing thrombotic thrombocytopenic purpura. *Blood* **65**, 1232–1236.

Moia, M., Vizzotto, L., Cattaneo, M., Mannucci, P.M., Casati, S. & Ponticelli, C. (1987) Improvement in the haemostatic defect of uraemia after treatment with recombinant human erythropoietin. *Lancet* **ii**, 1227–1229.

Monnens, L., van der Meer, W., Langernhuyson, C.,

van Munster, P. & van Oostrom, C. (1985) Platelet aggregating factor in the epidemic form of haemolytic uraemic syndrome. *Clin Nephrol* **24**, 135–137.

Mowbray, J.F. & Parayinanda, A. (1971) Platelet thrombi in rejection of renal allografts. In Duckert, R., Brinktous, K.M. & Hinnom, S. (eds) *Immunological Mechanisms of Blood Coagulation, Stuttgart* pp. 183–190. Shattauer, Stuttgart.

Munday, A.R. (1980) Prolongation of cat to dog renal xenografts survival with prostacyclin. *Transplantation* **30**, 226–228.

Munday, A.R., Bewick, M., Moncada, S. & Vane, J.R. (1980) Short term suppression of hyperacute allograft rejection in presensitized dogs with prostacyclin. *Prostaglandins* **19**, 595–603.

Murphy, W.G., Moore, J.C., Barr, R.D., Pai, M.K. & Kelton, J.G. (1987) Relationship between platelet aggregating factor and von Willebrand factor in thrombotic thrombocytopenic purpura. *Br J Haematol* **66**, 509–513.

Nachman, R.L. & Weksler, B.B. (1980) The platelet as an inflammatory cell. In Weissman, G. (ed.) *Cell Biology and Inflammation*, pp.145–162. Elsevier, Amsterdam.

Neild, G.H. (1987) The haemolytic uraemic syndrome: a review. *Q J Med* **63**, 367–376.

Neild, G.H. & Cameron, J.S. (1989) Glomerulonephritis. In Remuzzi, G. & Rossi, E.C. (eds) *Haemostasis and the Kidney*, pp. 56–79. Butterworth, London.

Neild, G.H. & Gordge, M.P. (1988) Platelet–endothelial interactions in renal injury. In Pittilo, R.M. & Machin, S.J. (eds) *Platelet–Vessel Wall Interactions*, pp. 121–153. Springer, Heidelberg.

Neild, G.H., Rocchi, G., Imberti, L., Fumagalli, F., Brown, Z., Remuzzi, G. & Williams, D.G. (1983) Effect of cyclosporin A on prostacyclin synthesis by vascular tissue. *Thromb Res* **32**, 373–379.

Neild, G.H., Reuben, R., Hartley, R.B. & Cameron, J.S. (1985) Glomerular thrombi in renal allografts associated with cyclosporin treatment. *J Clin Pathol* **38**, 253–258.

Nenci, G.G., Berrettini, M., Agnelli, G., Parise, P., Buoncristiani, V. & Bellatori, E. (1979) Effect of peritoneal dialysis, haemodialysis and kidney transplantation on blood platelet function. I: platelet aggregation by ADP and epinephrine *Nephron* **23**, 287–293.

Niwa, T., Maeda, K., Shibata, M. & Yamada, K. (1988) Clinical effects of selective thromboxane A2 sythetase inhibitor in patients with nephrotic syndrome. *Clin Nephrol* **30**, 276–281.

Nordoy, A., Svensson, V., Wiebe, D. & Hoak, J. (1978) Lipoproteins and the inhibitory effect of human endothelial cells on platelet function. *Circ Res 1978* **43**, 527–534.

Ozanne, P., Francis, R.B. & Meiselman, H.J. (1983) Red blood cell aggregation in nephrotic syndrome. *Kidney Int* **23**, 519–525.

Palosuo, T., Kano, K., Anthone, K., Gerbasi, J.R. & Milgrom, F. (1976) Circulating immune complexes after transplantation. *Transplantation* **21**, 312–316.

Parbtani, A. & Cameron, J.S. (1980) Platelet involvement in glomerulonephritis. In Remuzzi, G., Mecca, G. & de Gaetano, G. (eds) *Hemostasis, Prostaglandins and Renal Disease*, pp. 164–172. Raven Press, New York.

Parbtani, A., Frampton, G. & Cameron, J.S. (1979) Measurements of platelet release substances in glomerulonephritis. A comparison of beta thromboglobulin, platelet factor 4 and serotonin assays. *Thromb Res* **19**, 177–189.

Parbtani, A., Frampton, G. & Cameron, J.S. (1980a) Platelet and plasma serotonin concentrations in glomerulonephritis II. *Clin Nephrol* **14**, 112–123.

Parbtani, A., Frampton, G., Kasai, N., Yewdall, V. & Cameron, J.S. (1980b) Platelet and plasma serotonin concentrations in glomerulonephritis III. The nephritis of systemic lupus erythematosus. *Clin Nephrol* **14**, 164–172.

Perico, N. & Remuzzi, G. (1989) Thromboembolic complications during cyclosporin A therapy: possible causes and incidence. In Remuzzi, G. & Rossi, E.C. (eds) *Haemostasis and the Kidney*, pp. 321–330. Butterworths, London.

Pillay, V.K.G., Kurzman, N.A., Manaligod, J.R. & Jonasson, O. (1973) Selective thrombocytopenia due to localized microangiopathy of renal allografts. *Lancet* **ii**, 988–991.

Ponticelli, C., Imbasciati, E., Brancaccio, D., Tarantino, A. & Rivolta, E. (1974) Acute renal failure in systemic lupus erythematosus. *Br Med J* **iii**, 716–719.

Porter, K.A., Dossetor, J.B., Marchioro, T.L., Peart, W.S., Rendall, J.M., Starzl, T.E. & Terasaki, P.I. (1967) Human renal transplants. I. Glomerular changes. *Lab Invest* **16**, 153–181.

Pusineri, F., Gotti, E., Remuzzi, G., Mecca, G., Donati, M.B. & de Gaetano, G. (1980) Platelets from uraemic patients react normally to prostacyclin. *Int J Artific Organs* **3**, 125.

Rabiner, S.F. (1972) Bleeding in uremia. *Med Clin N Am* **56**, 221–233.

Rabiner, F.S. & Molinas, F. (1970) The role of phenol and phenolic acids on the thrombocytopathy and defective platelet aggregation of patients with renal failure. *Am J Med* **49**, 346–351.

Remuzzi, G. (1987) HUS and TTP: variable expressions of a single entity. (Nephrology forum) *Kidney Int* **32**, 292–308.

Remuzzi, G. (1988) Bleeding in renal failure. *Lancet* **i**, 1205–1208.

Remuzzi, G. & Pusineri, F. (1989) The uraemic platelet. In Remuzzi, G. & Rossi, E. (eds) *Haemostasis and the Kidney*, pp. 107–118. Butterworths, London.

Remuzzi, G. & Rossi, E.C. (1989) *Haemostasis and the Kidney*. Butterworth, London.

Remuzzi, G., Livio, M., Roncaglioni, M.C., Mecca, G., Donati, M.B & de Gaetano, G. (1977) Bleeding in renal failure: is von Willebrand factor implicated? *Br Med J* **ii**, 359–361.

Remuzzi, G., Misiani, R., Marchesi, D., Livio, M., Mecca, G., de Gaetano, G. & Donati, M.B. (1978) Haemolytic-uraemic syndrome: deficiency of plasma factor(s) regulating prostacyclin activity? *Lancet* **ii**, 871–872.

Remuzzi, G., Mecca, G., Marchesi, D., Livio, M., de Gaetano, G., Donati, M.B. & Silver, M.J. (1979a) Platelet hyperaggregability and the nephrotic syndrome. *Thromb Res* **16**, 345–54.

Remuzzi, G., Marchesi, D., Misiani, R., Mecca, G., de Gaetano, G. & Donati, M.B. (1979b) Familial deficiency of a plasma factor stimulating vascular prostacyclin synthesis. *Thromb Res* **16**, 517–525.

Remuzzi, G., Marchesi, D., Cavenaghi, A.E., Livio, M., Donati, M.B. & de Gaetano, G. (1979c) Bleeding in renal failure: a possible role of vascular prostacyclin (PGI2). *Clin Nephrol* **12**, 127–131.

Remuzzi, G., Benigni, A., Dodesini, P., Schiepatti, A., Livio, M., Poletti, E., Mecca, G. & de Gaetano, G. (1981) Parathyroid hormone inhibits human platelet function *Lancet* **ii**, 1321–1323.

Remuzzi, G., Benigni, A., Dodesini, P., Schiepatti, A., Gotti, E., Livio, M., Mecca, G., Donati, M.B. & de Gaetano, G. (1982) Platelet function in patients on maintenance haemodialysis: depressed or enhanced? *Clin Nephrol* **17**, 60–63.

Remuzzi, G., Benigni, A., Dodesini, P., Schiepatti, A., Livio, M., de Gaetano, G., Day, J.S., Smith, W.L., Pinca, E., Patrigiani, P. & Patrono, C. (1983) Reduced platelet thromboxane formation in uremia: evidence for a functional cyclooxygenase defect. *J Clin Invest* **71**, 762–768.

Richman, A.V. & Kasnic, G. (1982) Endothelial and platelet reactions in the idiopathic nephrotic syndrome. *Hum Pathol* **13**, 548–553.

Riella, M.C., George, C.R.P., Hickman, R.O., Striker, G.E., Slichter, S.J., Harker, L. & Quadracci, L.J. (1976) Renal microangiopathy of the haemolytic uraemic syndrome. *Nephron* **17**, 188–203.

Rigby, R.J., Driedger, A.A., Reid, B.D., Lindsay, R.M., Linton, A.L. & Clark, W.F. (1980) Failure to demonstrate renal uptake of labelled platelets in chronic glomerulonephritis. *Clin Sci* **59**, 147–150.

Rose, P.E., Enayat, S.M., Sunderland, R., Short, P.E., Williams, C.E. & Hill, F.G.H. (1985) Abnormalities of factor VIII related protein multimers in the haemolytic uraemic syndrome. *Arch Dis Child* **59**, 1135–1140.

Rosenberg, J.C., Broelsma, R.J., Bullener, G., Mammen, E.F., Lenaghan, R. & Rosenberg, B.F. (1969) Relationship of platelets, blood coagulation and fibrinolysis to hyperacute rejection of renal xenografts. *Transplantation* **8**, 152–161.

Rosner, E., Pauzner, R., Lusky, A., Modan, M. & Many, A. (1987) Detection and quantitative evaluation of lupus circulating anticoagulant activity. *Thromb Haemost* **57**, 144–147.

Rossi, E.C. (1989) Thrombotic thrombocytopenic purpura: a disseminated form of thrombotic microangiopathy. In Remuzzi, G. & Rossi, E.C. (eds) *Haemostasis and the Kidney*, pp. 237–258. Butterworth, London.

Rowlands, D.T., Hill, G.S. & Zmijewski, C.M. (1976) The pathology of renal homograft rejection. A review. *Am J Pathol* **85**, 774–804.

Rubin, K., Tingstrom, A., Hansson, G.K., Larsson, E., Ronnstrand, L., Klareskog, L., Claesson-Welsh, L., Heldin, C.-E., Fellstrom, B. & Terracio, L. (1988) Induction of B-type receptors for platelet-derived growth factor in vascular inflammation: possible implications for development of vascular proliferative lesions. *Lancet* **i**, 1353–1356.

Rylance, P.R., Gordge, M.P. & Weston, M.J. (1985) Platelet function is enhanced, not depressed in uraemia. *Proc Eur Dialysis Transpl Ass* **22**, 76–78.

Saito, H., Ideura, T. & Takeuchi, J. (1984) Effects of selective thromboxane A2 inhibitor on immune complex glomerulonephritis. *Nephron* **36**, 38–45.

Salzman, E.W. & Neri, L.L. (1966) Adhesiveness of blood platelets in uraemia. *Thromb Diath Haemorrh* **15**, 84–92.

Sanders, P.W., Taylor, N. & Curtis, J.J. (1985) Hemodialysis without anticoagulation. *Am J Kidney Dis* **5**, 32–35.

Scharschmidt, B.F., Martin, J.S., Shapiro, C.G., Plotz, P.H. & Berk, P.D. (1977) The use of calcium chelating agents and prostaglandin E1 to eliminate platelet and white blood cell losses resulting from hemoperfusion through charcoal, albumin, agarose gel and neutral cation exchange resins. *J Lab Clin Med* **89**, 110–119.

Schiepatti, A., Dodesini, P., Benigni, A., Massazza, M., Mecca, G., Remuzzi, G., Livio, M., de Gaetano, G. & Rossi, E.C. (1984) The metabolism of arachidonic acid by platelets in the nephrotic syndrome. *Kidney Int* **25**, 671–676.

Schlondorff, D. & Neuwirth, R. (1986) Platelet activating factor and the kidney. *Am J Physiol* **251**, F1–F11.

Schmitt, G.W., Moake, J.L., Rudy, C.K., Vicks, S.L. & Hamburger, R.J. (1987) Alterations in hemostatic parameters during hemodialysis with dialyzers of different membrane composition and flow design. *Am J Med* **83**, 411–418.

Schwab, S.J., Onorato, J.J., Sharar, L.R. & Dennis, P.A. (1987) Hemodialysis without anticoagulation. One-year prospective trial in hospitalized patients at risk for bleeding. *Am J Med* **83**, 405–410.

Sharma, H.M., Moore, S., Merrick, H.W. & Smith, M.R. (1972) Platelets in early hyperacute rejection and their modification by sulfinpyrazone (Anturan) therapy. *Am J Pathol* **66**, 445–453.

Shinkai, Y. & Cameron, J.S. (1987a) The effect of thromboxane synthetase inhibitor OKY-046 on the accelerated model of nephrotoxic nephritis in rabbits. *Nephron* **47**, 211–219.

Shinkai, Y. & Cameron, J.S. (1987b) Trial of platelet derived growth factor antagonist, trapidil, in accelerated nephrotoxic serum nephritis in rabbits. *Br J Exp Pathol* **68**, 847–852.

Shulman, H., Striker, G., Deeg, H., Kennedy, M., Storb,

R. & Donnall Thomas, E. (1981) Nephrotoxicity of cyclosporin A after allogeneic bone marrow transplantation. *New Engl J Med* **305**, 1392–1395.

Siddiqui, F.A. & Lian, E.C.-Y. (1985) Novel platelet agglutinating protein from a thrombotic thrombocytopenia purpura plasma. *J Clin Invest* **76**, 1330–1337.

Silberbauer, K., Sinzinger, H. & Winter, M. (1978) Increased prostacyclin availability of vascular tissue in experimentally induced acute uremia in rats. *Artery* **4**, 554–563.

Silver, M.J., Smith, J.B., Ingerman, C.M. & Kocsis, J.J. (1973) Arachidonic acid- induced human platelet aggregation and prostaglandin formation. *Prostaglandins* **4**, 863–875.

Sindrey, M., Marshall, T.L. & Naish, P. (1979) Quantitative assessment of the effects of platelet depletion in the autologous phase of nephrotoxic serum nephritis. *Clin Exp Immunol* **36**, 90–96.

Simpson, K.M., Bunch, D.C., Amemiya, H., Boehmig, H.J., Wilson, C.B., Dixon, F.J., Coburg, A.J., Hathaway, W.E., Giles, G.R. & Starzl, T.E. (1970) Humoral antibodies and coagulation mechanisms in the accelerated hyperacute rejection of renal homografts in sensitized canine recipients. *Surgery* **68**; 77–85.

Smith, M.C. & Dunn, M.J. (1981) Impaired platelet thromboxane production in renal failure. *Nephron* **29**, 133–137.

Sprandio, J.D., Shapiro, S., Thiagarajan, P. & McCord, S. (1988) Cultured human umbilical vein endothelial cells contain a membrane glycoprotein immunologically related to platelet glycoprotein Ib. *Blood* **71**, 234–237.

Stevens, P.E., Riley, B., Davies, S.P., Gower, P.E., Brown, E.A. & Kox, W. (1988) Continuous arteriovenous haemodialysis in critically ill patients. *Lancet* **ii**, 150–152.

Stewart, J.H. (1967) Platelet numbers and lifespan in acute and chronic renal failure. *Thromb Diath Haemorrh* **17**, 532–542.

Stewart, J.H. & Castaldi, P.A. (1967) Uraemic bleeding: a reversible platelet defect corrected by dialysis. *Q J Med* **36**, 409–423.

Stuart, M.J., Gerrard, J.M. & White, J.G. (1980) The influence of albumin and calcium on human platelet arachidonic acid metabolism. *Blood* **55**, 418–23.

Taylor, R.P., Kujala, G., Wilson, K., Wright, E. & Harbin, A. (1985) In vivo and in vitro studies of the binding of antibody/dsDNA immune complexes to rabbit and guinea pig platelets. *J Immunol* **134**, 2550–2558.

Tojo, S., Narita, M., Koyama, A., Sano, M., Suzuki, H., Tsuchiya, T., Tsuchida, H., Yamamoto, S. & Shishido, H. (1978) Dipyridamole therapy in the nephrotic syndrome. *Contr Nephrol* **9**, 111–127.

Tranqui, L., Duperray, A., Chenais, F., Alix, J.L. & Cordonnier, D. (1985) Effect of human platelet factors on the proliferation of rat mesangial cells. *Thromb Res* **39**, 245–252.

Turitto, V.T. & Weiss, H.J. (1980) Red blood cells: their dual role in thrombus formation. *Science* **207**, 541–543.

Turney, J.H., Williams, L.C., Fewell, M.R., Parsons, V. & Weston, M.J. (1980) Platelet protection and heparin sparing with prostacyclin during regular dialysis therapy. *Lancet* **ii**, 219–222.

Turney, J.H., Woods, H.F., Fewell, M.R. & Weston, M.J. (1981) Factor VIII complex in uraemia and effects of haemodialysis. *Br Med J* **282**, 1653–1656.

Ueda, N., Kawaguchi, S., Niinomi, Y., Nonoda, T., Ohnishi, M., Ito, S. & Yasaki, T. (1986) Effect of dipyridamole treatment on proteinuria in patients in pediatric renal disease. *Nephron* **44**, 174–179.

van Buren, D., van Buren, C.T., Flechner, S.M., Maddox, A.M., Verani, R. & Kahan, B.D. (1985) De novo hemolytic uremic syndrome in renal transplant recipients immunosuppressed with cyclosporine. *Surgery* **98**, 54–62.

van den Berg Wolf, M.G., Kootte, A.M.M., Weening, J.J. & Paul, L.C. (1988) Recurrent analytic uremic syndrome in a renal transplant recipient and review of the Leiden experience. *Transplantation* **45**, 248–251.

Vanhoutte, P.M. (1988) The endothelium- modulator of vascular smooth muscle tone. *New Engl J Med* **319**, 512–513.

Vanrenterghem, Y., Roels, L., Lerut, T., Gruwez, J., Michielsen, P., Gresele, P., Deckmyn, H., Colucci, M., Arnaout, J. & Vermylen, J. (1985) Thromboembolic complications and haemostatic changes in cyclosporin-treated cadaveric kidney allograft recipients. *Lancet* **i**, 999–1002.

Vicks, S.L., Gross, M.L. & Schmitt, G.W. (1983) Massive hemorrhage due to hemodialysis-associated thrombocytopenia. *Am J Nephrol* **3**, 30–33.

Viener, A., Aviram, M., Better, O.S. & Brook, J.G. (1986) Enhanced *in vitro* platelet aggregation in hemodialysis patients. *Nephron* **43**, 139–143.

Vlakoyannis, J. & Schoeppe, W. (1982) Adenylate cyclase activity and cAMP content of human platelets in uraemia. *Eur J Clin Invest* **12**, 379–381.

von Felten, A., Ermanni, M. & Binswanger, U. (1981) Immune complex associated platelet disorder in renal allograft recipients. *Acta Haematol* **65**, 221–228.

von Willebrand, E., Zola, H. & Hayry, P. (1985) Thrombocyte aggregates in renal allografts. Analysis with fine-needle aspiration biopsy and monoclonal antithrombocyte antibodies. *Transplantation* **39**, 258–262.

Walters, M.D.S., Levin, M., Smith, C., Nokes, T.J.C., Hardisty, R.M., Dillon, M.J. & Barratt, T.M. (1988) Intravascular platelet activation in the hemolytic uremic syndrome. *Kidney Int* **33**, 107–115.

Warrell, Jr R.P., Hultin, M.B. & Coller, B.S. (1979) Increased factor VIII/von Willebrand factor antigen and von Willebrand factor activity in renal failure. *Am J Med* **66**, 226–228.

Weinstein, M.J., Chute, L.E., Schmitt, G.W., Hamburger, R.H., Bauer, K.A., Troll, J.H., Janson, P.K. & Deykin, D. (1985) Abnormal factor VIII coagulant antigen in patients with renal dysfunction and in those with disseminated intravascular coagulation. *J Clin Invest* **76**, 1406–1411.

Winter, M., Frampton, G., Bennett, A., Machin, S.J. & Cameron, J.S. (1983a) Synthesis of thromboxane B2 in uraemia and the effects of dialysis. *Thromb Res* **30**, 265–272.

Winter, M., Seghatchian, M.J. & Cameron, J.S. (1983b) An abnormal factor VIII molecule in uraemia? *Lancet* **i**, 1112.

Winter, M., Needham, J., Mackie, L. & Cameron, J.S. (1984) Impaired vessel wall response to venous occlusion in patients with chronic renal failure on maintenance haemodialysis. *Clin Nephrol* **22**, 307–313.

Woo, K.T., Whitworth, J.A. & Kincaid-Smith, P. (1980) Effect of anti-platelet agents on circulating platelet aggregates in patients with glomerulonephritis. *Thromb Res* **20**, 663–668.

Woods, H.F., Ash, G., Parsons, V. & Weston, M.J. (1979) Reduction of dialyzer fibrin deposition with sulfinpyrazone. *Clin Nephrol* **12**, 122–127.

Yanigasawa, Y., Kurihara, H., Kimura, S., Tanobe, Y., Kobayashi, M., Mitsui, Y., Yazaki, Y., Goto, K. & Masaki, T. (1988) A novel potent vasoconstrictor peptide produced by vascular endothelial cells. *Nature* **332**, 411–415.

Yoshida, N. & Aoki, N. (1978) Release of arachidonic acid from human platelets. A key role for the potentiation of platelet hyperaggregability in normal subjects as well as those with a nephrotic syndrome. *Blood* **52**, 969–977.

Zimmerman, S.W., Moorthy, A.V., Dreher, W.H., Friedman, A. & Varanasi, U. (1983) Prospective trial of warfarin and dipyridamole in patients with membranoproliferative glomerulonephritis. *Am J Med* **75**, 920–927.

Zoja, C., Furci, L., Ghilardi, F., Zilio, P., Benigni, A. & Renmuzzi, G. (1986) Cyclosporin- induced endothelial cell injury. *Lab Invest* **55**, 455–462.

Zucker, M.B. (1979) Biological aspects of heparin action. Heparin and platelet function. *Fed Proc* **36**, 47–49.

12: Modulation of Platelet Function

Keith D. Butler

Introduction

To date the term antiplatelet drug has normally been a synonym for antithrombotic which is by no means proven in any clinical sense. The search for antiplatelet drugs has been focused within the area of thrombosis but as our knowledge of the roles that platelets can play in events such as inflammation, asthma and cancer broaden, hopefully the area of the search will also broaden, as it must not be expected that drugs developed to impair the onset of thrombosis will necessarily impair the platelet involvement, for example, in asthma. Since these other areas have been dealt with by previous authors the emphasis in this chapter will remain on the field of thrombosis.

An almost infinite number of compounds have been demonstrated over the last 30 years to inhibit platelet function *in vitro*. However, far fewer have been demonstrated to be antithrombotic or even platelet inhibitory *in vivo*. The demonstration of real clinical benefit has an even poorer record.

The range of the models of thrombosis used to test this array of pharmacological agents is extensive and has been reviewed previously (Philip, 1979, 1986; and in Chapter 4 of this volume). In general, arteries have been subjected to various forms of injury — electrical, chemical, thermal or mechanical. Foreign surfaces placed in the circulation or the injection of platelet aggregatory substances or a combination of these stimuli have also been utilized. Antithrombotic activity has been reported, although seldom with any consistency, for compounds such as aspirin, dipyridamole, phosphodiesterase inhibitors, cyclooxygenase and thromboxane synthase inhibitors. Receptor antagonists of thromboxane A_2, fibrinogen and thrombin have also been reported to have inhibitory activity. The variance of the many results with this range of compounds may well lie with the use of experimental systems in which the pathology of the events responsible for the generation of thrombosis are poorly defined or inappropriate for the drugs being studied. At present, it is clear that no one experimental model offers the best predictive value for clinical efficacy. This should hardly be surprising since the clinical pathology, where such evidence exists, varies greatly according to the type of thrombosis and the site involved. Experimental models need to be designed to match specific clinical events before they can be expected to have any chance of being predictive for pharmacological therapy or clinical benefit. Such models are being developed and the use of techniques such as angioplasty or arteriovenous grafts at least allows the potential use of active compounds, in such systems, to be considered for man, and allows some clinical evaluation of their antithrombotic properties before moving on to the more difficult areas to show clinical benefit in, such as myocardial infarction.

In general, the compounds currently of interest with respect to antithrombotic capability fall into four broad and frequently overlapping areas:

1 modulation of second messengers, e.g. calcium, cyclic adenosine monophosphate (cAMP);

2 modulation of prostanoid metabolism, e.g. cyclooxygenase inhibitors, thromboxane synthase inhibitors;

3 endogenous inhibitors or enhancement of their production, e.g. prostacyclin, endothelium derived relaxing factor (EDRF);

4 inhibition of thrombin formation or its action.

A full review of all the potential inhibitors of platelet function even within these four areas is far beyond that possible here and many aspects have been reviewed previously. All of those approaches have some problems. Modulation of the secondary messengers or prostaglandin metabolism involves interference with mechanisms common to all cell types and requires a way to target the effect to the platelet to avoid many of the undesirable side effects incurred with such compounds. As a result, much interest is concerned with the concept of inhibition at the level of the receptor. The success of this approach will be determined by whether the agonist targeted does indeed play a pivotal role in the clinical thrombotic disorder selected for treatment. There will be little point expecting a thromboxane receptor antagonist to be effective in a condition where thrombin plays the major pathological role and vice versa. In general with all of these pharmacological approaches, the resulting relevance to the clinic still remains to be proven but those with the widest clinical use and application are discussed below.

Modulation of second messengers

Calcium

Calcium is a central messenger in platelet activation (Gerrard *et al.* 1981; Rink *et al.* 1982; Johnson *et al.* 1985). In many disorders in which platelets appear to play an important role there has been demonstrated to be an elevation and/or abnormal handling of intracellular calcium (Ahn *et al.* 1987) which nifedipine has been shown to normalize. Others have also found that the abnormal handling of calcium is associated with increased sensitivity to aggregatory stimuli (Erne *et al.* 1985; Shanbaky *et al.* 1987).

Calcium modulators are utilized clinically for a wide range of cardiovascular disorders (e.g. cardiac dysrhythmias, hypertension, coronary and peripheral vasospastic events). Experimentally calcium modulators have been demonstrated to inhibit platelet aggregation *in vitro* (Ono & Kimura, 1981) and are capable of reducing the rate of platelet deposition and thrombus formation in polytetrafluorethylene (PTFE) grafts in dogs (Pumphrey *et al.* 1983). Clinical observations include reduction of circulating platelet aggregates (Chierchia *et al.* 1981) and the prolongation of bleeding time (Dale *et al.* 1983a). As yet, however, no conclusive evidence that the clinical benefit of these compounds is related to their platelet inhibitory activity is forthcoming. Considering the ubiquitous nature of their pharmacological profile this is not surprising.

More detailed reviews of the role of calcium and the effects of calcium modulators are available (Ellrodt & Singh, 1983; Murer, 1985; Tracy & Black, 1987).

Cyclic AMP

Sutherland and Robinson (Sutherland *et al.* 1966) proposed cyclic 3′,5′-adenosine monophosphate (cAMP) as a second messenger in the regulation of cell function. Exogenous cAMP had already been reported to be a weak inhibitor of platelet function (Marcus & Zucker, 1965) and since then both the synthetic and degradative enzymes for cAMP have been demonstrated (Zieve & Greenough, 1969; Amer & Mayol, 1973). Platelet cAMP levels are determined by the balance between synthesis and degradation as in other cell types. This balance will also regulate the level of free cytoplasmic Ca^{2+} within the cell (Fig. 12.1).

Blockade of the phosphodiesterases and/or stimulation of adenyl cyclase results in increased levels of platelet cAMP which stabilize the storage pool of calcium and promotes the movement of cytoplasmic Ca^{2+} into the intracellular stores. Decreased availability of free cytoplasmic divalent calcium impedes platelet activation which verapamil or nifedipine can induce by preventing extracellular calcium moving into the cell during activation. Stimulators of adenyl cyclase, e.g. prostaglandin E (PGE_1) and prostacyclin I_2 (PGI_2) as well as phosphodiesterase

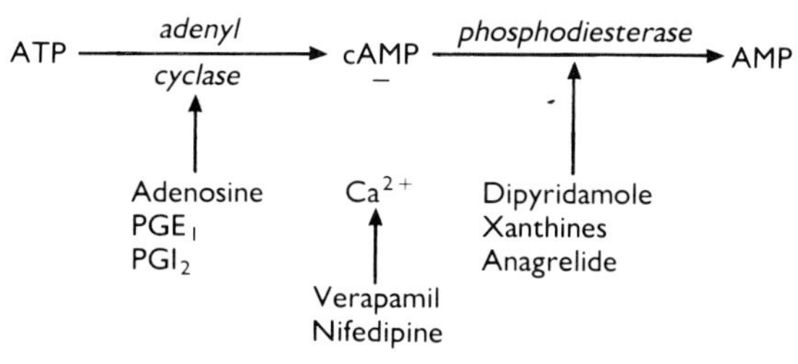

Figure 12.1

inhibitors (e.g. xanthines) have been demonstrated to be inhibitors of platelet function. Further synergy between these two classes of pharmacological agents has also been demonstrated (Ball *et al.* 1970; Mills & Smith, 1971).

Dipyridamole

Dipyridamole was originally introduced as a vasodilator and has been demonstrated to be a weak inhibitor of platelet function (Emmons *et al.* 1965a,b).

Two potential mechanisms of action have been considered for this compound which relate to its properties as a phosphodiesterase inhibitor (Mills & Smith 1971; Best *et al.* 1979) and also as an inhibitor of adenosine uptake (Summers *et al.* 1977; Gresele *et al.* 1983). The anti-aggregatory affect of adenosine on platelets was first demonstrated by Born and Cross (1963). This effect has since been shown to be associated with an increase in cAMP and to be mediated via receptors of the A_2 subtype (Haslam & Cusack, 1981). Thus the elevation of plasma levels of adenosine due to inhibition of uptake by dipyridamole (particularly by red cells) could lead to an inhibitory effect on platelets via the stimulation of adenyl cyclase. The neutralization of the platelet inhibitory effect of dipyridamole by adenosine deaminase or adenosine receptor antagonists (Gresele *et al.* 1986) together with potentiation of the action of dipyridamole by other phosphodiesterase inhibitors lends credence to this suggestion.

Dipyridamole activity, weak as it is, as a phosphodiesterase inhibitor and the discovery of PGI_2 led to the proposal that the antiplatelet effects could derive from synergism with endogenous PGI_2 (Moncada & Korbut 1978). Such an effect was demonstrated *in vitro* (Di Minno *et al.* 1978) but the theory seems at variance with the fact that aspirin, at doses which block PGI_2 production (Gresele *et al.* 1985; Hanson *et al.* 1985), is also synergistic with dipyridamole. Further, Gresele *et al.* (1985) and Hanson and Harker (1983) were both unable to demonstrate any synergism with dazoxiben, the latter compound being a selective thromboxane A_2 synthase inhibitor which causes redirection of prostanoid metabolism to increase the formation of prostanoids which stimulate adenyl cyclase (Bertele *et al.* 1984a,b). In addition a previous study by Groves *et al.* (1982) had failed to demonstrate synergy *in vivo* between dipyridamole and prostacyclin.

In vivo dipyridamole has been reported to inhibit platelet adhesion to rabbit aorta (Kinlough-Rathbone *et al.* 1978, 1983; Groves *et al.* 1982), collagen (Cazenave *et al.* 1978), artificial surfaces (Harker *et al.* 1979; Pumphrey *et al.* 1983) as well as prolonging platelet survival in homocystine-induced atherosclerosis in baboons (Harker *et al.* 1976). In combination with aspirin there is a potentiation of the effect of dipyridamole in the baboon (Harker *et al.* 1979; Hanson *et al.* 1985) and restenosis following balloon angioplasty in the pig has also been impaired (Steele *et al.* 1985).

Similar results with combinations of dipyridamole and aspirin have been obtained in man. Sinzinger *et al.* (1988) demonstrated a reduction in platelet deposition on atherosclerotic lesions and similar findings have been achieved by Goldman *et al.* (1983b) on prosthetic femoro-popliteal grafts. In addition, Barnathan *et al.* (1987) found the combination to prevent acute thrombosis following percutaneous transluminal coronary angioplasty (PTCA). In this situation, however, the results on restenosis rate remain equivocal with some workers reporting the rate to be unaltered (White *et al.* 1987b; Schwartz *et al.* 1988), although the latter workers did find a marked reduction in the incidence rate of transmural myocardial infarction. In contrast Chesebro *et al.* (1982) has reported a reduction in the re-occlusion rate in coronary artery grafts and dipyridamole has been demonstrated to inhibit smooth muscle cell proliferation in response to experimental vessel injury (Ingerman-Wojenski & Silver, 1988). In addition aspirin–dipyridamole combinations have also been reported to prolong shortened platelet survival in man (Harker Slichter, 1972; Steele *et al.* 1978; Tindall *et al.* 1982).

Despite these positive results both in animals and man it is still not clear whether the combination of dipyridamole and aspirin has any benefit over aspirin alone in man (Harker, 1986; Goldman *et al.* 1988; Sze *et al.* 1988).

Anagrelide

Anagrelide has been demonstrated to be a broad spectrum inhibitor of platelet function with an EC_{50} of 0.08 to 0.3 μg/ml, depending upon the platelet agonist used, being a highly selective inhibitor of phosphodiesterase (Gillespie, 1988). *In vivo* activity against arterial thrombus formation has been demonstrated with oral doses in the range 0.2–10 mg/kg (Fleming & Buyniski, 1979, 1983) and it has also been shown to prolong experimentally shortened platelet survival (Barrett & Butler, 1983). Unfortunately, in early preclinical studies, administration of the compound was accompanied by an asymptomatic fall in platelet count and a slight reduction in platelet survival in man. The effect appeared selective to platelet production (Andes *et al.* 1984) and has led to the compound being given orphan drug status by the Federal Drug Administration (FDA) for treatment of conditions involving thrombocytosis in man.

Modulation of prostanoid metabolism

Drugs which affect the arachidonate pathway do so by inhibiting either the cyclooxygenase (e.g. aspirin) or the thromboxane synthase (e.g. dazoxiben) which converts the endoperoxide to thromboxane (Fig. 12.2). All such compounds will thus inhibit thromboxane-dependent steps involved in platelet aggregation and release. However, where severe vessel injury occurs and mural thrombus formation is thrombin and/or fibrin mediated, thrombin inhibitor or anticoagulants may provide greater benefit (Harker & Fuster, 1986).

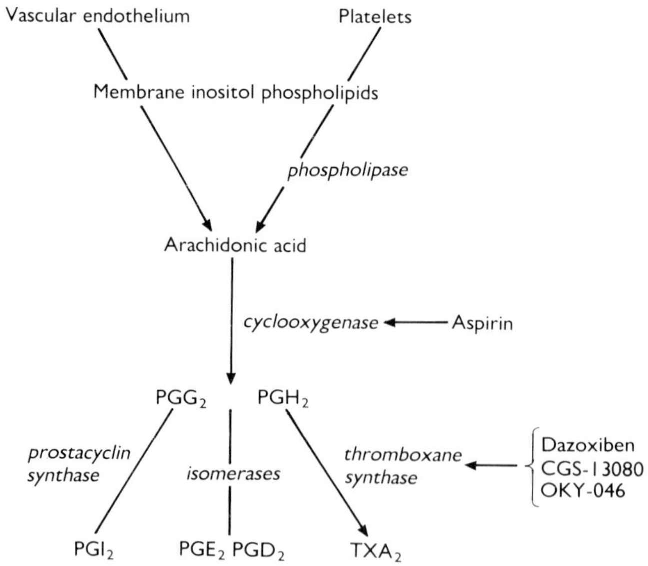

Figure 12.2 Modulation of prostanoid metabolism.

Cyclooxygenase inhibitors

Acetylsalicylic acid

Aspirin inhibits the platelet release reaction induced by adrenaline and collagen but has only a weak inhibitory effect on thrombin-induced platelet aggregation and secretion (Mustard & Packham, 1970). The drug itself is rapidly cleared from the circulation but the effect on platelet secretion can persist for 5–7 days (Weiss *et al.* 1968). The inhibitory effect on prostaglandin synthesis is associated with acetylation of the cyclooxygenase (Roth *et al.* 1975) and since this effect is irreversible, the effect persists for the lifetime of the platelet since it has no capacity for protein synthesis. This effect has been utilized as a non-isotopic method to measure platelet survival since aspirin does not have any protective function in conditions of reduced platelet survival (Stuart *et al.* 1975). The discovery of thromboxane A_2 (TXA_2) and PGI_2 led to the suggestion that it might be possible to obtain a differential inhibition between the platelet and the endothelium (Moncada & Vane, 1978). However, it has since been demonstrated that both cyclooxygenases are equally sensitive to inhibition by aspirin (Jaffe & Weksler, 1979; Preston *et al.* 1981). The endothelium can, by contrast with the platelet, resynthesize cyclooxygenase and this gave rise to the suggestion that a differential effect could be possible with respect to the duration of synthetic capacity for TXA_2 and PGI_2. Some evidence has been obtained from studies in man to support this concept. Vesterqvist (1986) has demonstrated that following a 500 mg dose of aspirin there was a long-lasting inhibition of thromboxane production whilst PGI_2 production was only inhibited significantly for a couple of hours. The debate as to what dosage regime should be used, however, continues. The debate has been enhanced by a number of observations that at high doses aspirin increased thrombus formation (Kelton *et al.* 1978; Buchanan *et al.* 1981) and did not increase bleeding time whilst low doses did increase bleeding time in man (O'Grady & Moncada, 1978). This has led to the assumption that the end result of the effect of aspirin may depend upon the TXA_2:PGI_2 ratio. More recently, de Gaetano and Cerletti (1988) have suggested that aspirin could also enhance the release of EDRF. This would also enhance the antiplatelet effect and could also cause an increase in bleeding time via a direction action of EDRF on the vessel wall.

Aspirin has been demonstrated to be effective in a wide range of animal models where thrombin does not play a major pathological role (Philip, 1979) and in recent years there has been a growing body of evidence demonstrating at least some degree of clinical benefit in certain thrombotic conditions.

There have been a number of reports of studies involving angioplasty in animals which demonstrate a reduction in platelet deposition and/or the subsequent restenosis rate (Wu *et al.* 1981; Faxon *et al.* 1984; Lam *et al.* 1987). This has been supported by clinical studies in which similar findings were reported on platelet deposition (Cunningham *et al.* 1984) but results on restenosis rates are inconsistent (Thornton *et al.* 1984; Kaltenbach *et al.* 1985).

In a model of stenosis-induced arterial thrombosis in femoral and coronary arteries in the dog, Folts *et al.* (1976, 1982) have demonstrated that the cyclic flow reductions observed were due to platelet aggregation which was susceptible to aspirin inhibition. Similar observations have been made in human subjects with stenosis in femoral or popliteal arteries (Folts *et al.* 1982). Clinical trials in unstable angina (Lewis *et al.* 1983; Cairns *et al.* 1985) have been reported and, whilst they differ in the duration of therapy and the dose used both showed clinical benefit with respect both to fatal and non-fatal cardiac events.

In other areas involving arterial damage or the presence of artificial thrombogenic surfaces in the vasculature aspirin has been ineffective. No benefit by aspirin alone has been demonstrated on platelet accumulation on atherosclerotic plaques in man (Sinzinger *et al.* 1988), A–V shunts in baboons (Hanson *et al.* 1985; Bjornsson *et al.* 1987) or autologous vein grafts in rabbits (Gershlick *et al.* 1985). Indeed in the latter study aspirin in high doses caused an increased platelet deposition in the graft as demonstrated in earlier studies by Buchanan *et al.* (1981) in crushed rabbit arteries. These experimental results contrast with those of Goldman *et al.* (1988) who demonstrated an increased early patency of saphenous vein grafts with aspirin therapy, but are in agreement with the results of Sharma *et al.* (1983) who found no benefit with aspirin alone. In all these situations, however, combination with dipyridamole was demonstrated to be beneficial.

Clinical evidence to date does appear to support a beneficial effect of aspirin, particularly in combination with dipyridamole, in reducing the rate of recurrent transient ischaemic attack (TIA), stroke and death in patients with TIA (Turpie, 1988). However Sze *et al.* (1988) are cautious as to whether dipyridamole does convey any real benefit to the effect of aspirin alone and most of the doses used in these studies would be considered as high, being around 1 g daily. Since then, Lee *et al.* (1988) have demonstrated that as little as 75 mg aspirin per day is sufficient to give complete inhibition of platelet function, and only marginally suppress prostacyclin production: whether the effect of aspirin demonstrated in TIA is truly related to an effect on platelet function still requires clarification. Unfortunately, there are no really good experimental models of occlusive stroke or TIA which have any relevance in their pathophysiology to the events which occur in man. With respect to platelet involvement in the development of TIA/stroke two models have been reported which utilize infusion of adenosine diphosphate (ADP) or arachidonic acid into the carotid (Fieschi *et al.* 1975; Fujimoto *et al.* 1984, 1985). The latter workers have reported increased thromboxane B_2 (TXB_2) production and the presence of platelet aggregates together with evidence of vascular damage, but to date no data relating to drug therapy have been forthcoming. More recently, the work of May *et al.* (1990) indicates that the platelet agonists chosen by previous workers may not have been the most suitable agents and that the use of thrombin may be more relevant to the clinical correlate but further studies will be required to establish the true value of the experimental model (see Chapter 4).

Thromboxane synthase inhibitors

Thromboxane A_2 is a major metabolite of arachidonic acid in the platelet. The discovery of prostacyclin synthetase in the vessel wall led to the proposal of redirection of prostanoid metabolism by inhibition of the thromboxane synthase (Bunting *et al.* 1983). Inhibition of thromboxane production, in theory, has the advantage of leaving prostacyclin production unimpaired but the disadvantage that there could be an accumulation of the endoperoxide metabolites (PGG_2 and PGH_2). This increased level of substrate for prostacyclin synthase could then result in increased production of PGI_2. In reality, however, the redirection tends to be less than specific with increases in other prostaglandins (e.g. PGE_2, PGD_2) also being found.

Dazoxiben

Dazoxiben is a potent inhibitor of thromboxane synthase, inhibition being reported at 3×10^{-9} M (IC_{50}) whilst concentrations of up to 10^{-4} M had little or no effect on cyclooxygenase or prostacyclin synthetase (Randall *et al.* 1981). Despite this potent ability to inhibit thromboxane production dazoxiben has only very weak activity on arachidonate-induced aggregation but will inhibit collagen-induced aggregation to some extent. This probably reflects the ability of the endoperoxides to sustain aggregation especially in the case of arachidonic acid (Parry, 1983). In addition, in man, the effect of dazoxiben is variable with the population being divided into 'responders' and 'non-responders' (Heptinstall *et al.* 1980, 1982). This has been suggested to be related to whether the patients prostanoid metabolism was directed to PGD_2 or other metabolites. However, Bertele *et al.* (1981) found that both groups of patients were capable of producing elevated levels of PGD_2 following dazoxiben treatment. Whatever the explanation of the difference in responsiveness between patients it is clear that, even with TXB_2 generation totally inhibited, aggregation can still occur (Bertele *et al.* 1981). Certainly dazoxiben inhibits TXB_2 production with a parallel enhancement of PGE_2, $PGF_{2\alpha}$, PGD_2 and 6-keto-$PGF_{1\alpha}$ (Maguire & Wallis, 1983; Bertele *et al.* 1984a; Patrignani *et al.* 1984) and although results on aggregation may be variable, bleeding time is prolonged in man (Dale *et al.* 1983b).

The combination of dazoxiben with a thromboxane antagonist (BM 13177) provides a greater inhibition of platelet aggregation and a more prolonged bleeding time. Under these conditions intracellular cAMP was increased although individually these compounds had no effect (Gresele *et al.* 1987). In addition the effects of dazoxiben on aggregation can be impaired by the use of an adenyl cyclase inhibitor (Bertele *et al.* 1984b) or enhanced by combination with calcium channel blockers (Onoda *et al.* 1984) or phosphodiesterase inhibitors (Smith, 1982; Sills *et al.* 1986).

In animal models of thrombosis dazoxiben has been shown to protect against sudden death in rabbits induced by intravenous administration of arachidonic acid (Lindsay *et al.* 1986) but not by azo-PGH_2 (Lefer *et al.* 1983). Further dazoxiben promotes deaggregation of aggregates induced by collagen (Butler *et al.* 1986) and inhibits increases in lung permeability induced by thrombin (Garcia-Szabo *et al.* 1983) and endotoxin-induced pulmonary hypertension (Ball *et al.* 1983). The short duration of action of dazoxiben (FitzGerald *et al.* 1983; Patrignani *et al.* 1984) necessitates adjusting the doseage regime to give an adequate level of TXB_2 inhibition for a suitable duration in order to demonstrate beneficial effects on more chronic models such as platelet survival in the hypercholesterolaemic rabbit (Butler *et al.* 1987).

In other models of arterial thrombosis the effectiveness of dazoxiben depends upon the model chosen. In those in which vessel injury has been induced by local electrical stimulation dazoxiben has been shown to reduce platelet deposition (Randall & Wilding, 1982), slow the rate of thrombus formation (Schumacher & Lucchesi, 1983) and abolish cyclic flow variations in stenotic coronary arteries (Bush *et al.* 1983). However, if thrombus formation or platelet deposition was studied on prosthetic arterial grafts, dazoxiben was ineffective (Goldman *et al.* 1983a; Hanson & Harker, 1983).

Dazoxiben has also been shown to have some cardioprotective actions, which may or may not be related to any action on platelets, in reducing ventricular fibrillation during reperfusion after coronary occlusion (Coker & Parratt, 1983) and providing a protective effect on energy metabolism in the reperfused heart (Pieper *et al.* 1988).

Clinical evaluations of dazoxiben have been attempted but studies with Raynauds phenomenon (Coffman & Rasmussen, 1984; Luderer *et al.* 1984; Tindall *et al.* 1985) have failed to show clinical benefit, whilst other studies have been with too few patients to allow meaningful evaluations to be made. Interestingly, a study on the ischaemic response during arterial pacing stress tests in patients with coronary artery disease did show a significant reduction compared with both the control response and aspirin treatment (Thaulow *et al.* 1984). However, to date the clinical usefulness of dazoxiben remains to be proven and results so far have been disappointing (FitzGerald *et al.* 1985).

Developmental compounds

Despite the failure to establish a clinical niche for dazoxiben a number of companies are still seeking to develop thromboxane synthase inhibitors and determine a clinical role for this type of compound.

OKY-046. Ono Pharmaceuticals have a series of OKY compounds which exhibit selective inhibition of thromboxane synthase. Of these OKY-046 and OKY-1581, have been evaluated on aggregation (Naito *et al.* 1983) and in various animal models with particular emphasis on models of lung shock (Garcia-Czabo *et al.* 1984; Nagai *et al.* 1987) and of cardiac ischaemia, particularly the effects following reperfusion (Ogura *et al.* 1988) or stenosis (Tomoda, 1986). In all cases these compounds displayed a beneficial protective effect for the target tissues (i.e. lung or heart). Other studies by Fukumori *et al.* (1984) on cerebral vasospasm in dogs displayed a reduction in basilar artery vasospasm together with an improvement in regional cerebral blood flow. This study was followed up clinically in patients suffering cerebral vasospasm after a ruptured cerebral aneurysm. Whilst the angiographs did not always display an impairement of vasospasm the authors claimed a reduction in the extent of cerebral ischaemia and infarction (Suzuki *et al.* 1985).

CGS 13080. Ciba-Geigy have reported compounds from two series of compounds which are selective inhibitors of thromboxane synthase: CGS 13080 which has a short duration of action (Ku *et al.* 1983) and a longer acting compound CGS 12970 (Ambler *et al.* 1985). Both entities have similar properties to those reported for this class of compound.

Redirection of prostanoid metabolism has been reported in both animal and human tissues (McNab *et al.* 1984; Mehta *et al.* 1985) and a review of the effects of CGS 13080 has been published previously (Lefer, 1984). As for the OKY compounds there is reported protection against the effects of ischaemia in the heart (O'Connor *et al.* 1986) and antithrombotic actions after angioplasty (Sanborn *et al.* 1986), electrical injury to the vasculature (Simpson *et al.* 1986) on re-occlusion of coronary arteries after thrombolytic therapy (Mickelson *et al.* 1987) in experimental situations. Reports of effects in man are limited, so far being restricted to effects on thromboxane B_2 formation, redirection of prostanoid metabolism and bleeding time (FitzGerald & Oates 1984; Reilly *et al.* 1986).

As with all the compounds with synthase-inhibiting activity as yet no clear clinical role has been ascertained. They all seem to exert some protection against ischaemia either of myocardial or cerebral siting. In addition they appear to have some useful properties which may be of benefit as an adjunct therapy to angioplasty or thrombolysis. In general, however, it does seem that to achieve any major effectiveness they may well have to be used in combination with a thromboxane receptor antagonist (Gresele *et al.* 1984; Reilly *et al.* 1986) which would augment the effects of synthase inhibition (Schrör & Thiemermann, 1986).

Endogenous inhibitors

Prostacyclin

The most potent platelet inhibitor described is PGI_2 (Moncada & Vane, 1977) being capable of inhibiting aggregation induced by arachidonic acid, ADP, collagen and the endoperoxides. In addition, it can cause deaggregation of platelets *in vitro* (Moncada *et al.* 1976), in extra corporeal shunts containing collagen strips (Gryglewski *et al.* 1978) and in man (Szczeklik *et al.* 1978). These actions result from the stimulation of adenyl cyclase (Gorman *et al.* 1977) which is probably also the explanation for the ability of PGI_2 to inhibit the expression of platelet prothrombinase activity on the platelet membrane following platelet activation (Zwaal *et al.* 1984).

Synergistic actions with both phosphodiesterase inhibitors and thromboxane synthase inhibitors have been demonstrated in reducing thrombin-induced ventricular thrombosis, thrombocytopenia and death, although the combinations also enhanced the hypotensive effects (Smith & Egan, 1987), all actions mediated via elevation of cAMP. More recently synergy has also been shown with EDRF or nitric oxide (Radomski *et al.* 1987a; MacDonald *et al.* 1988) and organic nitrates (Caterina *et al.* 1988), both of which increase intracellular levels of cyclic guanosine monophosphate (cGMP) (Rapoport & Murad, 1983). This synergy probably relates to the inhibitory action of EDRF on platelet adhesion (an action potentiated by selective inhibitors of cGMP phosphodiesterase) whilst prostacyclin does not have this ability (Radomski *et al.* 1987b). Since adhesion plays a primary role in haemostasis this interaction may well be more detrimental than beneficial but could play a valuable role in the control of vascular tone.

In vivo PGI_2 has been shown to inhibit platelet thrombus formation induced by venous stimuli (Higgs *et al.* 1977; Bourgain, 1979) but not platelet adhesion

(Ubatuba *et al.* 1979) except at very high doses (Adelman *et al.* 1981). Where prostacyclin may have a useful clinical role is possibly suggested by the experimental results with haemodialysis in dogs (Weston *et al.* 1979), cardiopulmonary bypass (Plachetka *et al.* 1980) and oxygenators (Coppe *et al.* 1979). This use of PGI_2 in extracorporeal circuits would avoid the side effects of hypotension and refractioness to the patient as little or no prostacyclin reaches the patients vascular tree (Mitchell, 1983). The effects demonstrated so far in man using infusions show a dose-related effect on bleeding time and platelet aggregation (Szczeklik *et al.* 1978; Machin *et al.* 1981) which disappears shortly after ending the infusion. The long-lasting clinical benefit observed particularly in peripheral vascular disease remains unexplained (Belch *et al.* 1983; Gryglewski *et al.* 1983).

Modulation of the effects of thrombin

Ticlopidine

Ticlopidine hydrochloride is chemically unrelated to other antiplatelet drugs and appears to have a unique mechanism of action (Gordon, 1984). The full pharmacological details of this compound have been published (Akashi *et al.* 1980a,b). The compound prolongs bleeding time, shortens platelet survival and inhibits aggregation to a wide range of stimuli (Panak *et al.* 1983; de Gaetano & Bertele, 1984) but is neither an inhibitor of cyclooxygenase nor cAMP phosphodiesterase. Ticlopidine will, however, potentiate the effects of PGI_2, PGD_2 and PGE_2 although not the synthesis of PGI_2 (Carrien *et al.* 1984; Frishman & Miller, 1986). The experimental evidence to date appears to suggest that ticlopidine impairs fibrinogen binding to the platelet by interacting with glycoproteins on the platelet membrane (Di Minno *et al.* 1985).

Ticlopidine does not, however, inhibit platelet adherence to chronic arterial injury in animals or to prosthetic surfaces (Smith & White, 1982; Stratton & Ritchie, 1984; Cattaneo *et al.* 1985) and neither did it decrease the rate of restenosis in pigs following angioplasty (Steele *et al.* 1984). In a recent study involving treatment prior to PTCA there was a significant reduction in the incidence of major immediate complications (White *et al.* 1987a) but no improvement in either the restenosis rate or the development of late complications (White *et al.* 1987b).

A number of other small clinical studies have been reported with ticlopidine and although in some studies aggregation was impaired (Kirstein *et al.* 1980) or platelet survival prolonged (Hawker & Aukland, 1984) no clinical benefit has been demonstrated in conditions of chronic stable angina (Khurmi *et al.* 1986), Raynaud's phenomenon (Destors *et al.* 1986), peripheral atherosclerosis (Kirestein *et al.* 1980) or intermittent claudication (Hawker & Aukland, 1984), the lack of effect being taken to indicate that platelets either play no part or only a secondary role in these clinical situations. Recently, a more detailed review on ticlopidine has become available (Saltiel & Ward, 1987).

Further clinical studies in stroke, peripheral arterial disease, diabetic retinopathy and coronary artery bypass grafts are currently being evaluated and these should allow a true judgement to be made as to the clinical usefulness of this compound.

Heparins

The effects and uses of heparin and low molecular weight derivatives have been extensively reviewed previously (Jaques & Mahadoo, 1978; Jaques, 1980, 1982; Levine & Hirsh, 1988; Ofosu & Gray, 1988).

Heparin has been demonstrated to be an effective treatment for venous thrombosis but the clinical use of the compound as an antithrombotic drug can be associated with clinically significant haemorrhagic side effects. The action of heparin on thrombin is indirect with heparin binding to and enhancing the activity of antithrombin III and at low heparin concentrations this would also cause the inactivation of Factor IXa as well as thrombin. Higher concentrations of heparin are necessary to cause inactivation of Factor Xa (Ofusu & Gray, 1988). A second hypothesis has been put forward by Jaques (1982) that heparin prevents thrombosis by being concentrated in, or on, the vascular endothelium, thus increasing the negative electropotential of the vessel wall.

The low-molecular-weight heparin fractions are as effective as unfractionated heparin in the prevention of venous thrombosis and they are claimed to produce less bleeding (Levine & Hirsh, 1988). Further it is suggested that the reduction in haemorrhagic tendency relates to the experimental observation that the low-molecular-weight heparins inhibit platelet function less than unfractionated heparin (Fernandez *et al.* 1986). However, to date, only one trial has clearly demonstrated a reduction in the clinical incidence of haemorrhage (Le Balc'h *et al.* 1987).

Certainly, the effects of heparin on platelets are paradoxical with Saba *et al.* (1984) demonstrating that heparin is capable of inhibiting aggregation to many agonists but also demonstrating an enhancement of thromboxane generation. In contrast many others observe enhancement of aggregation (e.g. Yamamoto *et al.* 1982) which is claimed to be due to the formation of fibrinogen aggregates (Yamamoto *et al.* 1984). These events may well be related to the clinical situation which can occur with heparin — that of systemic thrombocytopenia with associated thrombus formation, white clot syndrome (Stanton *et al.* 1988). As yet no such problems have been reported for the low-molecular-weight heparins.

Thrombin inhibitors

Thrombin is the ultimate serine protease of the coagulation cascade and plays a pivotal role in the generation of arterial and venous thrombosis together with platelet activation *in vivo*. Thrombin is a potent stimulus for inducing platelet shape change, secretion and aggregation at concentrations less than those required for the hydrolysis of fibrinogen (Shuman & Levine, 1978). The subsequent activation of the platelet allows initiation of the amplification pathways involving thromboxane synthesis and granule release. In addition, the platelet membrane can also play a catalytic role for further thrombus generation and subsequent fibrin formation (Zwaal & Hemker, 1982). These ramifications have been extensively reviewed (Greengard & Griffin, 1984; Hemker & Lindhout, 1984; Walsh, 1984).

Kinlough-Rathbone *et al.* (1977) suggested that thrombin may mediate its actions on platelets via two distinct mechanisms. At low thrombin concentrations via ADP release and the cyclooxygenase pathway and via a system involving internal shifts of ionic calcium at high thrombin concentrations. High, moderate and low affinity receptors for thrombin have been demonstrated on the platelet membrane, and occupancy of the high-affinity receptor, at low thrombin concentrations, correlates with platelet activation (Harmon & Jamieson, 1986).

The development of low-molecular-weight inhibitors of thrombin therefore opens the way to inhibition of arterial or venous thrombosis both by an indirect mechanism via impairment of the coagulation cascade and by a direct inhibition of platelet function.

Arginine derivatives

Workers at Mitsubishi have described a series of compounds, derived from arginine, which have both thrombin-inhibitory activity and are active *in vivo* (Hara *et al.* 1980; Kikumoto *et al.* 1980; Tonomura *et al.* 1980). All these compounds exhibit a potent and specific inhibition of thrombin-induced platelet aggregation being ineffective against other agonists. They also increase bleeding time in mice and suppress the development of disseminated intravascular coagulation (DIC) in rabbits. The most promising derivative (MC 19038) has an IC_{50} value in a thrombin clotting assay of 32 nM and a K_1 in a chromogenic substrate assay of 19 nM (Okamoto *et al.* 1981; Kikumoto *et al.* 1984). The compound inhibits thrombin-induced platelet aggregation at an IC_{50} of 9 nM and inhibits experimental models of arterial and venous thrombosis (Kumada & Abiko, 1981; Ikoma *et al.* 1982; Hara *et al.* 1987). This compound has been evaluated in some clinical situations and the results are suggestive that it could replace heparin during haemodialysis (Kumori *et al.* 1984; Higuchi *et al.* 1985; Matsuo *et al.* 1986). However, a full evaluation of the potential of this compound must await further reports.

Guanidine derivatives

The guanidine derivatives reported, FUT-175 (Aoyama *et al.* 1984) and Foy (Ohno *et al.* 1980, 1981), have not been demonstrated to have any specificity to thrombin being general serine protease inhibitors. They are, therefore, unlikely to have a future either as antithrombotic or platelet inhibitory compounds.

Benzamidine derivatives

A number of these derivatives have been examined for antithrombotic activity in animal models (Hauptman *et al.* 1983; Markwardt *et al.* 1983; Markwardt & Hauptmann, 1986; Cadroy *et al.* 1987). All are capable of inhibiting venous thrombosis or extracorporeal shunt thrombosis when given as infusions. In general their activities resemble that of heparin and no reports of clinical studies are available. Their usefulness would appear limited due to their short duration of action.

Peptidyl−arginine derivatives

GYKI 14451 (a tripeptide aldehyde) has been synthesized based on knowledge of the amino acid sequence of the active site of thrombin. This compound will inhibit coagulation in concentrations as low as 1 μM as well as inhibiting thrombin-induced platelet aggregation (Tremoli *et al.* 1984) and the thromboxane and malondialdehycle (MDA) production associated with this aggregation (Tremoli *et al.* 1981). Once again the duration of action of this compound is short but it has been demonstrated to inhibit models of venous stasis and to have oral activity when studied using thrombin time tests but not with standard coagulation tests. This compound has not yet been progressed to clinical situations as far as the author is aware.

D-Phenylalanyl-L-prolyl-L arginyl chloromethylketone (FPRCH$_2$Cl)

This compound binds irreversibly to thrombin (Kettner *et al.* 1979) and this complex can bind to and inactivate the high-affinity thrombin receptor on platelets (Harmon & Jamieson, 1986). It will inhibit fibrin formation (Hauptmann & Markwardt, 1980; Collen *et al.* 1982; Schaeffer *et al.* 1986) and totally inhibited thrombus growth in Dacron grafts in baboons (Hanson & Harker, 1988), this effect being accompanied by inhibition of platelet deposition, decreased release of platelet factor 4 (PF4), β-thromboglobulin (β-TG) and decreased fibrinopeptide A (FPA) levels, together with a prolongation of bleeding-time. Heparin under the same experimental conditions was ineffective.

Hirudin

Hirudin is a 65-amino-acid peptide found in the salivary gland of the leech (*Hirudo medicinalis*). The complete amino acid sequence is known and now several pharmaceutical companies with involvement in genetic engineering have produced a recombinant hirudin. This has permitted more detailed studies of the properties of this moiety to be conducted. Interest in this molecule is intense as it forms a tight ($K_1 = 8 \times 10^{-11}$ M) 1:1 complex with thrombin thereby inhibiting the cleavage of fibrinogen (Markwardt, 1970). Recombinant hirudin shows the same pharmacological characteristics to native hirudin (Markwardt *et al.* 1988) and the pharmacokinetics and pharmacodynamics of native hirudin in man have been evaluated (Bichler *et al.* 1988).

r-Hirudin inhibits experimental models of thrombin-induced DIC, coronary thrombosis induced by silver nitrate, venous stasis thrombosis, electrically induced arterial thrombosis and arteriovenous shunt thrombosis in the rat (Markwardt *et al.* 1988) and thrombosis following balloon angioplasty (Heras *et al.* 1990). The doses required are similar to those of native hirudin (Markwardt *et al.* 1982, 1983) and were lowest in models of venous thrombosis. It has been suggested that the higher concentrations of hirudin required to inhibit arterial thrombosis may reflect the higher affinity of thrombin for platelets compared with fibrinogen (Markwardt *et al.* 1988). In general, the effects of hirudin are similar to those of heparin but hirudin has additionally been shown to be effective in a model of platelet-dependent high shear rate arterial thrombosis in the baboon in which heparin is ineffective (Kelly *et al.* 1990). Further whilst hirudin caused an increase in bleeding time there was evidence of some preservation of haemostatic safety in comparison with other thrombin inhibitors and heparin. Hirudin also appears to allow a more controllable extension of activated partial thromboplastin time (APTT) then heparin and exerts a greater antithrombotic effects for comparable levels of anticoagulation than heparin (Talbot, 1990; Talbot *et al.* 1990).

At present hirudin provides an extremely useful tool to study the role of thrombin in both experimental and clinical situations. This should allow the elucidation of the major importance of thrombin in thrombosis, but evaluation of the full clinical potential of hirudin is probably still several years away.

Concluding remarks

To date little clinical benefit has been proven for any of the various inhibitors of platelet function. Those which interfere with the amplification loops show limited promise but do not deal with the central problem of the initial stimulus which results in platelet activation and the consequent clinical events. This area may show some resolution in the future with the concentration, emphasis and focus of many pharmaceutical companies into the development of specific thrombin inhibitors. This should show enormous clinical benefit provided that the concept of thrombin as the key stimulus in the generation of vascular pathological events is valid.

References

Adelman, B., Stemerman, M.B., Mennell, D. *et al.* (1981) The interaction of platelets with aortic subendothelium: inhibition of adhesion and secretion by prostaglandin I_2. *Blood* **48**, 198–205.

Ahn, Y.S., Jy, W., Harrington, W.J. *et al.* (1987) Increased platelet calcium in thrombosis and related disorders and its correction by nifedipine. *Thromb Res* **45**, 135–143.

Akashi, A., Tamura, K., Hirohashi, M. *et al.* (1980a) Pharmacological studies on ticlopidine, a new platelet aggregation inhibitor. Part 1: Cardiovascular effects. *Arzneim Forsch* **30**, 409–414.

Akashi, A., Hashizume, T., Tanaka, M. *et al.* (1980b) Pharmacological studies on ticlopidine, a new platelet aggregation inhibitor. Part II: General pharmacological properties. *Arzneim Forsch* **30**, 415–419.

Ambler, J.A., Butler, K.D., Ku, E.C. *et al.* (1985) CGS 12970: a novel, long acting thromboxane synthetase inhibitor. *Br J Pharmacol* **86**, 497–504.

Amer, M.S. & Mayol, R.F. (1973) Studies with phosphodiesterase. III Two forms of the enzyme from blood platelets. *Biochim Biophys Acta* **309**, 149–156.

Andes, W.A., Noveck, R.J. & Fleming, J.S. (1984) Inhibition of platelet production induced by an antiplatelet drug, anagrelide, in normal volunteers. *Thromb Haemost* **52**, 325–328.

Aoyama, T., Ino, Y., Ozeki, M. *et al.* (1984) Pharmacological studies of FUT-175, Nafamstat Mesilate. I. Inhibition of protease activity in *in vitro* and *in vivo* experiments. *Jap J Pharmacol* **35**, 203–227.

Ball, G., Brereton, G.G., Fulwood, M. *et al.* (1970) Effect of prostaglandin E, alone and in combination with theophylline or aspirin on collagen-induced platelet nucleotides including adenosine 3′5′-cyclic monophosphate. *Biochem J* **120**, 709–718.

Ball, H.A., Parratt, J.R. & Zeitlin, I.J. (1983) Effect of dazoxiben, a specific inhibitor of thromboxane synthetase, on acute pulmonary responses to *E.Coli* endotoxin in anaesthetised cats. *Br J Clin Pharmacol* **15**, 1275–1315.

Barnathan, E.S., Schwartz, J.S., Taylor, L. *et al.* (1987) Aspirin and dipyndamole in the prevention of acute coronary thrombosis complicating coronary angioplasty. *Circulation* **76**, 125–134.

Barrett, P.A. & Butler, K.D. (1983) Shortening of platelet survival by induced hypercholesterolaemia in rabbits and its prolongation by anagrelide. *Thromb Haemost* **50**, 656–659.

Belch, J.J.F., McKay, A., McArdle, B. *et al.* (1983) Epoprostenol (prostacyclin) and severe arterial disease. A double blind trial. *Lancet* **i**, 315–317.

Bertele, V., Corletti, C., Schieppati, A. *et al.* (1981) Inhibition of thromboxane synthetase does not necessarily prevent platelet aggregation. *Lancet* **i**, 1057–1058.

Bertele, V., Falanga, A., Tomasiak, M. *et al.* (1984a) Pharmacologic inhibition of thromboxane synthetase and platelet aggregation: Modulatory role of cyclooxygenase products. *Blood* **63**, 1460–1466.

Bertele, V., Falanga, A., Tomasiak, M. *et al.* (1984b) SQ 22536, an adenylate-cyclase inhibitor, prevents the antiplatelet effect of dazoxiben, a thromboxane-synthetase inhibitor. *Thromb Haemost* **51**, 125–128.

Best, L.C., McGuire, M.B., Jones, P.B.B. *et al.* (1979) Mode of action of dipyridamole on human platelets. *Thromb Res* **16**, 367–379.

Bichler, J., Fichtl, B., Siebeck, M. *et al.* (1988) Pharmacokinetics and pharmacodynamics of hirudin in man after single subcutaneous and intravenous bolus administration. *Arzneim-Forsch* **38**, 704–710.

Bjornsson, T.D., Hanson, S.R. & Harker, L.A. (1987) Effective antiplatelet drug concentrations in experimental arterial thromboembolism. *Thromb Res* **48**, 337–348.

Born, G.V.R. & Cross, M.J. (1963) The aggregation of blood platelets. *J Physiol* **168**, 178–195.

Bourgain, R.H. (1979) The inhibitory effect of PGI_2 (prostacyclin) on white platelet arterial thrombus formation. *Haemostasis* **8**, 117–119.

Buchanan, M.R., Dejana, E., Gent, M. *et al.* (1981) Enhanced platelet accumulation onto injured carotid arteries in rabbits after aspirin treatment. *J Clin Invest* **67**, 503–508.

Bunting, S., Moncada, S. & Vane, J.R. (1983) The prostacyclin–thromboxane A_2 balance: Pathophysiological and therapeutic implications. *Br Med Bull* **39**, 271–276.

Bush, L.R., Campbell, W.B., Tilton, C.D. *et al.* (1983) Effects of the selective thromboxane synthetase inhibitor, dazoxiben, on cyclic flow variations in stenosed canine coronary arteries. *Trans Assoc Am Physicians* **96**, 103–112.

Butler, K.D., Shand, R.A. & Wallis, R.B. (1986) The effects of modulation of prostanoid metabolism on the thoracic platelet accumulation induced by intravenous administration of collagen in the guinea-pig. *Thromb Haemostas* **56**, 263–267.

Butler, K.D., Butler, P.A., Shand, R.A. *et al.* (1987) Prolongation of platelet survival in hypercholesterolaemic rabbits by CGS-12970 (3-methyl-2-(3-pyridyl)-1-indoleoctanoic acid) and dazoxiben. *Thromb Res* **45**, 751–761.

Cadroy, Y., Caranobe, C., Bernat, A. *et al.* (1987) Antithrombotic and bleeding effects of a new synthetic direct thrombin inhibitor and of standard heparin in the rabbit. *Thromb Haemost* **58**, 764–767.

Cairns, J., Gent, M., Singer, J. *et al.* (1985) Aspirin, Sulphinpyrazone or both in unstable angina: Results of a Canadian Multicenter Trial. *New Engl J Med* **313**, 1369–1375.

Carrien, P., Orefice, G., Fioretti, A. *et al.* (1984) Effects of long term ticlopidine treatment on platelet function and its tolerability in cerebrovascular disease. *J Int Med Res* **12**, 286–291.

Caterina, R., Giannessi, D., Bernini, W. *et al.* (1988) Organic nitrates: direct antiplatelet effects and synergism with prostacyclin. *Thromb Haemostas* **59**, 207–211.

Cattaneo, M., Winocour, P.D., Somers, D.A. *et al.* (1985) Effect of ticlopidine on platelet aggregation, adherence to damaged vessels, thrombus formation and platelet survival. *Thromb Res* **37**, 29–43.

Cazenave, J.P., Packham, M.A., Kinlough-Rathbone, R.L., *et al.* (1978) Platelet adherence to the vessel wall and to collagen-coated surfaces. *Adv Exp Med Biol* **102**, 31–47.

Chesebro, J.H., Clement, I.P., Furster, V. *et al.* (1982) A platelet inhibitory trial in coronary by-pass operations: benefit of dipyridamole and aspirin in early graft patency. *New Engl J Med* **307**, 73–78.

Chierchia, S., Crea, F., Bernini, W. *et al.* (1981) Antiplatelet effects of verapamil in man. *Am J Cardiol* **47**, 399 (abstr).

Coffman, J.D. & Rasmussen, H.M. (1984) Effect of thromboxane synthetase inhibition in Raynaud's phenomenon. *Clin Pharmacol Ther* **36**, 369–373.

Coker, S.J. & Parratt, J.R. (1983) Effects of dazoxiben

on arrhythmias and ventricular fibrillation induced by coronary artery occlusion and reperfusion in anaesthetised greyhounds. *Br J Clin Pharmacol* **15**, 87S–95S.

Collen, D., Matsuo, O., Stassen, J.M. *et al.* (1982) *In vivo* studies of a synthetic inhibitor of thrombin. *J Lab Clin Med* **99**, 76–83.

Coppe, D., Wonders, T., Snider, M. *et al.* (1979) Preservation of platelet number and function during extracorporal membrane oxygenation by regional infusion of prostacyclin. In Vane, J.R. & Bergstrom, S. (eds) *Prostacyclin*, Ch 24, Raven Press, New York.

Cunningham, D.A., Kumar, B., Siegel, B.A. *et al.* (1984) Aspirin inhibition of platelet deposition at angioplasty sites: demonstration by platelet scintigraphy. *Radiology* **151**, 487–490.

Dale, J., Landmark, K.W. & Myhre, E. (1983a) The effects of nifedipine, a calcium antagonist, on platelet function. *Am Heart J* **105**, 103–105.

Dale, J., Thaulow, E., Myhre, E. *et al.* (1983b) The effect of a thromboxane synthetase inhibitor, dazoxiben, and acetylsaliylic acid on platelet function and prostaglandin metabolism. *Thromb Haemost* **50**, 703–706.

de Gaetano, G. & Bertele, V. (1984) Antiplatelet drugs and thrombosis prevention: ticlopidine in perspective. *Agents and Actions* **14**, 109–112.

de Gaetano, G. & Cerletti, C. (1988) Prolongation of bleeding-time by aspirin: a dual mechanism. *Thromb Res* **50**, 907–912.

Destors, J.M., Gauthier, E., Lelong, S. *et al.* (1986) Failure of a pure anti-platelet drug to decrease the number of attacks more than placebo in patients with Raynauds phenomenon. *Angiology* **37**, 565–569.

Di Minno, G., De Gaetano, D. & Garattini, S. (1978) Letter to Editor. *Lancet* **ii**, 1258.

Di Minno, G., Cerbone, A.M., Mattioli, P.L. *et al.* (1985) Functionally thrombastenic state in normal platelets following the administration of ticlopidine. *J Clin Invest* **75**, 328–338.

Ellrodt, A.G. & Singh, B.N. (1983) Clinical applications of slow channel blocking compounds. *Pharmacol Ther* **23**, 1–43.

Emmons, P.R., Harrison, M.J.G., Honour, A.J. *et al.* (1965a) Effect of dipyridamole on human platelet behaviour. *Lancet* **ii**, 603–606.

Emmons, P.R., Harrison, M.J.G., Honour, A.J. *et al.* (1965b) Effect of a pyrimidopyrimidine derivative on thrombus formation in the rabbit. *Lancet* **ii**, 255–257.

Erne, P., Resink, T.J., Burgisser, E. *et al.* (1985) Platelets and hypertension. *J. Cardiovasc Pharmacol* **7** (Suppl 6), S103–S108.

Faxon, D.P., Sanborn, T.A., Haudenschild, C.C. *et al.* (1984) Effect of antiplatelet therapy on restenosis after experimental angioplasty. *Am J Cardiol* **53**, 72C–76C.

Fernandez, F.A., N'guyen, P. & Van Ryn, J. *et al.* (1986) Hemorrhagic doses of heparin and other glycosaminoglycans induce a platelet effect. *Thromb Res* **43**, 491–495.

Fieschi, C., Battistini, N., Volante, F. *et al.* (1975) Animal model of TIA: An experimental study with intracarotid ADP infusion in rabbits. *Stroke* **6**, 617–621.

FitzGerald, G.A. & Oates, J.A. (1984) Selective and nonselective inhibition of thromboxane formation. *Clin Pharmacol Ther* **35**, 633–640.

FitzGerald, G.A., Brash, A.R., Oates, J.A. *et al.* (1983) Endogenous prostacyclin biosynthesis and platelet function during selective inhibition of thromboxane synthase in man. *J Clin Invest* **72**, 1336–1343.

FitzGerald, G.A., Reilly, I.A.G. & Pedersen, A.K. (1985) The biochemical pharmacology of thromboxane synthetase inhibition in man. *Circulation* **72**, 1194–1201.

Fleming, J.S. & Buyniski, J.P. (1979) A potent new inhibitor of platelet aggregation and experimental thrombosis, Anagrelide (BL 4162A). *Thromb Res* **15**, 373–388.

Fleming, J.S. & Buyniski, J.P. (1983) Anagrelide. In Scriabine, A. (ed.) *New Drugs Annual: Cardiovascular Drugs*, pp. 277–294. Raven press, New York.

Folts, J.D., Crowell, E.B. & Rowe, G.G. (1976) Platelet aggregation in partially obstructed vessels and its elimination with aspirin. *Circulation* **54**, 365–370.

Folts, J.D., Detmer, D.E. & Nadler, R. (1982) Possible platelet thrombi formation in dog and human femoral arteries. *Tex Heart Inst J* **9**, 19–26.

Frishman, W.H. & Miller, K.P. (1986) Platelets and antiplatelet therapy in ischemic heart disease. *Curr Probl Cardiol* **11**, 69–139.

Fukumori, T., Tani, E., Maeda, Y. *et al.* (1984) Effect of selective inhibitor of thromboxane A_2 synthetase on experimental cerebral vasospasm. *Stroke* **15**, 306–311.

Fujimoto, T., Suzuki, H., Aliga, S. *et al.* (1984) The role of platelets on the vascular injuries caused by arachidonic acid or ADP. *Ketsueki to Myakkan* **14**, 425–430.

Fujimoto, T., Suzuki, H., Tanoue, K. *et al.* (1985) Cerebrovascular injuries induced by activation of platelets *in vivo*. *Stroke* **16**, 245–250.

Garcia-Szabo, R.R., Peterson, M.B., Watkins, W.D. *et al.* (1983) Thromboxane generation after thrombin. Protective effect of thromboxane synthetase inhibition on lung fluid balance. *Circ Res* **53**, 214–222.

Garcia-Szabo, R., Kern, D.F. & Malik, A.B. (1984) Pulmonary vascular response to thrombin: Effects of thromboxane synthetase inhibition with OKY-046 and OKY-1581. *Prostaglandin* **28**, 851–866.

Gerrard, J.M., Peterson, D.A. & White, J.G. (1981) Calcium mobilisation in platelets. In Gordon, J.L. (ed.) *Platelets in Biology and Pathology*, pp. 407–436. Elsevier/North Holland Biomedical Press, Amsterdam.

Gershlick, A.H., Court, Y.D.S., Murday, A.J. *et al.* (1985) Adverse effects of high dose aspirin on platelet adhesion to experimental autogenous vein grafts. *Cardiovasc Res* **19**, 770–776.

Gillespie, E. (1988) Anagrelide: a potent and selective

inhibitor of platelet cyclic AMP phosphodiesterase enzyme activity. *Biochem Pharmacol* **37**, 2866–2868.

Goldman, M., Hall, C., Hawker, R.J. *et al.* (1983a) Dazoxiben examined for platelet inhibitory effect in an artificial circulation. *Br J Clin Pharmacol* **15**, 61S–65S.

Goldman, M.D., Simpsin, D., Hawker, R.J. *et al.* (1983b) Aspirin and dipyridamole reduce platelet deposition on prosthetic femoro-popliteal grafts in man. *Ann Surg* **198**, 713–716.

Goldman, S., Copeland, J., Moritz, T. *et al.* (1988) Improvement in early saphenous vein graft patency after coronary artery bypass surgery with antiplatelet therapy: results of a Veterans administration Cooperative study. *Circulation* **77**, 1324–1332.

Gordon, J.L. (1984) Ticlopidine: Quo Vadis? *Agents and Actions* **15** (Suppl 1), 108–115.

Gorman, R.R., Bunting, S. & Miller, O.V. (1977) Modulation of human platelet adenylate cyclase by prostacyclin (PGX). *Prostaglandins* **13**, 377–388.

Greengard, J.S. & Griffin, J.H. (1984) Platelet coagulant activity. *Meth Haematol* **8**, 144–157.

Gresele, P., Zoja, C., Deckmyn, H. *et al.* (1983) Dipyridamole inhibits platelet aggregation in whole blood. *Thromb Haemost* **50**, 852–856.

Gresele, P., Van Houtte, E., Arnout, J. *et al.* (1984) Thromboxane synthase inhibition combined with thromboxane receptor blockade: A step forward in antithrombotic strategy. *Thromb Haemost* **52**, 364.

Gresele, P., Deckmyn, H., Arnout, J. *et al.* (1985) Lack of synergism between dazoxiben and dipyridamole following administration to man. *Thromb Res* **37**, 231–236.

Gresele, P., Arnout, J., Deckmyn, H. *et al.* (1986) Mechanism of the antiplatelet action of dipyridamole in whole blood: Modulation of adenosine concentration and activity. *Thromb Haemost* **55**, 12–18.

Gresele, P., Arnout, J., Deckmyn, H. *et al.* (1987) Role of proaggregatory and antiaggregatory prostaglandins in hemostasis. Studies with combined thromboxane synthase inhibition and thromboxane receptor antagonism. *J Clin Invest* **80**, 1435–1445.

Groves, H.M., Kinlough-Rathbone, R.L., Cazenave, J.-P. *et al.* (1982) Effect of dipyridamole and prostacyclin on rabbit platelet adherence *in vitro* and *in vivo*. *J Lab Clin Med* **99**, 548–558.

Gryglewski, R.J., Korbut, R. & Ocetkiewicz, A.C. (1978) De-aggregatory action of prostacyclin in vivo and its enhancement by theophylline. *Prostaglandins* **15**, 637–644.

Gryglewski, R.J., Nowak, S., Kosta-Trabka, E. *et al.* (1983) Treatment of ischemic stroke with prostacyclin. *Stroke* **14**, 197–202.

Hanson, S.R. & Harker, L.A. (1983) Effect of dazoxiben on arterial graft thrombosis in the baboon. *Br J Clin Pharmacol* **15**, 57S–60S.

Hanson, S.R. & Harker, L.A. (1988) Interruption of acute platelet-dependent thrombosis by the synthetic antithrombin D-phenylalanyl-L-prolyl-L-arginyl chloromethyl ketone. *Proc Natl Acad Sci USA* **85**, 3184–3188.

Hanson, S.R., Harker, L.A. & Bjornsson, T.D. (1985) Effects of platelet-modifying drugs on arterial thromboembolism in Baboons: Aspirin potentiates the antithrombotic actions of dipyridamole and sulphinpyrazone by mechanism(s) independent of platelet cyclooxygenase inhibition. *J Clin Invest* **75**, 1591–1599.

Hara, H., Tamao, Y., Kikumoto, R. *et al.* (1980) Effect of a potent thrombin inhibitor No 407 on platelet function *in vitro* and *in vivo*. *Kobe J Med Sci* **26**, 47–60.

Hara, H., Tamao, Y., Kikumoto, R. *et al.* (1987) Effect of a synthetic thrombin inhibitor MCI-9038 on experimental models of disseminated intravascular coagulation in rabbits. *Thromb Haemost* **57**, 165–170.

Harker, L.A. (1986) Clinical trials evaluating platelet-modifying drugs in patients with atheroscherotic cardiovascular disease and thrombosis. *Circulation* **73**, 206–223.

Harker, L.A. & Fuster, V. (1986) Pharmacology of platelet inhibitors. *J Am Coll Cardiol* **8**, 21B–32B.

Harker, L.A. & Slichter, S.J. (1972) Platelet and fibrinogen consumption in man. *New Engl J Med* **287**, 999–1005.

Harker, L.A., Ross, R., Slichter, S.J. *et al.* (1976) Homocystine-induced arteriosclerosis. The role of endothelial cell injury and platelet response in its genesis. *J Clin Invest* **58**, 731–741.

Harker, L.A., Hanson, S.R. & Kirkman, R.R. (1979) Experimental arterial thromboembolism in baboons. Mechanism, quantification and pharmacologic prevention. *J Clin Invest* **64**, 559–560.

Harmon, J.T. & Jamieson, G.A. (1986) Activation of platelets by α-thrombin is a receptor-mediated event. *J Biol Chem* **261**, 15928–15923.

Haslam, R.J. & Cusack, N.J. (1981) Blood platelet receptors for adenylate cyclase. In Burnstock, G. (ed) *Purinergic Receptors*, pp. 221–286. Chapman and Hall, London.

Hauptmann, J. & Markwardt, F. (1980) Studies on the anticoagulant and antithrombotic action of an irreversible thrombin inhibitor. *Thromb Res* **20**, 347–351.

Hauptmann, J., Barth, A., Schönberger, F.-F. *et al.* (1983) Comparative study on the antithrombotic effects of a synthetic thrombin inhibitor and of heparin in animal models. *Biomed Bio-chim Acta* **42**, 959–965.

Hawker, R.J. & Aukland, A. (1984) Platelet survival, atheroscherotic intermittant claudication and ticlopidine. *Atherosclerosis* **50**, 147–158.

Hemker, H.C. & Lindhout, Th. (1984) A clotting scheme for 1984. *Nouv Rev Hematol* **26**, 227–31.

Heras, M., Chesebro, J.H., Penny, W.J. *et al.* (1990) Thrombin inhibition: A key step to prevent acute platelet-thrombus deposition during angioplasty on pigs. *Circulation* (in press).

Heptinstall, S., Bevan, J., Cockbill, S.R. *et al.* (1980) Effects of a selective inhibitor of thromboxane synthetase on human blood platelet behaviour. *Thromb Res* **20**, 219–230.

Heptinstall, S., Bientz, N., Cockbill, S.R. *et al.* (1982) Different effects of thromboxane synthetase inhibitors on platelets from different individuals. *Lancet* **ii**, 1156.

Higgs, G.A., Moncada, S. & Vane, J.R. (1977) Prostacyclin (PGI_2) inhibits the formation of platelet thrombi induced by adenosine diphosphate (ADP) *in vivo*. *Br J Pharmacol* **61**, 137P.

Higuchi, M., Kunitomi, O., Nishida, Y. *et al.* (1985) Effect of MD 805, a synthetic thrombin inhibitor, on disseminated intravascular coagulation developed on hematological disorders. *Jap J Clin Haemotol* **26**, 1754–1762.

Ikoma, H., Ohtsu, K., Tamao, Y. *et al.* (1982) Effect of a potent thrombin inhibitor, MCI-9038, on novel experimental arterial thrombosis. *Blood and Vessel* **13**, 72–77.

Ingerman-Wojenski, C.M. & Silver, M.J. (1988) Model system to study interaction of platelets with damaged arterial wall. II. Inhibition of smooth muscle cell proliferation by dipyridamole and AH-P719. *Exp Mol Pathol* **48**, 116–134.

Jaffe, E. & Weksler, B.B. (1979) Recovery of endothelial cell prostacyclin production after inhibition by low doses of aspirin. *J Clin Invest* **63**, 532–535.

Jaques, L.B. (1980) Heparins-anionic polyelectrolyte drugs. *Pharmacol Rev* **31**, 99–166.

Jaques, L.B. (1982) Heparin: a unique misunderstood drug. *Trends Pharmacol Sci* **4**, 289–291.

Jaques, L.B. & Mahadoo, J. (1978) Pharmacodynamics and clinical effectiveness of heparin. *Sem Thromb Haemost* **4**, 298–325.

Johnson, P.C., Ware, A.J., Cliveden, P.B. *et al.* (1985) Measurement of ionized calcium in blood platelets with the photoprotein aequorin. *J Biol Chem* **260**, 2069–2076.

Kaltenbach, M., Kober, G., Scherer, D. *et al.* (1985) Recurrence rate after successful coronary angioplasty, *Eur Heart J* **6**, 276–281.

Kelly, A.B., Marzec, U.M., Hanson, S.R. *et al.* (1990) Hirudin inhibition of platelet dependent thrombus formation *in vivo*. *J Clin Invest* (in press).

Kelton, J.G., Hirsh, J., Carter, C.J. *et al.* (1978) Thrombogenic effect of high-dose aspirin in rabbits. *J Clin Invest* **62**, 892–895.

Kettner, C., Shaw, E. *et al.* (1979) D-Phe–pro–arg CH_2 C1 – A selective affinity label for thrombin. *Thromb Res* **14**, 969–973.

Khurmi, N.S., Bowles, M.J. & Raftery, E.B. (1986) Are anti-platelet drugs of value in the management of patients with chronic stable angina? A study with ticlopidine. *Clin Cardiol* **9**, 493–498.

Kikumoto, R., Tamao, Y., Ohkubo, K. *et al.* (1980) Thrombin inhibitors 3. Carboxyl-containing amide derivatives of N^{α}-substituted L-Arginine. *J Med Chem* **23**, 1293–1299.

Kikumoto, R., Tamao, Y., Tazuka, T. *et al.* (1984) Selective inhibition of thrombin by (2R,4R)-4-methyl-1-N^{α}-[3methyl-1,2,3,4-tetrahydro-8-quinoline-sulphonyl] – L]arginyl)-2 piperidinecarboxylic acid. *Biochemistry* **33**, 85–90.

Kinlough-Rathbone, R.L., Packham, M.A., Reimers, H.J. *et al.* (1977) Mechanisms of platelet shape change, aggregation and release induced by collagen, thrombin or A 23187. *J Lab Clin Med* **90**, 707–719.

Kinlough-Rathbone, R.L., Groves, H.M., Cazenave, J.P. *et al.* (1978) Effect of dipyridamole and aspirin on platelet adherence to damaged rabbit aortas *in vitro* and *in vivo*. *Fed Proc* **37**, 260.

Kinlough-Rathbone, R.L., Packham, M.A. & Mustard, J.F. (1983) Vessel injury, platelet adherence and platelet survival *Arteriosclerosis* **3**, 529–546.

Kirstein, P., Jogestrand, T., Johnsson, H. *et al.* (1980) Antiaggregatory, physiological and clinical effects of ticlopidine in subjects with peripheral atherosclerosis. *Atherosclerosis* **36**, 471–480.

Ku, E.C., McPherson, S.E., Signor, C. *et al.* (1983) Characterisation of imidazo [1,5-a] pyridine-5-hexanoic acid (CGS-13080) as a selective thromboxane synthetase inhibitor using *in vitro* and *in vivo* biochemical models. *Biochem Biophys Res Commun* **112**, 899–906.

Kumada, T., & Abiko, Y. (1981) Comparative study on heparin and a synthetic thrombin inhibitor No. 805 (MD 805) in experimental antithrombin III-deficient animals. *Thromb Res* **24**, 285–298.

Kumori, K., Tanaka, K., Nakajima, N. *et al.* (1984) Anticoagulation with a synthetic thrombin inhibitor after cardiovascular surgery and for treatment of disseminated intravascular coagulation. *Critical Care Med* **12**, 1039–1043.

Lam, J.Y.T., Chesebro, J.H., Steele, P.M. *et al.* (1987) Is vasospasm related to platelet deposition? Relationship in a porcine preparation of arterial injury *in vivo*. *Circulation* **75**, 243–248.

Le Balc'h, T., Laudais, A., Butel, J. *et al.* (1987) Enoxaparine (Lovenox), versus standard heparin in prophylaxis of deep vein thrombosis after total hip replacement. *Thromb Haemost* **1**, (Suppl), 892a.

Lee, T.-K., Chen, Y.-C., Lien, I.-N. *et al.* (1988) Inhibitory effect of acetylsalicylic acid on platelet function in patients with completed stroke or reversible ischemic neurologic deficit. *Stroke* **19**, 566–570.

Lefer, A.M. (1984) Basic properties and indications for CGS 13080, a new selective thromboxane synthetase inhibitor. *Drugs of the Future* **9**, 437–442.

Lefer, A.M., Burke, S.E. & Smith, J.B. (1983) Role of thromboxane and prostaglandin endoperoxides in the pathogenesis of eicosanoid induced sudden death. *Throm Res* **32**, 311–320.

Levine, M.N. & Hirsh, J. (1988) Clinical use of Low Molecular weight heparins and heparinoids. *Sem Thromb Haemost* **14**, 116–125.

Lewis, H.D., Davis, J.W., Archibald, D.G. *et al.* (1983) Protective effects of aspirin against acute myocardial infarction and death in men with unstable angina. *New Engl J Med* **309**, 396–404.

Lindsay, L.A., Olson, R.W., Sakane, Y. *et al.* (1986)

Dazoxiben, UK 38 485 and aspirin: Duration of effect for preventing thrombotic sudden death in rabbits. *Thromb Res* **43**, 177–186.

Luderer, J.R., Nicholas, G.G., Neumyer, M.N. *et al.* (1984) Dazoxiben, a thromboxane synthetase inhibitor, in Raynaud's phenomenon. *Clin Pharmacol Ther* **36**, 105–115.

MacDonald, P.S., Read, M.A. & Dusting, G.J. (1988) Synergistic inhibition of platelet aggregation by endothelium-derived relaxing factor and prostacyclin. *Thromb Res* **49**, 437–449.

Machin, S.J., Chamone, D.A.F., Defreyn, G. *et al.* (1981) The effect of clinical prostacyclin infusions in advanced arterial disease on platelet function and plasma 6-keto-PGF_1 levels. *Brit J Haematol* **47**, 413–422.

MacNab, M.W., Foltz, E.L., Graves, B.S. *et al.* (1984) The effects of a new thromboxane synthetase inhibitor, CGS 13080, in man. *J Clin Pharmacol* **24**, 76–83.

Maguire, E.D. & Wallis, R.B. (1983) *In vivo* redirection of prostaglandin endoperoxides into 6-keto $PGF_{1\alpha}$ formation by thromboxane synthetase inhibitors in the rat. *Thromb Res* **32**, 15–27.

Marcus, A.J. & Zucker, M.B. (1965) *The Physiology of Blood Platelets: Recent Biochemical, Morphological and Clinical Research*. Grune and Stratton, New York.

Markwardt, F. (1970) Hirudin as an inhibitor of thrombin. *Meth Enzymol* **19**, 924–932.

Markwardt, F. & Hauptmann, J. (1986) Synthetische thrombininhibitoren als antithrombotika. *Z Klin Med* **41**, 540–543.

Markwardt, F., Hauptmann, J., Nowak, G. *et al.* (1982) Pharmacological studies on the antithrombotic action of hirudin in experimental animals. *Thromb Haemost* **47**, 226–229.

Markwardt, F., Nowak, G. & Hoffmann, J. (1983) Comparative studies on thrombin inhibitors in experimental microthrombosis. *Thromb Haemost* **49**, 235–237.

Markwardt, F., Fink, G., Kaiser, B. *et al.* (1988) Pharmacological survey of recombinant hirudin. *Pharmazie* **43**, 202–207.

Matsuo, T., Nakao, K., Yamada, T. *et al.* (1986) A new thrombin inhibitor MD 805 and thrombocytopenia encountered with heparin hemodialysis. *Thromb Res* **44**, 247–251.

May, G.R., Herd, C., Butler, K.D. & Page, C.P. (1990) A radioisotopic model of platelet aggregation in the rabbit *in vivo*. *J Pharmacol Methods* **24**, 19–35.

Mehta, J., Mehta, P., Lawson, D.L. *et al.* (1985) Influence of selective thromboxane synthetase blocker CGS-13080 on thromboxane and prostacyclin biosynthesis in whole blood: Evidence for synthesis of prostacyclin by leukocytes from platelet-derived endoperoxides. *Lab Clin Med* **106**, 246–252.

Mickelson, J.K., Simpson, P.J., Gallas, M.T. *et al.* (1987) Thromboxane synthetase inhibition with CGS-13080 improves coronary blood flow after streptokinase-induced thrombolysis. *Am Heart J* **113**, 1345–1352.

Mills, D.C.B. & Smith, J.B. (1971) The influence on platelet aggregation of drugs that affect the accumulation of 3′5′-cylic monophosphate in platelets. *Biochem J* **121**, 185–196.

Mitchell, J.R.A. (1983) Clinical aspects of the arachidonic acid–thromboxane pathway. *Br Med Bull* **39**, 289–295.

Moncada, S. & Korbut, R. (1978) Dipyridamole and other phosphodiesterase inhibitors act as antithrombotic agents by potentiating endogenous prostacyclin. *Lancet* **i**, 1286.

Moncada, S. & Vane, J.R. (1977) The discovery of prostacyclin (PGX) — a fresh insight into arachidonic acid metabolism. In Karsh, K. & Fried, F. (eds) *Biochemical Aspects of Prostaglandin and Thromboxanes*, pp. 155–177. Academic press. London, New York.

Moncada, S., Gryglewski, R.J., Bunting, S. *et al.* (1976) A lipid peroxide inhibits the enzyme in blood vessels microsomes that generates from prostaglandin endoperoxide the substance (prostaglandin x) which prevents platelet aggregation. *Prostaglandins* **12**, 715–733.

Murer, E.H. (1985) The role of platelet calcium. *Sem Hematol* **22**, 313–323.

Mustard, J.F. & Packham, M.A. (1970) Factors influencing platelet function: adhesion, release and aggregation. *Pharmacol Rev* **22**, 97–187.

Nagai, H., Yakuo, I., Inagaki, N. *et al.* (1987) Role of thromboxane (TX) A_2 in guinea-pig Forssman shock and the effect of OKY-046, TXA_2 synthetase inhibitor. *Prostaglandins Leukotrienes Med* **26**, 133–141.

Naito, J., Komatsu, H., Ujie, A. *et al.* (1983) Effects of thromboxane synthetase inhibitors on aggregation of rabbit platelets. *Eur J Pharmacol* **91**, 41–48.

O'Connor, K.M., Friehling, T.D., Kelliher, G.J. *et al.* (1986) Effect of thromboxane synthetase inhibition on vulnerability to ventricular arrhythmia following coronary occlusion. *Am Heart J* **111**, 683–688.

Ofusu, F.A. & Gray, E. (1988) Mechanisms of action of heparin: Applications to the development of derivatives of heparin and heparinoids with antithrombotic properties. *Sem Thromb Haemost* **14**, 9–17.

O'Grady, J. & Moncada, S. (1978) Aspirin: A paradoxical effect on bleeding time. *Lancet* **ii**, 780.

Ogura, T., Watanabe, I., Saito, T. *et al.* (1988) Effects of OKY-046 a selective thromboxane A_2 synthetase inhibitor on ventricular arrhythmias and prostaglandins during coronary artery ligation and reperfusion in anesthetized dogs. *Jap J Pharmacol* **47**, 95–98.

Ohno, H., Kosaki, G., Kambayashi, J. *et al.* (1980) FOY: [Ethyl *p*-(6-guanidinohexanoyloxy) benzoate] methanesulfonate as a serine proteinase inhibitor. 1. Inhibition of thrombin and factor Xa *in vitro*. *Thromb Res* **19**, 579–588.

Ohno, H., Kambayashi, J., Chang, S.W. *et al.* (1981) FOY: [Ethyl *p*-(6-guanidinohexanoyloxy) benzoate] methanesulfonate as a serine proteinase inhibitor. II. *In vivo* effect on coagulo-fibrinolytic system in comparison with heparin or aprotinin. *Thromb Res* **24**, 445–452.

Okamoto, S., Hijikata, A., Kikumoto, R. *et al.* (1981) Potent inhibition of thrombin by the newly synthesized arginine derivative No. 805. The importance of stereostructure of its hydrophobic carboxyamide portion. *Biochem Biophys Res Commun* **101**, 440–446.

Ono, H. & Kimura, M. (1981) Effect of calcium-antagonistic vasodilators, diltiazem, nifedipine, perhexiline and verapamil on platelet aggregation *in vitro*. *Arzneimittelforschung* **31**, 1131–1134.

Onoda, J.M., Sloane, B.F. & Honn, K.V. (1984) Antithrombogenic effects of calcium channel blockers: Synergism with prostacyclin and thromboxane synthase inhibitors. *Thromb Res* **34**, 367–378.

Panak, E., Maffrand, J.P., Picard-Fraire, C. *et al.* (1983) Ticlopidine: a promise for the prevention and treatment of thrombosis and its complications. *Haemostasis* **13** (Suppl 1), 1–54.

Parry, M. (1983) Effects of thromboxane synthetase inhibition on arachidonate metabolism and platelet behaviour. *Br J Clin Pharmacol* **15**, 23S–29S.

Patrignani, P., Filabozzi, P., Catella, F. *et al.* (1984) Differential effects of dazoxiben, a selective thromboxane-synthase inhibition, on platelet and renal prostaglandin-endoperoxide metabolism. *J Pharmacol Exp Ther* **228**, 472–477.

Philip, R.B. (1979) Experimental models of arterial thrombosis and the screening of platelet-inhibiting, antithrombotic drugs: a review. *Meth Find Exp Clin Pharmacol* **1**, 197–224.

Philip, R.B. (1986) Possible drug strategies in combating atheroembolic disorders. In Warren, B.A. (ed.) *Atheroembolism*, pp. 103–155. CRC Press, Boca Raton.

Pieper, G.M., Farber, N.E. & Gross, G.J. (1988) Metabolic protection of the reperfused canine endocardium by the thromboxane synthetase inhibitor, dazoxiben. *Prostaglandins, Leukotrienes and Essential Fatty Acids* **33**, 13–22.

Plachetka, J.R., Salomon, N.W., Larson, D.F. *et al.* (1980) Platelet loss during experimental cardiopulmonary by pass and its prevention with prostacyclins. *Ann Thorac Surg* **30**, 58–63.

Preston, F.E., Whipps, S., Jackson, C.A. *et al.* (1981) Inhibition of prostacyclin and platelet thromboxane A_2 after low dose aspirin. *New Engl J Med* **304**, 76–79.

Pumphrey, C.W., Fuster, V., Dewanjee, M.K. *et al.* (1983) Comparison of the antithrombotic action of calcium antagonist drugs with dipyridamole in dogs. *Am J Cardiol* **51**, 591–595.

Radomski, H.W., Palmer, R.M.J. & Moncada, S. (1987a) The anti-aggregatory properties of vascular endothelium: Interactions between prostacyclin and nitric oxide. *Br J Pharmacol* **91**, 639–646.

Radomski, H.W., Palmer, R.M.J. & Moncada, S. (1987b) The role of nitric oxide and cGMP in platelet adhesion to vascular endothelium. *Biochem Biophys Res Commun* **148**, 1482–1489.

Randall, H.J. & Wilding, R.I.R. (1982) Acute arterial thrombosis in rabbits: reduced platelet accumulation after treatment with thromboxane synthetase inhibitor dazoxiben hydrochloride (UK 37248–01). *Thromb Res* **28**, 607–616.

Randall, H.J., Parry, M.J., Hawkeswood, E. *et al.* (1981) UK 37248, a novel, selective thromboxane synthetase inhibitor with platelet anti-aggregatory and anti-thrombotic activity. *Thromb Res* **23**, 145–162.

Rapoport, R.M. & Murad, F. (1983) Endothelium-dependent and nitrovasodilator-induced relaxation of vascular smooth muscle: role of cyclic GMP. *J Cycl Nucl Prot Phos Res* **9**, 281–296.

Reilly, I.A.G., Doran, J.B., Smith, A.B. *et al.* (1986) Increased thromboxane biosynthesis in a human preparation of platelet activation: biochemical and functional consequences of selective inhibition of thromboxane synthase. *Circulation* **73**, 1300–1309.

Rink, T.J., Smith, S.W. & Tsien, R.Y. (1982) Cytoplasmic free Ca^{2+} in human platelets: Ca^{2+} threshold and Ca^{2+} independent activation for shape-change and secretion. *FEBS Lett* **148**, 21–26.

Roth, G.J., Stanford, N. & Majerus, P.W. (1975) Acetylation of prostaglandin synthase by aspirin. *Proc Natl Acad Sci USA* **72**, 3073–3076.

Saba, H.I., Saba, S.R. & Morelli, G.A. (1984) Effect of heparin on platelet aggregation. *Am J Hematol* **17**, 295–306.

Saltiel, E. & Ward, A. (1987) Ticlopidine: A review of its pharmacodynamic and pharmacokinetic properties, and therapeutic efficacy in platelet-dependent disease states. *Drugs* **34**, 222–262.

Sanborn, T.A., Ballelli, L.M., Faxon, D.P. *et al.* (1986) Inhibition of ^{51}Cr-labelled platelet accumulation after balloon angioplasty in rabbits: Comparison of heparin, aspirin and CGS-13080, a selective thromboxane synthetase inhibitor. *J Amer Coll Cardiol* **7**, 213A.

Schaeffer, R.C., Briston, C., Chilton, S.-M. *et al.* (1986) Disseminated intravascular coagulation following Echis carinatus venom in dogs: Effects of a synthetic thrombin inhibitor. *J Lab Clin Med* **107**, 488–497.

Schrör, K. & Thiemermann, C. (1986) Treatment of acute myocardial ischaemia with a selective antagonist of thromboxane receptors (BM 13.177). *Br J Pharmacol* **87**, 631–637.

Schumacher, W.A. & Lucchesi, B.R. (1983) Effect of the thromboxane synthetase inhibitor UK 37248 (Dazoxiben) upon platelet aggregation, coronary artery thrombosis and vascular reactivity. *J Pharmacol Exp Ther* **227**, 790–796.

Schwartz, L., Bourassa, M.G., Lesperance, J. *et al.* (1988) Aspirin and dipyridamole in the prevention of restenosis after percutaneous transluminal coronary angioplasty. *New Eng J Med* **318**, 1714–1719.

Shanbaky, N.M., Ahn, Y., Jy, W. *et al.* (1987) Abnormal aggregation accompanies abnormal platelet Ca^{2+} handling in arterial thrombosis. *Thromb Haemost* **57**, 1–10.

Sharma, G.U.R.K., Khuri, S.E., Josa, M. *et al.* (1983) The effect of antiplatelet therapy on saphenous vein coronary artery bypass graft patency. *Circulation* **68** (Suppl II), 218–221.

Shuman, M.A. & Levine, S.P. (1978) Thrombin generation and secretion of platelet factor 4 during blood clotting. *J Clin Invest* **61**, 1101–1106.

Sills, T., Cowley, A.J. & Heptinstall, S. (1986) Aspirin and dazoxiben as inhibitors of platelet behaviour: modification of their effects by agents that alter cAMP production. *Thromb Res* **42**, 91–98.

Simpson, P.J., Smith, C.B., Rosenthal, G. *et al.* (1986) Reduction in the incidence of thrombosis by the thromboxane synthetase inhibitor CGS-13080 in a canine model of coronary artery injury. *J Pharmacol Exp Ther* **238**, 497–501.

Sinzinger, H., O'Grady, J. & Fitscha, P. (1988) Platelet deposition on human atheroscherotic lesions is decreased by low-dose aspirin in combination with dipyridamole. *J Int Med Res* **16**, 39–43.

Smith, E.F. & Egan, J.W. (1987) Comparison of the effects of a thromboxane synthase inhibitor or prostacyclin in combination with a phosphodiesterase inhibitor for prevention of experimental thrombosis and sudden death in rabbits. *J Pharmacol Exp Ther* **241**, 855–860.

Smith, J.B. (1982) Effect of thromboxane synthetase inhibitors on platelet function: enhancement by inhibition of phosphodiesterase. *Thromb Res* **28**, 477–485.

Smith, J.R. & White, A.M. (1982) Fibrin, red cell and platelet interaction in an experimental model of thrombosis. *Br J Pharmacol* **77**, 29–38.

Stanton, P.E., Evans, J.R., Lefemine, A.A. *et al.* (1988) White Clot syndrome. *South Med J* **81**, 616–620.

Steele, P., Rainwater, J., Vogel, R. *et al.* (1978) Platelet suppressant therapy in patients with coronary artery disease. *Am Med Assocy* **240**, 228–231.

Steele, P.M., Chesebro, J.H., Holmes, D.R. *et al.* (1984) Balloon angioplasty in pigs: comparative effects of platelet-inhibitor drugs. *Circulation* **70** (Suppl II), 361 (abstr).

Steele, P.M., Chesebro, J.H., Stanson, A.W. *et al.* (1985) Balloon angioplasty: natural history of the pathophysiological response to injury in a pig model. *Circ Res* **57**, 105–112.

Stratton, J.R. & Ritchie, J.L. (1984) Failure of ticlopidine to inhibit deposition of indium-111-labelled platelets on Dacron prosthetic surfaces in humans. *Circulation* **69**, 677–683.

Stuart, M.J., Murphy, B.S. & Oski, F.A. (1975) A simple nonradioisotope technic for the determination of platelet life-span. *New Engl J Med* **292**, 1310–1313.

Summers, A., Subbarao, K., Rucinski, B. *et al.* (1977) The effect of dipyridamole on adenosine uptake by platelets *ex vivo*. *Thromb Res* **11**, 611–618.

Sutherland, E.W., Robinson, G.A. *et al.* (1966) The role of 3′,5′-AMP in response to catecholamines and other hormones. *Pharmacol Rev* **18**, 145–161.

Suzuki, S., Iwabuchi, T., Tanaka, T. *et al.* (1985) Prevention of cerebral vasospasm with OKY-046 an imidazole derivative and a thromboxane synthetase' inhibitor. A preliminary co-operative clinical study. *Acta Neurochirurgica* **77**, 133–141.

Szczeklik, A., Gryglewski, R.J., Nizankowski, R. *et al.* (1978) Circulatory and antiplatelet effects of intravenous prostacyclin in man. *Pharmacol Res Commun* **10**, 545–556.

Sze, P.C., Reitman, D., Pincus, M.D. *et al.* (1988) Antiplatelet agents in the secondary prevention of stroke: Meta-analysis of the randomized control trials. *Stroke* **19**, 436–442.

Talbot, M. (1990) The biology of recombinant hirudin (CGP-39393) — a new prospect in the treatment of thrombosis. *Sem Haematol Thromb* (in press).

Talbot, M.D., Ambler, J., Butler, K.D. *et al.* (1990) Recombinant desulphatohirudin (CGP–39393): anticoagulant and antithrombotic properties *in vivo*. *Thromb Haemost* (in press).

Thaulow, E., Dale, J. & Myhre, E. (1984) Effects of a selective thromboxane synthetase inhibitor, dazoxiben, and of acetylsalicylic acid on myocardial ischemia in patients with coronary artery disease. *Am J Cardiol* **53**, 1255–1258.

Thornton, M.A., Gruentzig, A.R., Hollman, J. *et al.* (1984) Coumadin and aspirin in prevention of recurrence after transluminal coronary angioplasty. *Circulation* **69**, 721–727.

Tindall, H., Paton, R.C., McNicol, M. *et al.* (1982) Aspirin, dipyridamole and platelet survival in patients with diabetes mellitus. *Clin Sci* **63**, 205–209.

Tindall, H., Tooke, J.E., Menys, V.C. *et al.* (1985) Effect of dazoxiben, a thromboxane synthetase inhibitor on skin-blood flow following cold challenge in patients with Raynaud's phenomenon. *Eur J Clin Invest* **15**, 20–23.

Tomoda, H. (1986) Development of an experimental model of acute myocardial infarction and the effects of a thromboxane synthetase inhibitor (OKY-046) *Am Heart J* **112**, 696–704.

Tonomura, S., Kikumoto, R., Tamao, Y. *et al.* (1980) A novel series of synthetic thrombin inhibitors II relationships between structure of modified OM-inhibitors and their thrombin inhibitory effect. *Kobe J Med Sci* **26**, 1–9.

Tracy, T.S. & Black, C.D. (1987) Calcium modulators: Future agents, future uses. *Drug Intell Clin Pharmacol* **21**, 575–583.

Tremoli, E., Maderna, P., Colli, S. *et al.* (1981) CYKI 14451, a synthetic tripeptide inhibitor of thrombin: activity on platelet aggregation and arachidonic acid metabolism. *Pharmacol Res Commun* **13**, 339–349.

Tremoli, E., Colli, S. & Paoletti, R. (1984) GYKI 14451, a synthetic tripeptide inhibitor of thrombin '*in vitro*' and '*in vivo*' studies. *Adv Exp Med Biol* **164**, 187–192.

Turpie, A.G.G. (1988) Clinical studies: Evidence for intervention with specific antiplatelet drugs in arterial thromboembolism. *Sem Thromb Hemost* **14**, 41–49.

Ubatuba, F.B., Moncada, S., Vane, J.R. *et al.* (1979) The effect of prostacyclin (PGI_2) on platelet behaviour, thrombus formation *in vivo* and bleeding time. *Thromb Haemost* **41**, 425–434.

Vesterqvist, O. (1986) Rapid recovery of in vivo prostacyclin formation after inhibition by aspirin: Evidence from measurements of the major urinary metabolic of prostacyclin by CG–MS. *Eur J Clin Pharmacol* **30**, 69–73.

Walsh, P.N. (1984) Activation of coagulation factors on the surface of platelets. *Haemotologia* **17**, 57–66.

Weiss, H.J., Aledort, L.M. & Kochwa, S. (1968) The effect of salicylates on the hemostatic properties of platelets in man. *J Clin Invest* **47**, 2169–2180.

Weston, M.J., Woods, H.F., Ash, G. *et al.* (1979) Prostacyclin as an alternative to heparin for hemodialysis in dogs. In Vane, J.R. & Bergstroms, J. (eds) *Prostacyclin,* Ch 32. Raven Press, New York.

White, C.W., Chastman, B., Lassar, T.A. *et al.* (1987a) Antiplatelet agents are effective in reducing the immediate complications of PTCA: Results from the ticlopidine multicentre trial. *Circulation* **76**, IV–400 (abstr).

White, C.W., Knudson, M., Schmidt, D. *et al.* (1987b) Neither ticlopidine no aspirin-dipyridamole prevents restenosis post PTCA: Results from a randomised placebo-controlled multicentre trial. *Circulation* **76**, IV–213 (abstr).

Wu, K.K., Chen, Y.C., Fordham, E. *et al.* (1981) Differential effects of two doses of aspirin on platelet-wall interaction *in vivo*. *J Clin Invest* **68**, 382–387.

Yamamoto, N., Watanabe, K., Ando, Y. *et al.* (1982) On the mechanism of heparin-induced potentiation of platelet aggregation. *Thromb Res* **26**, 159–164.

Yamamoto, N., Tanoue, K. & Yamazaki, H. (1984) Appearance of platelet-clumping activity in heparinized plasma after acidification — its mainly due to aggregation of fibrinogen. *Thromb Res* **36**, 103–112.

Zieve, P.D. & Greenough, W.B. (1969) III, Adenyl cyclase in human platelets: activity and response. *Biochem Biophys Res Commun* **35**, 462–468.

Zwaal, R.F.A. & Hemker, H.C. (1982) Blood cell membranes and haemostasis. *Haemostasis* **11**, 12–39.

Zwaal, R.F.A., Comfurius, P., Hemker, H.C. *et al.* (1984) The inhibition of platelet prothrombinase activity by prostacyclin. *Haemostasis* **14**, 320–324.

Index